PHYSICAL EXAMINATION
OF THE
SPINE AND
EXTREMITIES

PHYSICAL EXAMINATION OF THE SPINE AND EXTREMITIES

STANLEY HOPPENFELD, M.D.

Associate Clinical Professor of Orthopedic Surgery, Director of Scoliosis Service, Albert Einstein College of Medicine, Bronx, New York; Deputy Director of Orthopedic Surgery, Attending Physician, Bronx Municipal Hospital Center, Bronx, New York; Associate Attending Physician, Hospital for Joint Diseases, New York, New York

In collaboration with
RICHARD HUTTON

Medical illustrations by
HUGH THOMAS

APPLETON & LANGE
Norwalk, Connecticut

Library of Congress Cataloging in Publication Data
Hoppenfeld, Stanley
   Physical examination of the spine and extremities.

   Bibliography
   Includes index.
   1. Spine—Examination. 2. Extremities
(Anatomy)—Examination. I. Title. [DNLM:
1. Extremities. 2. Spine. 3. Physical exami-
nation—Methods. WE800 H798p]
RD734.H66   617'.375'075   76-1486
ISBN 0-8385-7853-5 A&L
       0-8385-7867-5 Syntex Edition

97 98 99 / 34 33

Prentice-Hall International, Inc., London
Prentice-Hall of Australia, Pty. Ltd., Sydney
Prentice-Hall of India Private Limited, New Delhi
Prentice-Hall of Japan, Inc., Tokyo
Prentice-Hall of Southeast Asia (Pte.) Ltd., Singapore
Whitehall Books, Wellington, New Zealand

PRINTED IN THE UNITED STATES OF AMERICA

cover illustration: Hugh Thomas
page layout: Jean Taylor

ISBN 0-8385-7853-5

DEDICATION

To my wife *Norma*, who has added a very
special dimension to my life.

To my parents, my most devoted teachers.

To all the men who preserved this body of
knowledge, added to it, and passed it
on for another generation.

Acknowledgments

No book is written without help. I would like to say thank you to a host of wonderful people.

Leading all acknowledgments must be mine to Richard Hutton and Hugh Thomas, my associates for six years. They and I worked together on this book from start to finish. Whatever success it earns, I share with them.

To my orthopedic colleagues at the Albert Einstein College of Medicine for all their personal help: Elias Sedlin, Robert Schultz, Uriel Adar, David Hirsh, and Rashmi Sheth.

To the attending physicians at the Hospital for Joint Diseases who during my residency passed on most of this knowledge to me. I express my appreciation by preserving it for yet another generation.

To the orthopedic residents at the Albert Einstein College of Medicine whom it has been a pleasure teaching the material contained in this volume.

To Joseph Milgram who has been a friend and teacher during these many years of education.

To Arthur J. Helfet for making the opportunity available for writing this book and for his teachings on the knee.

To the British Fellows who have participated in the teaching of physical examination of the spine and extremities during their stay in the United States and for their suggestions in the writing of this book: Clive Whalley, Robert Jackson, David Gruebel-Lee, David Reynolds, Roger Weeks, Fred Heatley, Peter Johnson, Richard Foster, Kenneth Walker, Maldwyn Griffiths, and John Patrick.

To Nathan Allan Shore, D.D.S. for his teachings of the temporomandibular joint and for the continued spark of inspiration he has always provided me.

To Arthur Merker, D.D.S. for his friendship and for providing his house by the sea as a place to hide away and work.

To Paul Bresnick for his help in initiating the writings of the Lower Extremity.

To Mr. Allan Apley for his friendship and valuable suggestions in the rewriting of the book.

To Frank Ferrieri for watching "the store" when I was working on the book.

To Laurel Courtney in appreciation for her time in reviewing the manuscript and for her positive approach.

To Sis and David for their unwaivering friendship during the midst of preparing the book.

To Ed Delagi for listening to my many thoughts and for reviewing the Gait Chapter.

To Morton Spinner for reviewing the Wrist and Hand Chapter and making appropriate suggestions.

To Mel Jahss for reviewing the Foot and Ankle Chapter and giving it a sure "footing."

My deep gratitude to Muriel Chaleff our Executive Secretary and long term friend who so generously participated in the production of this book.

To Joan Nicosia in appreciation for her help in the preparation of the Wrist and Hand Chapter.

To Lauretta White who extended friendship, typed and kept files, thereby holding back chaos for six long years.

To Anthea Blamire for her secretarial support.

To Carol Halpern for going out of her way to help with the typing production of this book.

To Sabina DeFraia who worked long and productive hours in typing the many drafts of these pages.

To Doreen Berne for her professionalism in handling the manuscript at Appleton-Century-Crofts.

To Steven Abramson for his valuable assistance in the production of the book and its slide package.

To Laura Jane Bird for her help in the design of the book.

To our Publisher who has brought our team effort to a happy conclusion.

Contents

Preface

During my residency and subsequent teaching years, the need for a clear, concise manual concerning the process of physical examination of the spine and extremities became increasingly apparent. As I conceived it, such a manual would direct the clinician or student in a logical, efficient, and thorough search for relevant anatomy and pathology. A book of this type would also incorporate three important features: a tight consistent organization, an abundance of constructive illustrations, and an effective teaching method. It is truly said that necessity is the mother of invention, for the following material certainly represents the product of the above-expressed need.

In accordance with our original concept, the organization of the following text is consistent. Each chapter conforms to the clinical process of examination of the specific area, yet the format is not inflexible, and may vary according to the dictates of the particular examination.

To increase perspective, the book contains over 600 illustrations. The drawings are a result of constant teaching and refinement. They were designed specifically to add clarity and dimension to the written word, and have been brought to fruition over a three-year period. Many are oversimplified to impress basic concepts upon the clinician, while others convey accurate anatomic detail. Most illustrations are drawn from the examiner's point of view, thereby showing the reader how to learn, by imitation, the most effective techniques of physical examination.

In regard to the teaching method presented herein, the basic principles of physical examination are applied to each area discussed, a format which is followed consistently throughout the text. This procedure has been used successfully for seven years at The Albert Einstein School of Medicine, in the instruction not only of residents, medical students, and physicians of diverse specialties, but also of physical therapists and other professionals. While the level of the material presented may vary from group to group, the method of presentation does not.

It must be emphasized that there can be no substitute for the actual experience of conducting a physical examination under the direct guidance of knowledgeable personnel. A mere book cannot be presumed to take the place of the tutelage of a skilled senior physician, nor can it guide the clinician on a personal basis. However, this manual can relieve the physician of many of the burdensome tasks of transmitting basic, crucial concepts and techniques of examination, allowing him valuable time to work with the subtler details. To quote Sir William Osler: "To study medicine without books is to sail an uncharted sea, while to study medicine only from books is not to go to sea at all."

It is my sincere hope that this volume will serve as a functional guidebook through which clinicians and students can rapidly assimilate the basic knowledge essential to physical examination of the spine and extremities.

STANLEY HOPPENFELD, M.D.

1
Physical Examination of the Shoulder

INSPECTION

BONY PALPATION
    Suprasternal Notch
    Sternoclavicular Joint
    Clavicle
    Coracoid Process
    Acromioclavicular Articulation
    Acromion
    Greater Tuberosity of the Humerus
    Bicipital Groove
    Spine of the Scapula
    Vertebral Border of the Scapula

SOFT TISSUE PALPATION BY CLINICAL ZONES
    Zone I — Rotator Cuff
    Zone II — Subacromial and Subdeltoid Bursa
    Zone III — The Axilla
    Zone IV — Prominent Muscles of the Shoulder
            Girdle

RANGE OF MOTION
    Active Range of Motion Tests
      Quick Tests
    Passive Range of Motion Tests
      Abduction _____ 180°
      Adduction _____ 45°
      Flexion _____ 90°
      Extension _____ 45°
      Internal Rotation _____ 55°
      External Rotation _____ 40°–45°

NEUROLOGIC EXAMINATION
    Muscle Testing
    Reflex Testing
    Sensation Testing

SPECIAL TESTS
    The Yergason Test
    Drop Arm Test
    Apprehension Test for Shoulder Dislocation

EXAMINATION OF RELATED AREAS

1

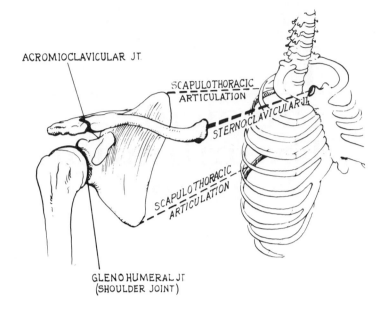

Fig. 1. The shoulder girdle.

The shoulder girdle is composed of three joints and one "articulation":

1) the sternoclavicular joint
2) the acromioclavicular joint
3) the glenohumeral joint (the shoulder joint)
4) the scapulothoracic articulation

All four work together in a synchronous rhythm to permit universal motion (Fig. 1). Unlike the hip, which is a stable joint having deep acetabular socket support, the shoulder is a mobile joint with a shallow glenoid fossa (Fig. 2). The humerus is suspended from the scapula by soft tissue, muscles, ligaments, and a joint capsule, and has only minimal osseous support.

Examination of the shoulder begins with a careful visual inspection, followed by a detailed palpation of the bony structures and soft tissues comprising the shoulder girdle. Range of motion determination, muscle testing, neurologic assessment, and special tests complete the examination.

INSPECTION

Inspection begins as the patient enters the examining room. As he walks, evaluate the evenness and symmetry of his motion; the upper extremity, in normal gait, swings in tandem with the opposite lower extremity. As the patient disrobes to the waist, observe the rhythm of his shoulder movement. Normal motion has a smooth, natural, bilateral quality; abnormal motion appears unilaterally jerky or distorted, and often represents the patient's attempt to substitute an inefficient, painless movement for one that was once efficient but has since become painful. Initial inspection should, of course, include a topical scan for blebs, discoloration, abrasions, scars, and other signs of present or previous pathology.

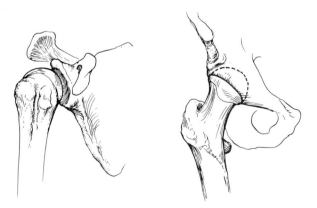

Fig. 2. The humerus has very minimal osseous support. Notice the shallow glenoid fossa in the shoulder as compared to the deep acetabular socket of the hip.

As you inspect, compare each area bilaterally, noting any indications of pathology as well as the condition and general contour of the anatomy. The easiest way to determine the presence of abnormality is by bilateral comparison, for such comparison more often than not reveals any variation that may be present. This method is one of the keys to good physical examination, and holds true not only for inspection, but for the palpation, range of motion testing, and neurologic portions of your examination as well.

Asymmetry is usually quite obvious. For example, one arm may hang in an unnatural position, either adducted (toward the midline) across the front of the body, or abducted away from it, leaving a visible space in the axilla. Or, the arm may be internally rotated and adducted, in the position of a waiter asking for a tip (Erb's palsy) (Fig. 3).

Now, turn your attention to the most prominent bone of the shoulder's anterior aspect, the clavicle (Fig. 4). The clavicle is a strut bone that keeps the scapula on the posterior aspect of the thorax and prevents the glenoid from turning

anteriorly. It rises medially from the manubrial portion of the sternum and extends laterally to the acromion. Only the thin platysma muscle crosses its superior surface. The clavicle is almost subcutaneous, clearly etching the overlying skin, and a fracture or dislocation at either terminal is usually quite obvious. In the absence of the clavicle, the normal ridges on the skin which define it (clavicular contour) are also absent, and exaggerated rounded shoulders are a visible result.

Next inspect the deltoid portion of the shoulder, the most prominent mass of the shoulder girdle's anterior aspect. The rounded look of the shoulder is a result of the draping of the deltoid muscle from the acromion over the greater tuberosity of the humerus. Normally, the shoulder mass is full and round, and the two sides are symmetrical (Fig. 4). However, if the deltoid has atrophied, the underlying greater tuberosity of the humerus becomes more prominent, and the deltoid no longer fills out the contours of the shoulder mass. Abnormality of shoulder contour may also be caused by shoulder dislocation if the greater tuberosity is

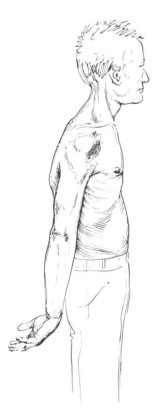

Fig. 3. Erb's palsy.

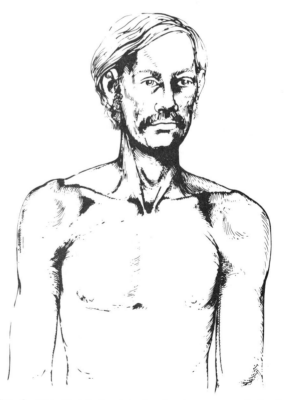

Fig. 4. The clavicle is almost subcutaneous and clearly etches the overlying skin.

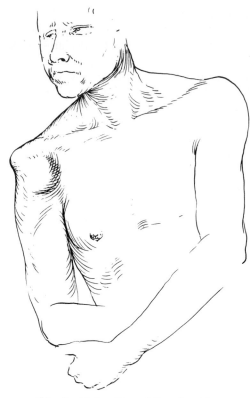

Fig. 5. Dislocation of the shoulder.

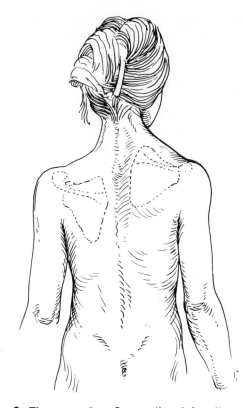

Fig. 6. The scapulae—Sprengel's deformity—partially undescended scapula.

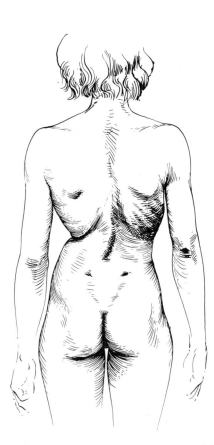

Fig. 7. Lateral curvature of the spine (scoliosis).

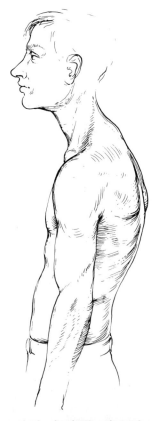

Fig. 8. Excessively kyphotic thoracic spine—Scheuermann's disease or juvenile kyphosis.

displaced forward, as is usually the case; the shoulder loses its full lateral contour and appears indented under the point of the shoulder. The arm is held slightly away from the trunk (Fig. 5).

The deltopectoral groove lies medial to the shoulder mass and just inferior to the lateral concavity of the clavicle (Fig. 4). The groove is formed by the meeting of the deltoid muscle fibers and the pectoralis major muscle and is one of the most efficient locations in the shoulder's anterior region for surgical incision. It also represents the surface marking for the cephalic vein, used for a venous cut-down if no other vein is easily accessible.

Now, direct your attention to the posterior aspect of the shoulder girdle (Fig. 21). The most prominent bony landmark is the scapula, a triangular bone that rests upon the thoracic cage. The outline of its ridges upon the skin makes the scapula easy to locate. In its resting position, it covers ribs two to seven; its medial border lies approximately two inches from the spinous processes (Fig. 22). The smooth, triangular area of the spine of the scapula is opposite spinous process T3. The scapula conforms to the shape of the rib cage, contributing to the slightly kyphotic shape of the thoracic spine. Any asymmetry in the relationship between the scapulae and the thorax may indicate weakness or atrophy of the serratus anterior muscle and may

present as a winged effect (Fig. 66). Another cause of scapular asymmetry is Sprengel's deformity, wherein the scapula has only partially descended from the neck to the thorax. This high-riding scapula may cause an apparent webbing or shortening of the neck (Fig. 6).

The posterior midline of the body, with its visible spinous processes, lies midway between the scapulae. Notice whether the spine is straight, without lateral curvature (scoliosis) (Fig. 7). A spinal curvature may make one shoulder appear lower than the other, with the dominant side being more muscular. Occasionally, the thoracic spine is excessively rounded or kyphotic, usually a result of Scheuermann's disease or juvenile kyphosis (Fig. 8).

BONY PALPATION

For the examiner, the palpation of bony structures provides a systematic and orderly method of evaluating the relevant anatomy. Position yourself behind the seated patient; place your hands upon the deltoid and acromion. This first contact with the patient should be gentle but firm to instill a feeling of security. A natural cupped position for your hands is most efficient and allows the fingertips to gauge skin temperature.

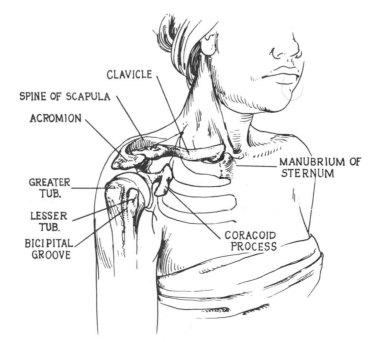

Fig. 9. Anterior aspect of the shoulder's bone structure.

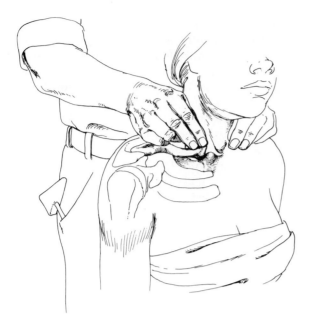

Fig. 10. The suprasternal notch and sternoclavicular joint.

Suprasternal Notch. Move your hands medially from their position on the deltoid and acromion (Figs. 9, 10) until you feel the suprasternal notch.

Sternoclavicular Joint. This joint is immediately lateral to the suprasternal notch and should be palpated bilaterally. Remember that the clavicle is slightly superior to the manubrial portion of the sternum, and that the joint itself is very shallow. The clavicle normally rises above the manubrium and is held in position by the sternoclavicular and the interclavicular ligaments. Dislocation of the clavicle usually manifests as a medial and superior displacement; the clavicle will have moved well onto the top of the manubrium sternum, and its new position will be obviously asymmetrical when compared to the opposite side.

Clavicle. Move laterally from the sternoclavicular joint and palpate in a sliding motion along the smooth anterior superior surface of the clavicle (Fig. 11). Muscles attach to the clavicle solely from the inferior and posterior aspects, leaving the anterior superior strip bare, except for the overlying platysma muscle. First, palpate along the convex medial two-thirds, then along the concave lateral one-third of the clavicle, noting any protuberances, crepitation, or loss of continuity which might indicate a fracture (Fig. 12). In a thin patient, you may be able to feel the supraclavicular nerves as they cross the clavicle at various points.

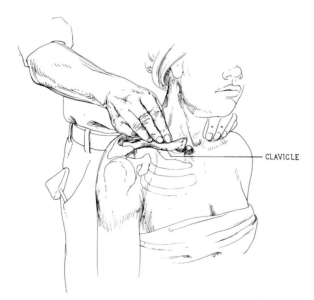

Fig. 11. Palpation of the clavicle: the medial two-thirds is convex and tubular.

CLAVICLE

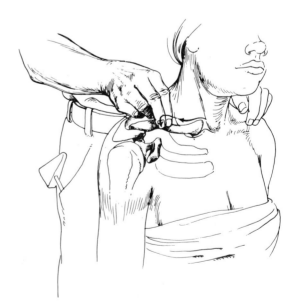

Fig. 12. The concave lateral one-third of the clavicle.

Coracoid Process. At the deepest portion of the clavicular concavity, lower the fingers distally about one inch from the anterior edge of the clavicle, and press laterally and posteriorly in an oblique line until you feel the coracoid process (Fig. 13). The process faces anterolaterally; only its medial surface and tip are palpable. It lies deep under the cover of the pectoralis major muscle, but it may be felt if you press firmly into the deltopectoral triangle.

Acromioclavicular Articulation. Return to the clavicle and continue palpation laterally for approximately one inch to the subcutaneous acromioclavicular articulation (Fig. 14). Although the clavicle begins to flatten out in its lateral one-third, it never fully loses its round contour and protrudes slightly above the acromion. The acromioclavicular joint is thus easier to palpate if you push in a medial direction against the thickness at the end of the clavicle (Fig. 15). Motion of the shoulder girdle causes the acromioclavicular joint to move and makes it easier to identify. Therefore, ask the patient to flex and extend his shoulder several times; you will be able to feel the movement of the joint under your fingers (Fig. 15). The acromioclavicular joint may be tender to palpation with associated crepitation, secondary to osteoarthritis or to dislocation of the lateral end of the clavicle.

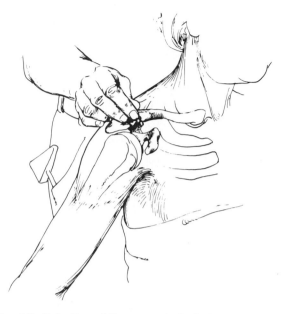

Fig. 15. Palpation of the acromioclavicular articulation is easier if the patient rotates his arm.

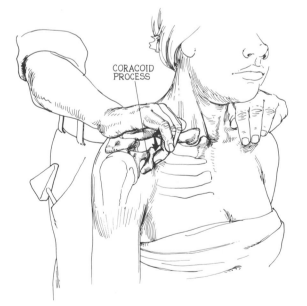

Fig. 13. The coracoid process.

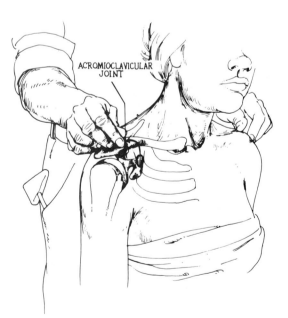

Fig. 14. The acromioclavicular articulation.

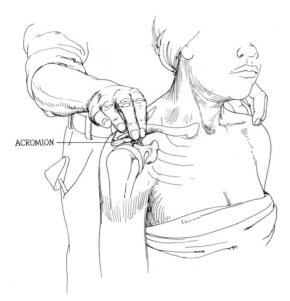

Fig. 16. The anterior aspect of the acromion.

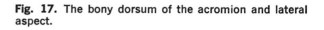

Fig. 17. The bony dorsum of the acromion and lateral aspect.

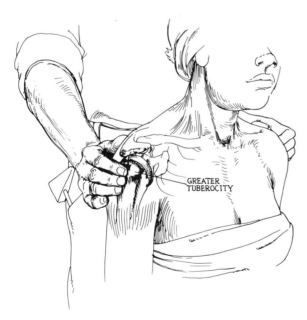

Fig. 18. The greater tuberosity of the humerus.

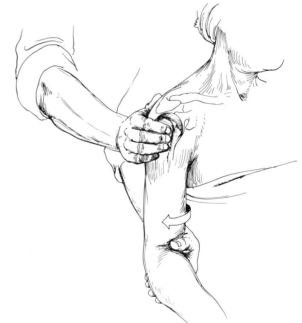

Fig. 19. The bicipital groove and the lesser tuberosity.

Acromion. The rectangular acromion, sometimes referred to as the shoulder's summit, contributes to its general contour. Palpate its bony dorsum and anterior portion (Figs. 16, 17).

Greater Tuberosity of the Humerus. From the lateral lip of the acromion, palpate laterally to the greater tuberosity of the humerus, which lies inferior to the acromion's lateral edge (Fig. 18). There is a small step-off between the lateral acromial border and the greater tuberosity.

Bicipital Groove. The bicipital groove is located anterior and medial to the greater tuberosity and is bordered laterally by the greater tuberosity and medially by the lesser tuberosity. It is more easily palpable if the arm is externally rotated. External rotation presents the groove in a more exposed position for palpation, and reveals in smooth succession the greater tuberosity, the bicipital groove, and the lesser tuberosity (Figs. 19, 20). Palpation of the bicipital groove should be undertaken carefully, for the tendon of the long head of the biceps, with its synovial lining, lies within it. Too much digital pressure may not only hurt the patient, but is likely to cause him to become tense, making further examination more difficult. Note that the lesser tuberosity is at the same level as the coracoid process.

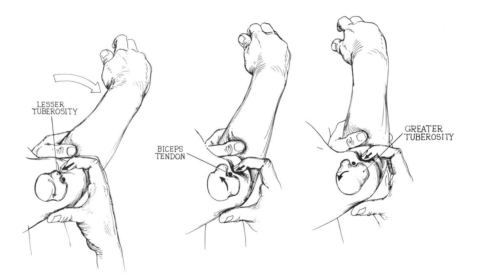

Fig. 20. Palpation of the bicipital groove should be done carefully. Too much pressure may hurt the patient. Rotation of the humerus allows for palpation of the walls of the bicipital groove.

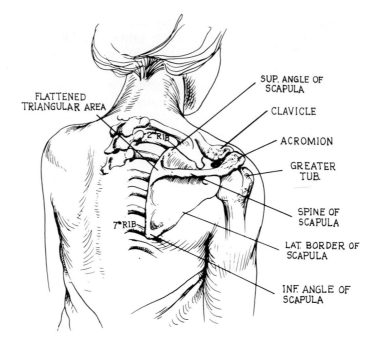

Fig. 21. The posterior aspect of the shoulder's bone structure.

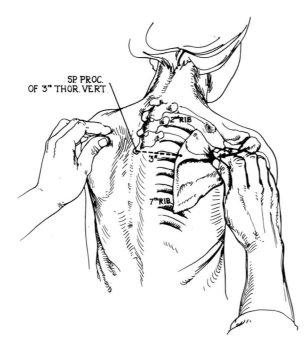

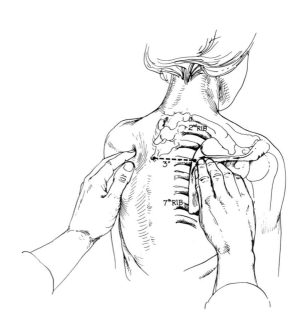

Fig. 22. The scapula in its resting position covers ribs 2 to 7, with its medial border approximately 2 to 3 inches from the spinous processes.

Fig. 23. The spine of the scapula is opposite the spinous process of the third thoracic vertebra.

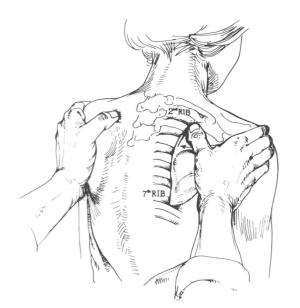

Fig. 24. Palpation of the superior medial angle on the medial border of the scapula.

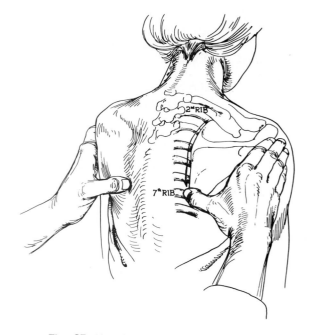

Fig. 25. Vertebral border of the scapula.

Spine of the Scapula. Move posteriorly and medially and palpate the acromion as it tapers to the spine of the scapula (Fig. 21). Remember that the acromion and the spine of the scapula form one continuous arch (Fig. 22). The spine of the scapula then extends obliquely across the upper four-fifths of the scapular dorsum and ends in a flat, smooth triangle at the medial border of the scapula (Fig. 23). Probe up the scapula's medial border to its superior medial angle (Fig. 24). This scapular angle is not as distinct as the subcutaneous inferior angle, since it is covered by the levator scapula muscle and loses definition because of its anterior curve. It is clinically important, however, for it is frequently the site of referred pain from the cervical spine.

Vertebral Border of the Scapula. As you trace down the medial border of the scapula (Fig. 25), notice that it is approximately two inches (about the width of three fingers) from the spinous processes of the thoracic vertebrae and that the triangle at the vertebral end of the spine of the scapula is at the level of T3. From the inferior angle of the scapula, palpate the lateral border to the point where the scapula disappears beneath the latissimus dorsi, teres major, and teres minor muscles (Fig. 26).

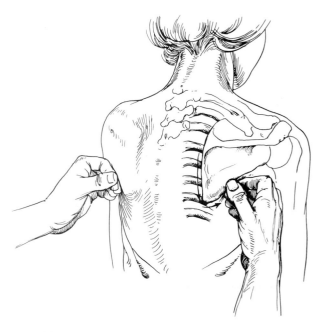

Fig. 26. Palpation of the lateral border of the scapula.

SOFT TISSUE PALPATION BY CLINICAL ZONES

The examination of the soft tissue structures of the shoulder has been divided into four clinical zones:

1) Rotator Cuff
2) Subacromial and Subdeltoid Bursa
3) Axilla
4) Prominent Muscles of the Shoulder Girdle.

The discussion of each area contains the specific pathology and clinical significance that pertains to it. The purpose of palpation of these anatomic configurations is threefold: (1) to establish the normal soft tissue relationships within the shoulder girdle, (2) to detect any variations from normal anatomy, and (3) to discover any pathology which may be manifested as unusual lumps or masses. During palpation of the muscles of the shoulder girdle, the examiner should assess the tone, consistency, size, and shape of the individual muscles, in addition to their condition (whether they are hypertrophic or atrophic). Any tenderness elicited during palpation should be located precisely, and its cause discovered.

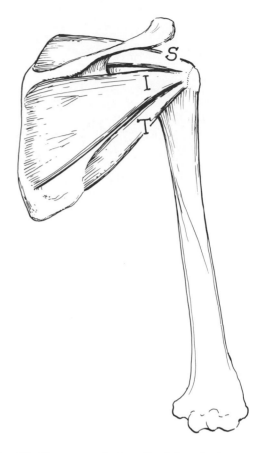

Fig. 27. The supraspinatus, the infraspinatus, and the teres minor muscles—the SIT muscles.

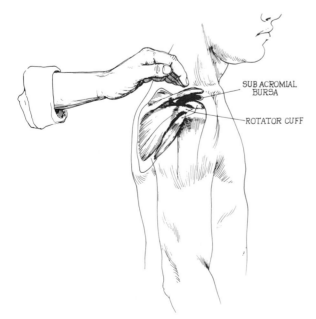

Fig. 28. The rotator cuff lies underneath the acromion.

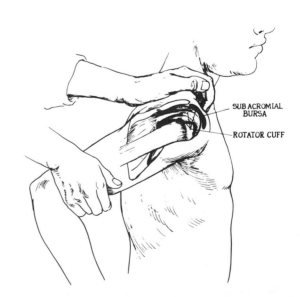

Fig. 29. Passive extension of the shoulder moves the rotator cuff into a palpable position.

Zone I—Rotator Cuff

The rotator cuff has clinical importance because degeneration and subsequent tearing of its tendon of insertion is a rather common pathology which results in restriction of the shoulder movement, especially in abduction. The cuff is composed of four muscles, three of which are palpable at their insertions into the greater tuberosity of the humerus. These three, the supraspinatus, the infraspinatus, and the teres minor, are called the SIT muscles, since, in the order of their attachment, their initials spell "sit" (Fig. 27). In a modified anatomic position (with the arm hanging at the side), the supraspinatus lies directly under the acromion; the infraspinatus is posterior to the supraspinatus; and the teres minor is immediately posterior to the other two muscles. The fourth muscle in the rotator cuff, the subscapularis, is located anteriorly and is not palpable.

Since the rotator cuff lies directly below the acromion, it must be rotated out from underneath before it can be palpated (Fig. 28). Passive extension of the shoulder moves the rotator cuff into a palpable position; therefore, hold the patient's arm just proximal to the elbow joint and lift the elbow posteriorly. Palpate the roundness of the exposed rotator cuff slightly inferior to the anterior border of the acromion (Fig. 29). The SIT muscles cannot be distinguished from each other, but they can be palpated as a unit at and near their insertion into the greater tuberosity of the humerus. Any tenderness elicited during palpation may be due to defects or tears, or to the detachment of the tendon of insertion from the greater tuberosity. Of the muscles of the rotator cuff, the supraspinatus is the most commonly ruptured, especially near its insertion.

Zone II—Subacromial and Subdeltoid Bursa

Subacromial or subdeltoid bursitis is a frequent pathologic finding which can cause much tenderness and restriction of the shoulder motion. The subacromial bursa has been rotated anteriorly with the rotator cuff from under the acromion during passive extension. The bursa has essentially two major sections: subacromial and subdeltoid. However, several portions of the bursa are palpable at points just below the edge of the acromion (Fig. 30). From the anterior edge of the acromion, the bursa may extend as far as the bicipital groove. From the lateral edge of the acromion, the bursa extends under the deltoid muscle, separating it from the rotator cuff and allowing each to move freely (Fig. 31). The subacromial bursa, like the rotator cuff, should be palpated very carefully,

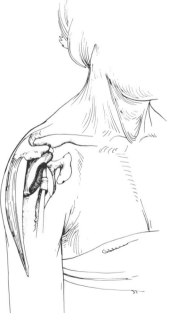

Fig. 30. Portions of the subacromial and subdeltoid bursa are palpable where they extend out from under the acromial edge.

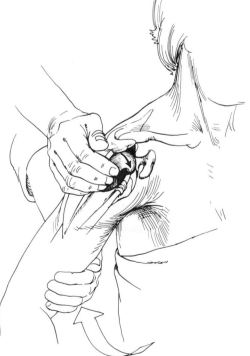

Fig. 31. Palpation of the subdeltoid bursa.

because the area can be very tender if there is bursitis present. The bursa should be palpated for any additional thickening, masses, or specific tenderness. Bursal thickening may be accompanied by crepitation as the shoulder moves.

Zone III—Axilla

The axilla (armpit) is a quadrilateral pyramidal structure through which vessels and nerves pass to the upper extremity (Fig. 32). Stand in front of the patient and abduct his arm with one hand as you gently insert your index and middle fingers into the axilla (Fig. 33). Then return the patient's arm to his side to relax the skin at the base of the axilla so that additional cephalad pressure will allow your fingers to penetrate higher. Probe for any lymph node enlargements, which feel like small, discrete nodules and may be tender (Fig. 34).

The fleshy anterior wall of the axilla is formed by the pectoralis major muscle, and the posterior wall, also fleshy, by the latissimus dorsi muscle. The medial wall is defined by ribs two to six and the overlying serratus anterior muscle, and the lateral wall by the bicipital groove of the humerus. The glenohumeral joint represents the apex of the pyramid, and the webbed skin and fascia of the armpit, the base. The anterior and posterior walls converge laterally on the bicipital groove of the humerus and diverge medially against the thoracic

wall. The major nerve supply (the brachial plexus) and the major blood supply (the axillary artery) to the upper extremity enter via the apex of the axilla.

Move to the medial wall of the axilla, press your fingertips firmly over the ribs, and palpate the serratus anterior muscle (Fig. 34). Note its condition in comparison to its counterpart on the opposite side. Next, palpate the lateral wall, the bicipital groove of the humerus. The brachial artery is the most obvious palpable structure in the lateral quadrant. Its pulse can be felt when gentle pressure is applied against the shaft of the humerus between the ropelike coracobrachialis muscle and the long head of the triceps (Fig. 35).

The anterior and posterior walls of the axilla can be palpated when the patient's arm is abducted (away from the midline). Abduction accentuates the pectoralis major and the latissimus dorsi, making them easier to palpate. To palpate the posterior wall, grasp the latissimus dorsi between your thumb and your index and middle fingers (Fig. 36). Then palpate the latissimus dorsi cephalad and caudad over its broad expanse. Move to the anterior wall and palpate the pectoralis major muscle in a similar manner (Fig. 37). Remember that the pectoralis major muscle has a broad, sweeping origin from the clavicle and the sternum, and tapers to a narrow insertion into the humerus. Palpate the latissimus dorsi and the pectoralis major muscles for tone and condition, and compare them to the opposite side.

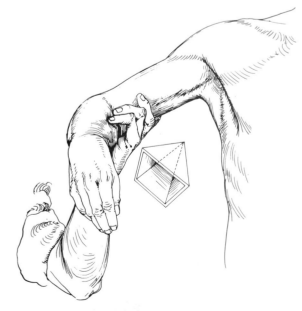

Fig. 32. The axilla is pyramidal in shape.

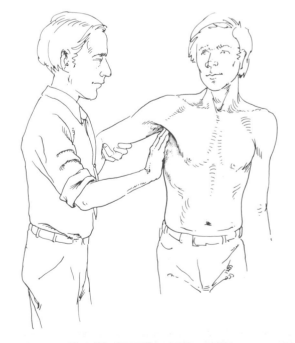

Fig. 33. Palpation of the axilla.

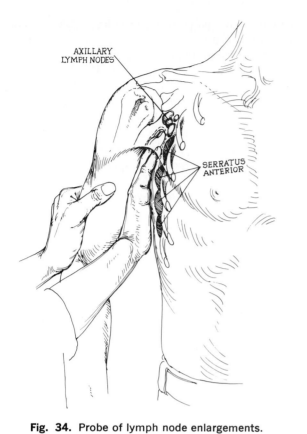

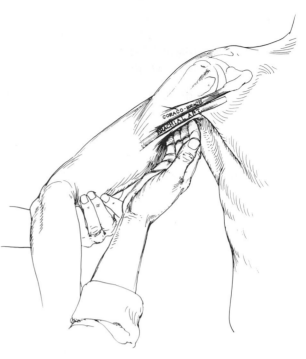

Fig. 35. Palpation of the brachial artery.

Fig. 34. Probe of lymph node enlargements.

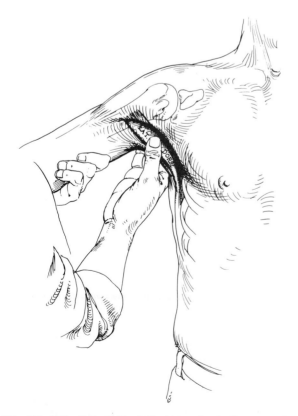

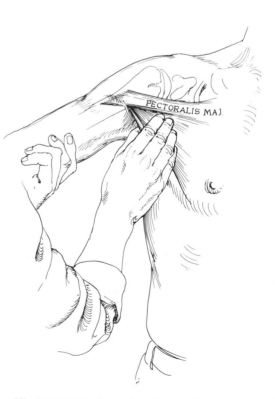

Fig. 36. Palpation of the latissimus dorsi—the posterior wall of the axilla.

Fig. 37. The pectoralis major muscle—the anterior wall of the axilla.

Zone IV—Prominent Muscles of the Shoulder Girdle

The muscles of the shoulder girdle should be palpated bilaterally to determine relationships of size, shape, consistency, and tone. Bilateral comparison may not only unearth any deviations from normal anatomy, such as abnormal contour, bumps, gaps, or the absence of a muscle, but will also define the patient's topical anatomy.

Note any tenderness that you may elicit, but remember that tenderness is a subjective symptom given by the patient, whereas a palpable defect is an objective finding, both verifiable and reproducible.

Palpate the muscles in the anterior aspect of the shoulder first, from the superior to the inferior regions. Then palpate the muscles in the posterior aspect in a similar fashion.

Sternocleidomastoid. This muscle is clinically important for three reasons: (1) It is frequently the site of hematomas, which may cause the neck to turn to one side (wry neck); (2) lymph nodes near its anterior and posterior borders often become enlarged as a result of infection; (3) it is frequently traumatized in hyperextension injuries of the neck, such as whiplash injury.

Grasp the sternocleidomastoid at its base and palpate the length of the muscle (both sternocleidomastoids should be palpated simultaneously) (Figs. 38, 39). Note that this muscle has a dual origin, medially on the manubrium and laterally on the medial third of the clavicle. As you palpate the muscle toward its insertion into the mastoid process of the skull, check for lymph node enlargement along its borders. The sternocleidomastoids

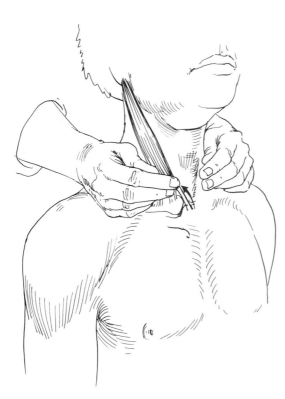

Fig. 38. The sternocleidomastoid.

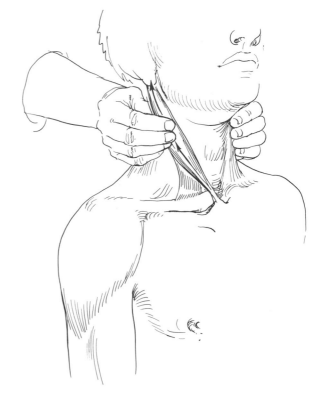

Fig. 39. The sternocleidomastoids should be palpated simultaneously.

become more prominent on the side opposite that to which the head is turned, and the muscle can be palpated at its distal origin more easily if the patient turns his head first to one side, then to the other. With experience, the origin of this muscle can be palpated during the palpation of the sternoclavicular joint.

Pectoralis Major. The pectoralis major is clinically important as the muscle most frequently absent congenitally, either wholly or in part. The two heads of the pectoralis major have an origin which sweeps in an almost continuous arc from the entire sternum onto the medial two-thirds of the clavicle. The origin ends at the lateral concavity of the clavicle, where it defines the medial border of the deltopectoral groove. The pectoralis major then inserts into the lateral lip of the bicipital groove of the humerus after forming the anterior wall of the axilla.

You have palpated near the insertion of the pectoralis major while examining the axilla. Palpate the entire pectoralis major bilaterally, concentrating on the muscle's medial portions and using a five-finger sweeping action over its surface (Fig. 40). The costrochondral junctions lie just lateral to the sternum, and are palpable through the pectoralis major muscle (Fig. 41). The junctions may become tender or enlarged from trauma or from Tietze's syndrome (costochondritis). Move toward the insertion of the pectoralis major and note that it crosses the bicipital groove of the humerus on the way to its insertion into the lateral lip of the groove. If tenderness exists, be sure to distinguish between tenderness in the groove and tenderness in the muscle itself. Note that breast tissue overlies the pectoralis major and attaches to its anterior fascia. Check the tissue as you palpate for lumps or masses.

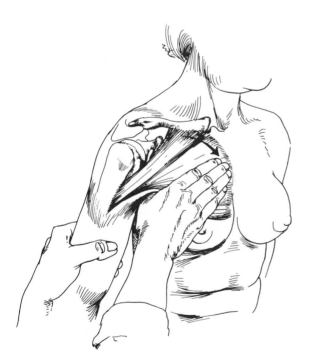

Fig. 40. Palpation of the pectoralis major muscle.

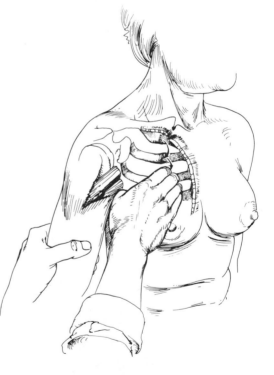

Fig. 41. The costochondral junctions.

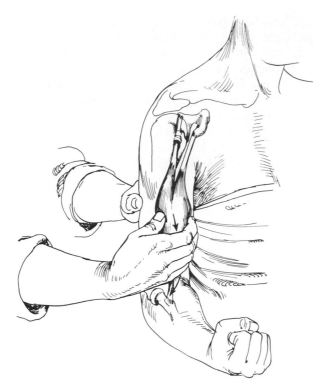

Fig. 42. Palpation of the biceps.

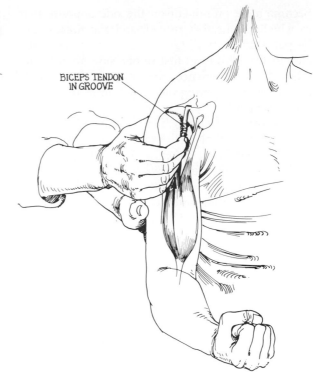

BICEPS TENDON
IN GROOVE

Fig. 43. The tendon of the long head of the biceps.

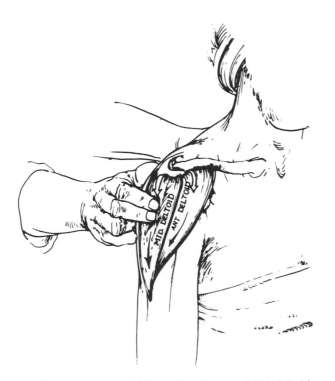

Fig. 44. The anterior and middle portions of the deltoid.

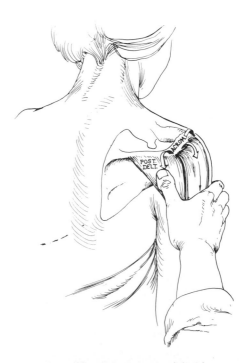

Fig. 45. The posterior deltoid.

Biceps. The biceps becomes more prominent and more easily palpable when the elbow is flexed. Occasionally, the long head of the biceps may be torn from its origin, curling like a ball at the midpoint of the humerus and giving the muscle a different form and shape compared to the opposite side. Begin palpation distally where the muscle becomes tendinous and crosses the elbow joint on the way to its insertion into the bicipital tuberosity of the radius (Fig. 42). Then palpate proximally until you feel the bicipital groove and the tendon of the long head of the biceps which runs through it (Fig. 43). The proximal end of the biceps is frequently involved in tenosynovitis and dislocation of the long head of the biceps from the bicipital groove. Note that the tendon is easier to palpate in the groove when the shoulder is externally rotated.

Deltoid. This muscle, in conjunction with the subdeltoid bursa and the rotator cuff, has clinical importance because of its relation to the common pathology of bursitis. The deltoid may also become atrophic secondary to shoulder injury.

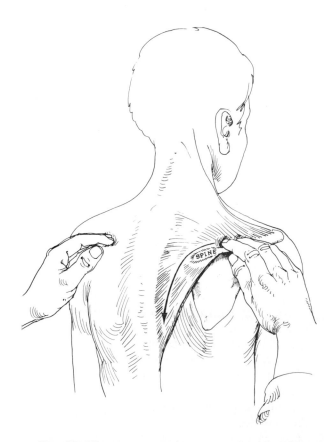

Fig. 46. The lower angle of the trapezius muscle.

Axillary nerve damage from shoulder dislocation can cause muscle atrophy and loss of tone.

The deltoid has a broad, uninterrupted, curved origin which rises from the lateral one-third of the clavicle, crosses the acromioclavicular joint, follows the anterior, lateral, and posterior borders of the acromion, and sweeps down the spine of the scapula. The clavicular portion of the origin begins in the lateral concavity of the clavicle where the pectoralis major muscle ends; the mass of the muscle contributes to the shoulder's full contour. It then tapers down the arm to a point about halfway down the humerus, where it converges at its insertion into the deltoid tuberosity. Palpate the deltoid muscle, using the bony landmarks of the acromion as reference points, in a linear fashion from the anterior, lateral, and posterior borders of the acromion to its insertion into the deltoid tuberosity (from points of origin to point of insertion) (Figs. 44, 45). Notice that the anterior portion of the deltoid covers the bicipital groove; tenderness in the groove may be difficult to distinguish from tenderness in the deltoid's anterior portion since the site of tenderness may be common to both structures. The lateral area should be carefully and thoroughly palpated for specific points of tenderness that may be associated with bursitis. As your technique improves, soft tissue palpation of the deltoid can be combined with the bony palpation of the acromion, head of the humerus, and spine of the scapula.

Trapezius. The superior portion of the trapezius is frequently involved in neck injuries during auto accidents or from other strains on the neck region which may result in hematomas.

Hold the sloping superior lateral portion of the trapezius gently between your thumb and four fingers and palpate from its origin in the occipital region as it plays out onto the clavicle and the acromion. The trapezius muscle blends with the deltoid along most of its insertion into the clavicle, acromion, and spine of the scapula, and distinguishing between the two at this location is difficult. Palpate along the upper portion of the spine of the scapula (one of the areas of insertion for the trapezius and of origin for the deltoid), noting any tenderness or difference in the size, contour, or consistency of the two muscles. From the spine of the scapula, palpate the lower angle of the trapezius (Fig. 46), running your fingers bilaterally in a converging line down to the muscle's most distal insertion at spinous process T12. The trapezius is less distinct in this area, in comparison to its more prominent cervical portion.

Rhomboid Minor and Major. The rhomboids are postural muscles which retract the scapulae and bring the shoulders to a position of "attention." Quite often, secretaries who sit and type for long periods of time will complain of pain in the substance and the insertions of the rhomboids. This pain is usually the result of simple muscle strain and is easily reproducible.

The rhomboids, which originate along the spine (C7–T5), extend obliquely downward and laterally, inserting into the medial border of the scapula. Because it is difficult to differentiate between the two rhomboids, they should be palpated together.

Orient yourself for the palpation of the rhomboids by locating the smooth, triangular area at the medial border of the scapula. This area opposite T3 serves as the point of insertion for the rhomboid minor muscle.

The rhomboids can be made to stand out so that they are distinguishable from the overlying trapezius muscle. To accomplish this, ask the patient to put his arm behind his back with the elbow flexed and the shoulder internally rotated (Fig. 47). Then have him push posteriorly while you resist his motion; the rhomboids will become palpable. First, palpate the belly of the muscles

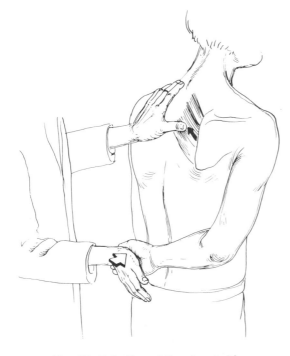

Fig. 47. Palpation of the rhomboids.

obliquely and downward across the two-inch space between the spinous processes and the medial border of the scapula. Then palpate the rhomboids on the other side to provide a means for comparison.

Latissimus Dorsi. This muscle tapers from its broad origin at the iliac crest toward the shoulder, and then twists upon itself before inserting into the floor of the bicipital groove of the humerus.

You have palpated near the insertion of the latissimus dorsi while examining the posterior wall of the axilla. Abduction of the arm will make the latissimus dorsi more prominent along the flank fold of the axilla. Place your thumb in the axilla as a base for palpation and move your four fingers in a sweeping fashion across the posterior aspect of the muscle. Continue palpation caudad, moving toward the iliac crest until the latissimus dorsi becomes indistinct. Palpate the opposite latissimus dorsi and compare findings. The latissimus dorsi is rarely clinically implicated; although a patient may complain of "pulled muscles," they are usually of little clinical significance.

Serratus Anterior. You have palpated the serratus anterior during palpation of the medial (chest) wall of the axilla. Now, palpate it again. As you run your fingers across the muscle, notice that it is serrated (along ribs one through eight) like the edge of a knife. The serratus anterior muscle prevents winging of the scapula by anchoring the vertebral border of the scapula to the thoracic cage (Fig. 66).

RANGE OF MOTION

Both active and passive testing methods are used to determine if a patient's range of motion is limited. In active testing, the patient uses his own muscles to complete the range of motion, while in passive testing, the examiner moves the patient's limbs through the range of motion. Passive testing should be carried out whenever a patient has difficulty performing the active tests. As a general rule, if a patient is able to perform a complete range of active motion without pain or discomfort, there is no need to conduct the passive tests.

The range of motion of the shoulder girdle involves six motions: (1) abduction, (2) adduction, (3) extension, (4) flexion, (5) internal rotation, and (6) external rotation. These specific motions combine to provide a wide variety of motion for the shoulder.

Active Range of Motion Tests

The Apley "Scratch" test is the quickest active way to evaluate a patient's range of motion. First, to test abduction and external rotation, ask the patient to reach behind his head and touch the superior medial angle of the opposite scapula (Fig. 48). Next, to determine the range of internal rotation and adduction, instruct the patient to reach in front of his head and touch the opposite acromion (Fig. 49). Third, to further test internal rotation and adduction, have the patient reach behind his back to touch the inferior angle of the opposite scapula (Fig. 50). Observe the patient's movement during all phases of testing for any limitation of motion or for any break of normal rhythm or symmetry.

To test the patient's range of motion another way, instruct him to abduct his arms to 90°, keeping his elbows straight. Then ask him to turn his palms up in supination and continue abduction

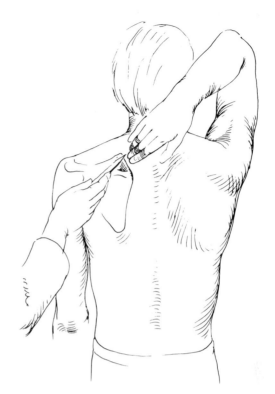

Fig. 48. The Apley Scratch Test: External rotation and abduction.

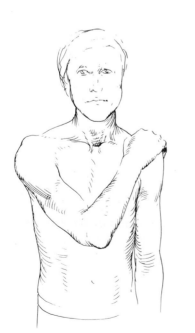

Fig. 49. Test for internal rotation and adduction.

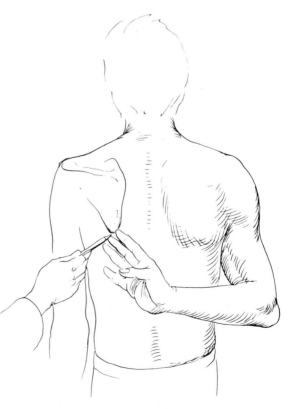

Fig. 50. Internal rotation and adduction.

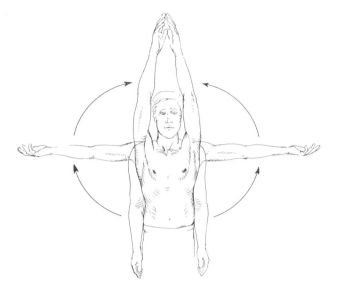

Fig. 51. Range of motion.

until his hands touch over his head (Fig. 51). This will demonstrate full bilateral abduction and provide instant bilateral comparison. Next, have the patient place his hands behind his neck and push his elbows out posteriorly to test abduction and external rotation. Finally, to test adduction and internal rotation, ask the patient to place both hands behind his back as high as they will go as if he were scratching the inferior scapular angle. The chief advantage of this quick range of motion tests is that the patient demonstrates motion on both sides simultaneously, making it easy to examine for symmetry of motion and to note even small losses on the abnormal side.

Passive Range of Motion Tests

If a patient is unable to perform fully any of the motions of the shoulder girdle, passive testing should be conducted. A patient may not be able to demonstrate full active range of motion for a variety of reasons: he may have muscle weakness, soft tissue contractures (in the joint capsule or ligaments, or as a result of muscle contractures), or bony blockage (bony fusion or excrescences). Passive testing eliminates the patient's own muscle strength from consideration as a variable, since the examiner supplies the power. A passive test, then, is used to detect whether a limitation in range of motion is consistent both with and without muscle power. If the joint moves through a full range of motion under passive testing conditions, but has restricted active motion, you may assume that muscle weakness is the cause of restriction. If

restriction is consistent under passive test conditions, muscle weakness can usually be eliminated as the direct cause, and bony (intra-articular) or soft tissue (extra-articular) blockage is most likely, although muscle weakness may also exist as a result of nonutilization of the joint.

To distinguish between intra-articular and extra-articular blockage, check the quality and feel of the blockage within the joint. If the blockage has a rubbery feel and gives slightly under pressure, there is probably extra-articular (soft tissue) blockage. If, on the other hand, the blockage seems inflexible and range of motion ends abruptly, there is probably an intra-articular (bony) blockage.

It must be emphasized that the patient should be totally relaxed during these tests, for if he is tense, afraid, or insecure in your hands, his muscles will tense and splint the joint, not allowing a full passive range of motion. It is essential, therefore, that these tests be administered gently. Passive testing can be conducted with the patient either standing or sitting. His elbow should be bent during testing because flexion of the elbow cuts down on the sweep of the arm, making movement in the shoulder girdle easier and more precise. In passive testing, one of your hands should stabilize the extremity while the other manipulates the limb.

When testing for range of motion of the shoulder girdle (especially in abduction), remember that motion should be broken down into three categories: (1) pure glenohumeral motion, (2) scapulothoracic motion, and (3) a combination of glenohumeral and scapulothoracic motion.

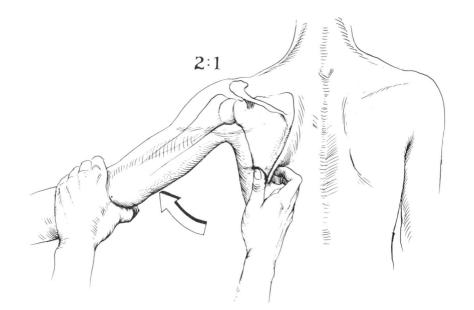

2:1

Fig. 52. Test for abduction: Motion occurs at the glenohumeral and scapulothoracic articulation in a two to one ratio.

ABDUCTION—180°
ADDUCTION— 45°

Abduction of the arm occurs in the glenohumeral joint and scapulothoracic articulation in a two to one ratio (2:1); for every 3° of abduction, 2° occur in the glenohumeral joint, and 1° occurs at the scapulothoracic articulation. Stand behind the patient and anchor the scapula by holding its inferior angle (Fig. 52). With your free hand abduct the patient's arm. The scapula should not move until the arm is abducted to approximately 20° (indicating free glenohumeral motion). At that point, the humerus and scapula move together in a 2:1 ratio to complete abduction. If the glenohumeral joint does not move in its normal ratio with the scapulothoracic articulation but seems to be fixed in adduction, the patient may have frozen shoulder syndrome (Fig. 53). If this is the case, he may be able to shrug his shoulder to nearly 90° of abduction using pure scapulothoracic motion.

An effective alternate method of testing abduction is to anchor the scapula by placing your hand firmly upon the acromion of the extremity being tested. This ensures that relatively little scapulothoracic action enters into glenohumeral motion. Place your other hand immediately superior to the elbow joint (thereby isolating the glenohumeral joint with your two hands). Then, move the arm slowly laterally and upward as far as it will comfortably go.

As you test the range of abduction, watch the patient for any sign of hesitation or pain. Normal

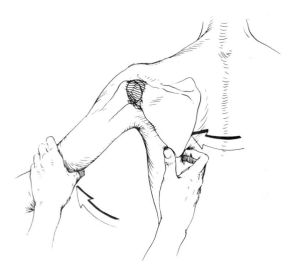

Fig. 53. Frozen Shoulder Syndrome: No glenohumeral motion—only scapulothoracic motion.

pure glenohumeral abduction is approximately 90°. As the scapula begins to move, you will feel scapular motion through the hand resting on its tip. Abduction will continue to approximately 120°. At this point, the surgical neck of the humerus strikes the acromion (Fig. 54). Full abduction can be completed only when the humerus is externally rotated to increase the articulating surface of the humeral head and to turn the surgical neck away from the tip of the acromion (Figs. 55, 56).

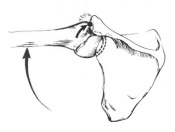

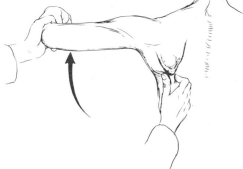

Fig. 54. Abduction continues to approximately 120°, where the surgical neck of the humerus strikes the acromion.

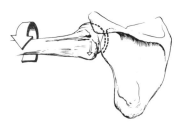

Fig. 55. Full abduction is possible only when the humerus is externally rotated.

Fig. 56. External rotation increases the articulating surface of the humeral head and turns the surgical neck away from the tip of the acromion.

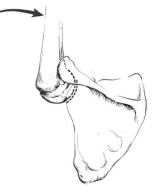

Now, bring the patient's arm back to his side and begin moving it across the front of his body in adduction. Normal adduction allows the arm to swing about 45° across the front of the body. Test the other shoulder and compare results. Adduction may be limited by bursitis or by tears in the rotator cuff (especially in the supraspinatus).

FLEXION —90°
EXTENSION—45°

In the more extreme degrees of extension, the patient will tend to lean away from the movement of his arm. Therefore, cup your hand over his acromion both to stabilize the scapula and to fix the entire body. Your hand will prevent or at least sense this movement. Place your other hand proximal to the elbow joint and move the arm into extension. Normally the arm will extend to approximately 45°. Then move the arm forward through the anatomic position into flexion. Normal flexion is about 90°. Repeat the procedures of flexion and extension on the other side and compare results. A limited range of flexion and extension may indicate bicipital tendinitis or bursitis in the shoulder.

INTERNAL ROTATION —55°
EXTERNAL ROTATION—40°–45°

To test internal and external rotation, stand in front of the patient and hold his elbow to his waist to prevent the substitutions of abduction for internal rotation and adduction for external rotation. Take the patient's wrist in your other hand, and, keeping his elbow bent to about 90°, externally rotate the arm, using the shoulder as the point and the forearm as the indicator of motion. External rotation should range about 40° to 45°. Bursitis is one cause of limitation. Then return the arm to its starting position and move it into internal rotation. The arm will normally rotate about 55° before its motion is interrupted by the body.

NEUROLOGIC EXAMINATION

The neurologic portion of the examination permits assessment of the strength of each group of muscles that motors the shoulder joint. It may also indicate the degree of motor weakness that might restrict range of motion. In addition to muscle testing, reflex and sensation tests allow for further determination of the integrity of the nerve supply to the shoulder.

Muscle Testing

Muscle testing in the shoulder involves nine motions: (1) flexion, (2) extension, (3) abduction, (4) adduction, (5) external rotation, (6) internal rotation, (7) scapular elevation (shoulder shrug), (8) scapular retraction (position of attention), and (9) shoulder protraction (reaching).

For the purposes of this discussion, these motions have been divided into distinct categories. However, it is far simpler to continue the flow of testing by moving from one test to the next without interruption. For example, since the arc of motion is continuous from flexion through extension, you may proceed directly from the test for flexion to the test for extension.

For the neurologic examination, the patient may either sit or stand, depending solely upon his comfort. The muscles of the shoulder girdle are tested by functional groups.

FLEXION

Primary Flexors:
  1) Anterior portion of the deltoid
     axillary nerve, C5
  2) Coracobrachialis
     musculocutaneous nerve, C5–C6
Secondary Flexors:
  1) Pectoralis major (clavicular head)
  2) Biceps
  3) Anterior portion of the deltoid

Stand behind the patient and place your hand palm downward upon the acromion so that you can stabilize the scapula and palpate the anterior portion of the deltoid as you test. Place your other hand just proximal to the elbow, wrapping your fingers around the anterior aspect of the arm and the biceps muscle (Fig. 57).

When the elbow is flexed to 90°, instruct the patient to begin flexion of the shoulder. As he begins, gradually increase your resisting pressure until you determine the maximum resistance he can overcome. Test the opposite shoulder to provide a means for comparison, and evaluate your findings in accordance with the muscle grading chart (Table 1).

Table 1. Muscle Grading Chart	
Muscle Gradations	**Description**
5—Normal	Complete range of motion against gravity with full resistance
4—Good	Complete range of motion against gravity with some resistance
3—Fair	Complete range of motion against gravity
2—Poor	Complete range of motion with gravity eliminated
1—Trace	Evidence of slight contractility. No joint motion
0—Zero	No evidence of contractility

EXTENSION

Primary Extensors:
1) Latissimus dorsi
   thoracodorsal nerve, C6, C7, C8
2) Teres major
   lower subscapular nerve, C5, C6
3) Posterior portion of the deltoid
   axillary nerve, C5, C6

Secondary Extensors:
1) Teres minor
2) Triceps (long head)

Stay behind the patient and keep your stabilizing hand upon his acromion. Place your thumb on the posterior aspect of the shoulder so that during active extension you can palpate the posterior portion of the deltoid for tone. Place your resisting hand just proximal to the posterior aspect of the elbow joint with the thenar eminence and palm against the posterior portion of the humerus. During the muscle test for extension, palpate the triceps with the thumb. To maintain a smooth transition from testing flexion to extension, simply turn your resisting hand from its anterior position to a position of resistance posterior to the arm.

Ask the patient to flex his elbow and to slowly extend his arm posteriorly. As his shoulder moves into extension, gradually increase pressure until you determine the maximum amount of resistance that he can overcome (Fig. 58).

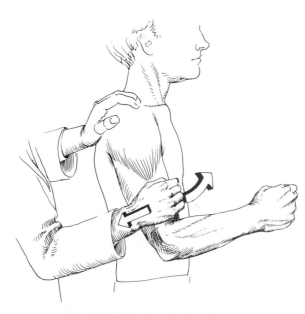

Fig. 57. Test for shoulder flexion.

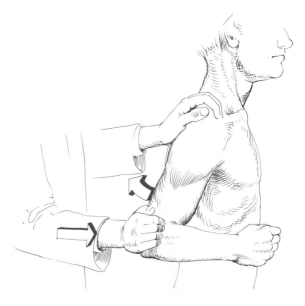

Fig. 58. Test for shoulder extension.

ABDUCTION

Primary Abductors:
1) Middle portion of the deltoid
   axillary nerve, C5, C6
2) Supraspinatus
   suprascapular nerve, C5, C6

Secondary Abductors:
1) Anterior and posterior portions of the deltoid
2) Serratus anterior (by direct action on the scapula)

Remain behind the patient. Continue to stabilize the acromion, but slide your hand slightly laterally so that while you stabilize the shoulder girdle you can also palpate the middle portion of the deltoid. Keep your other hand proximal to the elbow joint, but move it from the posterior aspect of the humerus to the lateral aspect so that maximum resistance can be applied. Your palm should now be pressed against the lateral epicondyle and supracondylar line of the humerus, with your fingers wrapped around the anterior aspect of the arm.

Ask the patient to abduct his arm, and, as he moves it into abduction, gradually increase resisting pressure until you determine the maximum resistance that he can overcome (Fig. 59).

ADDUCTION

Primary Adductors:
1) Pectoralis major
   medial and lateral anterior thoracic nerve, C5, C6, C7, C8, T1
2) Latissimus dorsi
   thoracodorsal nerve, C6, C7, C8

Secondary Adductors:
1) Teres major
2) Anterior portion of the deltoid

Remain behind the patient, with your stabilizing hand upon the acromion and your resisting hand proximal to the elbow joint. Since the pectoralis major muscle is a primary adductor, move your stabilizing hand anteriorly and inferiorly on the acromion so that you can palpate the pectoralis major as it is tested. Instruct the patient to place his arm in a few degrees of abduction and shift your resisting hand so that your thumb rests against the medial aspect of his humerus.

Then ask him to begin adduction while you gradually increase the degree of resisting pressure, until you determine the maximum amount of resistance he can overcome (Fig. 60).

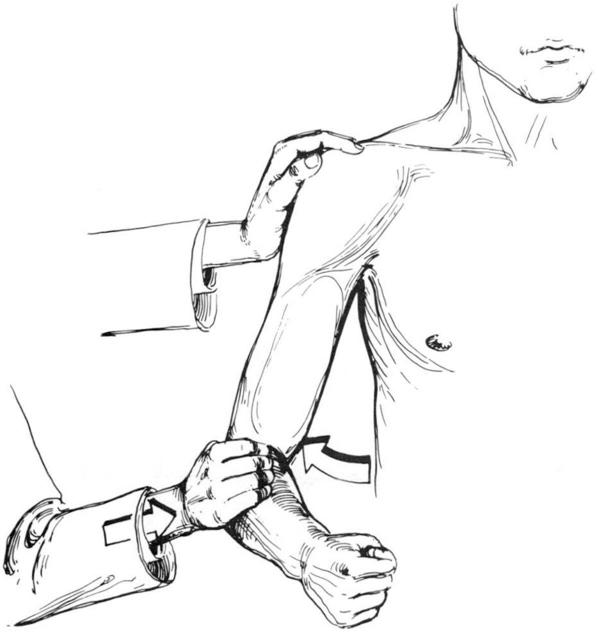

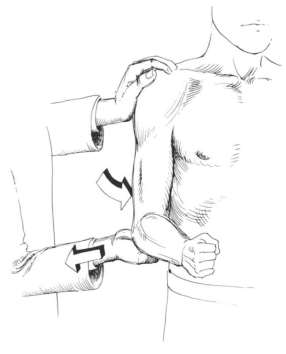

Fig. 59. Test for shoulder abduction.

Fig. 60. Test for shoulder adduction.

EXTERNAL ROTATION

Primary External Rotators:
  1) Infraspinatus
      suprascapular nerve, C5, C6
  2) Teres minor
      branch of the axillary nerve, C5

Secondary External Rotator:
  1) Posterior portion of the deltoid

Move to the patient's side and have him bend his elbow to 90°, with his forearm in a neutral position. Stabilize the extremity by holding his flexed elbow into his waist. This will prevent him from substituting adduction for pure external rotation. Move your resisting hand to his wrist, so that your thenar eminence rests upon its dorsal surface to provide maximum resistance. Because of the need for stabilization and resistance far from the location of the muscles used in external rotation, you will not be able to palpate them during the test. The muscles of external rotation are in a deep layer and are not normally palpable anyway.

Instruct the patient to rotate his arm outward. As he moves into external rotation, gradually increase the pressure of resistance until you determine the maximum resistance he can overcome (Fig. 61).

INTERNAL ROTATION

Primary Internal Rotators:
  1) Subscapular
      upper and lower subscapular nerves, C5, C6
  2) Pectoralis major
      medial and lateral anterior thoracic nerves, C5, C6, C7, C8, T1
  3) Latissimus dorsi
      thoracodorsal nerve, C6, C7, C8
  4) Teres major
      lower subscapular nerve, C5, C6

Secondary Internal Rotator:
  1) Anterior portion of the deltoid

Remain at the patient's side and instruct him to maintain his elbow in 90° of flexion as you continue to stabilize his upper arm by holding his elbow firmly against his waist. Stabilization of the elbow will prevent the patient from substituting abduction for the desired motion of pure internal rotation. Maintain your stabilizing hand just proximal to the wrist, but shift it so that the fingers wrap around the volar surface of the wrist, with your palm over the radial styloid process.

Ask the patient to gradually rotate his arm around the front of his body and, as he does so, slowly increase resistance against his wrist (Fig. 62).

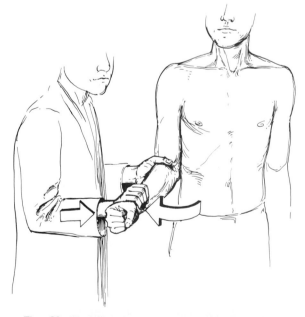

Fig. 61. Test for external rotation of the shoulder.

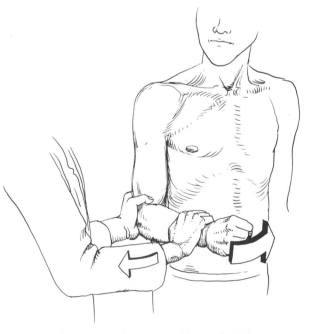

Fig. 62. Test for internal rotation of the shoulder.

SCAPULAR ELEVATION
(Shoulder Shrug)

Primary Elevators:
1) Trapezius
   spinal accessory nerve, or cranial nerve XI
2) Levator scapulae
   C3, C4 and frequently branches from the dorsal scapula nerve, C5

Secondary Elevators:
1) Rhomboid major
2) Rhomboid minor

Stand behind the patient and place one hand upon each acromion. The lateral position of your hand allows the trapezius to work freely and gives your hands a firm, bony base of support. Each hand, while resisting the shrugging mechanism, also provides balance for the other side. Place your thumb posteriorly over the lateral portion of the trapezius muscle, so that you can palpate it during the test. The levator scapulae muscle originates at the superior medial angle of the scapula deep below the trapezius and is not palpable.

Instruct the patient to shrug his shoulders, and slowly increase downward resisting pressure until you determine the maximum resistance he can overcome (Fig. 63). Normally the scapular elevators can hold scapular elevation beyond the maximum pressure you can muster. They should be tested bilaterally and any difference between the elevation of the two sides should be noted.

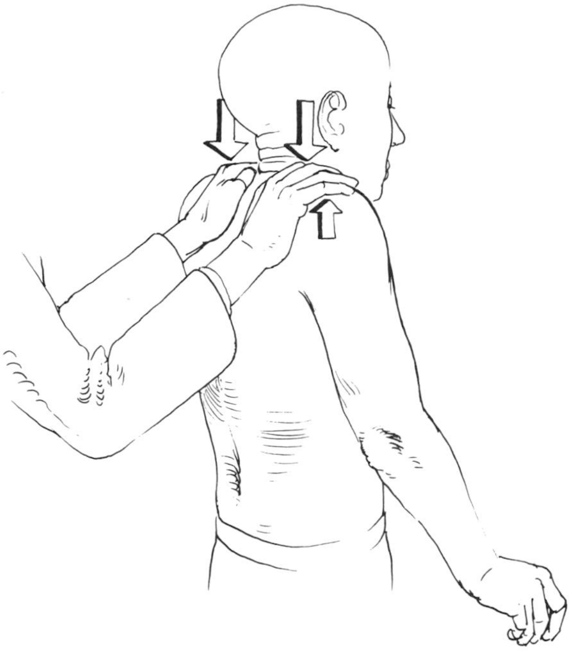

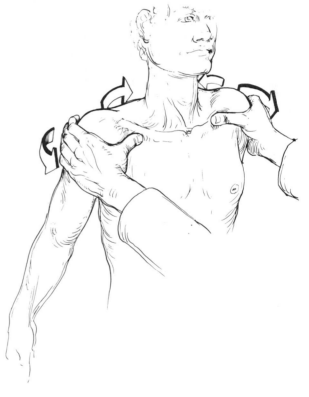

Fig. 63. Test for scapular elevation (shoulder shrug).

Fig. 64. Test for scapular retraction (position of attention).

SCAPULAR RETRACTION
(Position of Attention)

Primary Retractors:
1) Rhomboid major
   dorsal scapular nerve, C5
2) Rhomboid minor
   dorsal scapular nerve, C5

Secondary Retractor:
1) Trapezius

Stand in front of the patient and place your hands upon his shoulders with the palms anterior to the acromion and the fingers on the shoulder's posterior aspect. Your fingers should be behind the shoulder so that they can provide the moving force when you attempt to push or bend the shoulders around the fulcrum of your thumb (Fig. 64).

Ask the patient to throw his shoulders back to the "position of attention" (maximum retraction), then slowly apply pressure with your fingers trying to bend the shoulders forward around your thumb. Take care not to dig your fingers into the patient's musculature.

SCAPULAR PROTRACTION
(Reaching)

Primary Protractor:
1) Serratus anterior
   long thoracic nerve, C5, C6, C7

Scapular protraction refers to the anterior movement of the scapula on the thorax, especially in the last few degrees of reaching.

To prepare the patient, instruct him to flex his arm to 90° (parallel to the floor), then to flex his elbow so that his hand touches his shoulder. Place one hand over his spine to stabilize the trunk and to prevent substitution of trunk rotation for pure shoulder protraction. Place your resisting hand under the patient's elbow, cupping it in your palm. Then ask him to force his bent arm forward, as if he were trying to touch the wall with his elbow. As he protracts his shoulder, gradually increase your resistance against this forward movement until the maximum resistance he can overcome becomes apparent (Fig. 65). While testing shoulder protraction, check the motion of the scapula for any winging that might take place. In this instance, winging indicates weakness of the serratus anterior muscle. Such weakness may also become evident when the patient pushes against a wall, or does a regular push-up (Fig. 66).

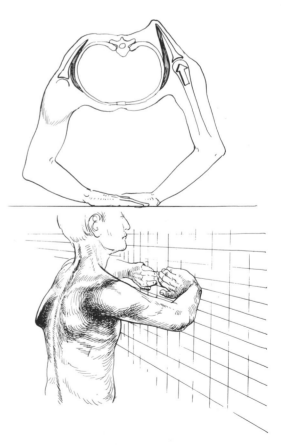

Fig. 66. Scapular winging indicates weakness of the serratus anterior muscle and is evident when the patient does a push-up or pushes against the wall.

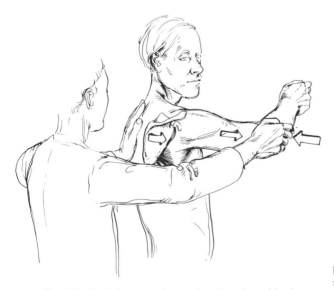

Fig. 65. Test for scapular protraction (reaching).

Reflex Testing

The biceps and the triceps, both of which cross the glenohumeral joint, may be tested for reflexes. However, since they are primarily elbow muscles, instructions for eliciting the biceps and triceps reflexes are given on page 55 in the examination of the elbow.

Sensation Testing

Innervation for sensation in the upper extremity is delineated in dermatomes, or bands, by neurologic levels. In the shoulder region, sensation is provided as follows:

1) the lateral arm—C5 nerve root—pure sensation in a round patch on the lateral aspect of the deltoid muscle (axillary nerve) (Fig. 67);
2) the medial arm—T1 nerve root;
3) the axilla—T2 nerve root;
4) from the axilla to the nipple—T3 nerve root;
5) the nipple—T4 nerve root (Fig. 68).

The sensation of the shoulder region dermatomes should be tested and evaluated bilaterally to provide a means for comparison. It is important to determine the number of dermatomes involved in any neurologic damage. The findings from the muscle tests as well as the results of sensation tests can be used to determine whether or not any neurologic levels are involved in pathology.

To test the integrity of sensation around the shoulder, prick each dermatome lightly with a pin, asking the patient if he feels the pinprick. Then prick the opposite side. Each dermatome should then be tested similarly, using a brush. Again, ask the patient if the sensations in the two shoulders are similar or dissimilar. Abnormal sensation (paresthesia) may either be increased (hypesthesia), decreased (hypoesthesia), or altogether absent (anesthesia).

The axillary nerve is frequently damaged secondary to shoulder dislocation, leaving an anesthetic patch on the lateral aspect of the deltoid muscle.

Remember that results from the sensation tests are subjective findings reported to you by the patient, and, as such, are neither objective nor

Fig. 67. Sensation test—Lateral arm.

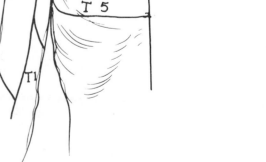

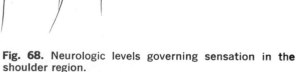

Fig. 68. Neurologic levels governing sensation in the shoulder region.

verifiable. If, for some reason, the patient is unable to give appropriate responses to your questions, sensations tests are of little value.

SPECIAL TESTS

Certain special tests pertain to the anatomy and pathologic condition of each joint. They are structured to uncover a specific type of pathology, and are most helpful when previous portions of your examination have led you to suspect the nature of the pathology. Three such tests for the shoulder are: (1) the Yergason test for long head of the biceps tendon stability, (2) the drop arm test for rotator cuff tear, and (3) the apprehension test for shoulder dislocation.

THE YERGASON TEST. This test determines whether or not the biceps tendon is stable in the bicipital groove. To conduct this test, instruct the patient to fully flex his elbow. Then grasp his flexed elbow in one hand while holding his wrist with your other hand. To test the stability of the biceps tendon, externally rotate the patient's arm as he resists, and, at the same time, pull downward on his elbow (Fig. 69). If the biceps tendon is

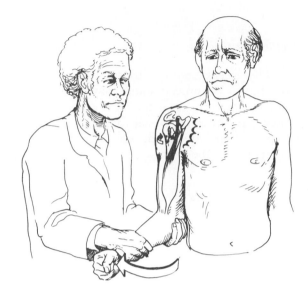

Fig. 69. The Yergason test: to determine the stability of the long head of the biceps tendon in the bicipital groove.

unstable in the bicipital groove, it will pop out of the groove and the patient will experience pain. If the tendon is stable, it will remain secure and the patient will experience no discomfort (Fig. 70).

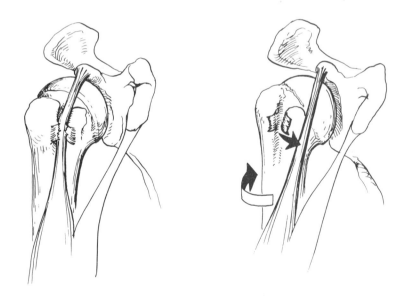

Fig. 70. The unstable biceps tendon.

DROP ARM TEST. This test detects whether or not there are any tears in the rotator cuff (Fig. 71). First, instruct the patient to fully abduct his arm (Fig. 72). Then ask him to slowly lower it to his side. If there are tears in the rotator cuff (especially in the supraspinatus muscle), the arm will drop to the side from a position of about 90° abduction (Fig. 73). The patient still will not be able to lower his arm smoothly and slowly no matter how many times he tries. If he is able to hold his arm in abduction, a gentle tap on the forearm will cause the arm to fall to his side.

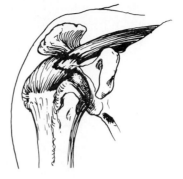

Fig. 71. Tears in the rotator cuff.

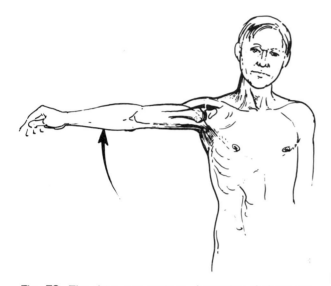

Fig. 72. The drop arm test: to determine if there are tears in the rotator cuff.

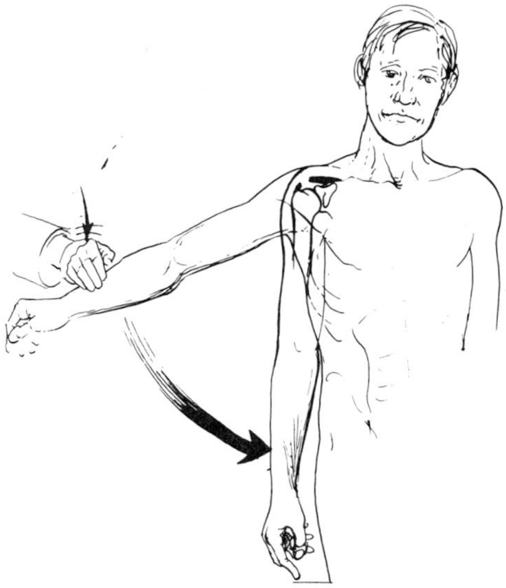

Fig. 73. If there are tears in the rotator cuff, the arm drops and the patient is unable to lower his arm slowly to his side.

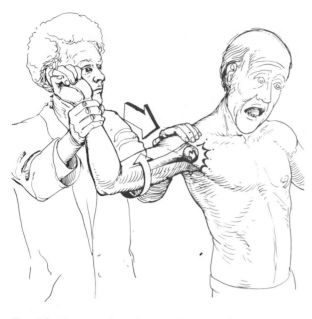

Fig. 74. The apprehension test for shoulder dislocation.

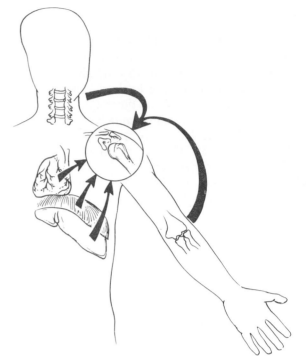

Fig. 75. Areas around the shoulder sometimes refer or radiate pain to the shoulder.

APPREHENSION TEST FOR SHOULDER DISLOCATION. To test for chronic shoulder dislocation, abduct and externally rotate the patient's arm to a position where it might easily dislocate. If his shoulder is ready to dislocate, the patient will have a noticeable look of apprehension or alarm on his face and will resist further motion (Fig. 74). This test is similar to the patella apprehension test for dislocation of the patella.

EXAMINATION OF RELATED AREAS

Since the shoulder is a classic area for referred pain, it is necessary in a complete examination to include an examination of those areas known to refer pain to it.

A coronary (myocardial infarction) may radiate pain to the left shoulder. Shoulder symptoms may also be related to irritation of the diaphragm, which shares the same root innervation (C4, C5) as the dermatome covering the shoulder's summit. Therefore, the chest and upper abdomen should be carefully examined to determine if symptoms of pathology associated with them are being referred to the shoulder (Fig. 75).

Problems of the neck, such as a herniated cervical disc or other general trauma, may also radiate pain to the shoulder or scapula. This type of radiating pain from the neck area is often felt at the superior medial angle of the scapula (Fig. 75).

Sometimes, a spinal fracture, in addition to causing local pain, may radiate pain to the shoulder along the course of any muscle affected by the fracture. For example, if there is a fracture of the cervical spine, the rhomboids may transmit pain to the scapula (Fig. 75).

The shoulder may also be affected by pathology of the elbow and the distal end of the humerus, where a fracture can radiate pain proximally to the shoulder (Fig. 75). This is, however, a rather uncommon finding.

2
Physical Examination of the Elbow

INSPECTION
    Carrying Angle
    Swelling
    Scars

BONY PALPATION
    Medical Epicondyle
    Medial Supracondylar Line of the Humerus
    Olecranon
    Ulnar Border
    Olecranon Fossa
    Lateral Epicondyle
    Lateral Supracondylar Line of the Humerus
    Radial Head

SOFT TISSUE PALPATION
    Zone I   — Medial Aspect
    Zone II — Posterior Aspect
    Zone III — Lateral Aspect
    Zone IV — Anterior Aspect

RANGE OF MOTION
    Active Range of Motion Tests
        Flexion _____ 135°+
        Extension _____ 0°–5°
        Supination ____ 90°
        Pronation ____ 90°
    Passive Range of Motion Tests
        Flexion and Extension
        Supination and Pronation

NEUROLOGIC EXAMINATION
    Muscle Testing
    Reflex Testing
        Biceps Reflex _____ C5
        Brachioradialis Reflex __ C6
        Triceps Reflex _____ C7
    Sensation Testing

SPECIAL TESTS
    Tests for Ligamentous Stability
    Tinel Sign
    Tennis Elbow Test

EXAMINATION OF RELATED AREAS

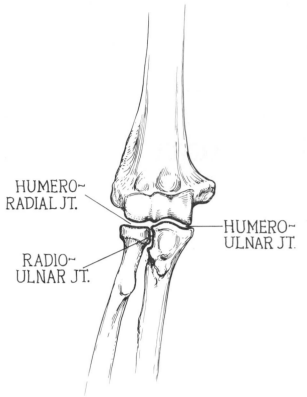

Fig. 1. The three elbow articulations.

HUMERO- RADIAL JT.

RADIO- ULNAR JT.

HUMERO- ULNAR JT.

The elbow, a ginglymus (hinge) joint, is a relatively stable joint, with firm osseous support. It is composed of three articulations:

1) the humeroulnar joint
2) the humeroradial joint
3) the radioulnar joint (Fig. 1).

Examination of the elbow will include these articulations and the soft tissues surrounding them.

INSPECTION

Carrying Angle

When the arm is extended in the anatomic position (palms facing anteriorly), the longitudinal axes of the upper arm and forearm form a lateral (valgus) angle at the elbow joint known as the "carrying angle." (Valgus, meaning "away from the midline" or "lateral," is easily remembered if the "L" in valgus is associated with the "L" in lateral) (Fig. 2).

A normal carrying angle measures approximately 5° in males and between 10° and 15° in females. The carrying angle allows the elbow to fit closely into the depression at the waist, immediately superior to the iliac crest. The angulation is particularly noticeable when the hand is carrying something heavy (Fig. 3).

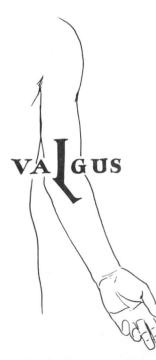

VA**L**GUS

Fig. 2. A valgus angle.

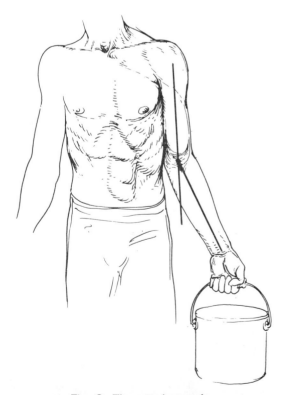

Fig. 3. The carrying angle.

CUBITUS VALGUS. The carrying angle is abnormal if the forearm stands out further than the normal 5° to 15° described. Such increased angulation can be caused by epiphyseal damage secondary to lateral epicondylar fracture and may cause a delayed nerve palsy, which presents in the ulnar nerve distribution in the hand.

CUBITUS VARUS. A decrease in the carrying angle is called a varus angle, or more descriptively, a "gunstock deformity" (Fig. 4). It is often a result of trauma, such as a supracondylar fracture in a child, where the distal end of the humerus is subject to either malunion or growth retardation at the epiphyseal plate. Its incidence is more frequent than that of the cubitus valgus.

Initially, the elbow joints should be inspected while the patient's arms are in full extension, since the carrying angle and any valgus or varus deformities are not evident in flexion. The carrying angles should be symmetrical bilaterally. If they are not, their degree of deviation from the norm should be measured.

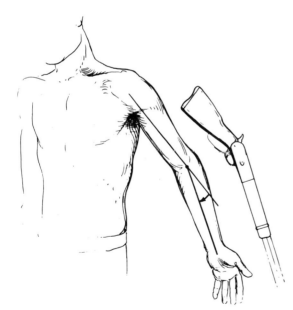

Fig. 4. A "gunstock" deformity (varus angulation).

Swelling

Swelling may be of a local or a diffuse nature. Localized swelling most often presents as a bump or a small, specific mass under the skin, such as a swollen olecranon bursa, where swelling is confined to the limited area of the bursa (Fig. 5). Diffuse swelling of the elbow may fill the entire joint; the patient may have to hold his elbow in a flexed position (about 45°) so that the joint can reach its maximum volume and accommodate the swelling with minimal pain. A supracondylar fracture at the humerus' distal end or a crush injury of the elbow are two traumatic injuries that can cause diffuse swelling.

As a general rule, localized swelling is contained within the joint capsule or bursa and does not extravasate into nearby tissues, whereas diffuse swelling is widespread and involves the entire elbow region. In both types of swellings, some of the normally visible creases in the region are lost to view.

Scars

Burn patients may have general surface scarring, and may develop joint contractures restricting elbow movement. Needle-puncture scarring is seen in the upper forearm and cubital fossa secondary to multiple injections from intravenous infusion by a physician, or perhaps by the enterprising patient himself.

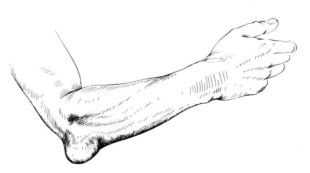

Fig. 5. Localized swelling of the olecranon bursa.

BONY PALPATION

Stand at the patient's side and hold the anterior lateral aspect of his arm. With your other hand around the biceps, abduct and extend the arm further until the olecranon process becomes clearly visible; have the patient flex the elbow to approximately 90° (Fig. 6).

The precise location of any crepitation heard or felt during movement of the elbow joint should, if possible, be determined. Crepitation may be caused by synovial or bursal thickening, by a fracture, or by osteoarthritis. Check also for pain, swelling, and temperature elevation.

Medial Epicondyle. The medial epicondyle is located on the medial side of the distal end of the humerus (Fig. 7). It is rather large and subcutaneous, and its bony contours stand out conspicuously from the surrounding tissue. The medial epicondyle is frequently fractured in children.

Medial Supracondylar Line of the Humerus. Move upward in linear fashion from the epicondyle, and palpate this short bony ridge, even though it is covered by the thick origin of the wrist flexor muscles and is not very distinct (Fig. 8). As you

trace up the line, check for bony excrescences along its surface. Occasionally, a small bony process may develop on the medial supracondylar line, trapping the median nerve and causing symptoms of median nerve compression. Palpate back down the medial supracondylar line and return to the medial epicondyle. Note that much of the elbow can be palpated in this linear fashion; both the olecranon process and its associated ulnar border and the lateral epicondyle and its supracondylar line are most efficiently palpated in this way.

Olecranon. The olecranon is the large process at the upper end of the ulna (Fig. 9). It is conical in shape and has a relatively sharp apex which is covered by the loose, tractable skin that permits extreme elbow flexion. Flexion moves the olecranon out of the depth of its fossa, making it available for palpation. Although it feels subcutaneous to the touch, the olecranon is actually covered by the olecranon bursa and the triceps tendon and aponeurosis. The bursa and the tendon are very thin at the apex of the olecranon and do not hinder palpation.

Ulnar Border. Hold the patient's arm in abduction and palpate from the olecranon down the subcutaneous posterior ulnar border which runs in a relatively straight line to the ulnar styloid process at the wrist (Fig. 10). Then return to the olecranon process over the same route (Fig. 11).

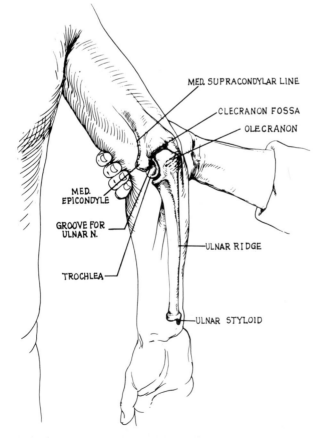

Fig. 6. Anatomy of the elbow (posterior view).

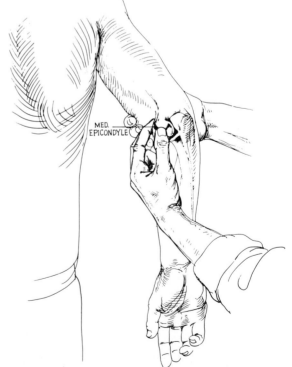

Fig. 7. Palpation of the medial epicondyle of the humerus.

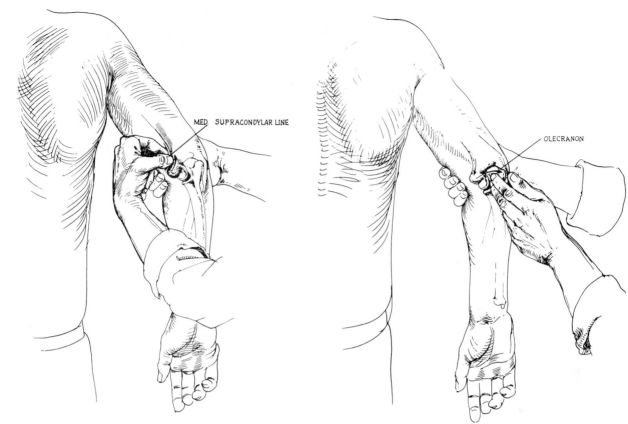

Fig. 8. Palpation of the medial supracondylar line of the humerus.

Fig. 9. The olecranon.

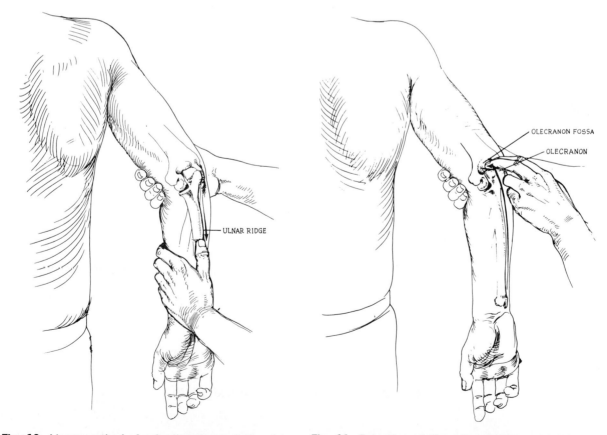

Fig. 10. Linear method of palpating the posterior ulnar border.

Fig. 11. Palpation of the ulnar border and olecranon fossa.

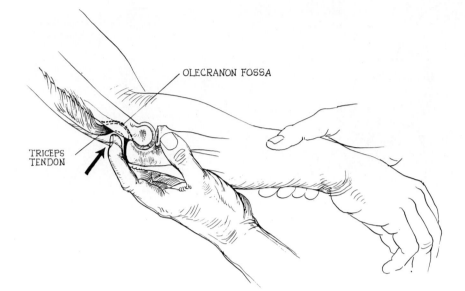

Fig. 12. The olecranon fossa.

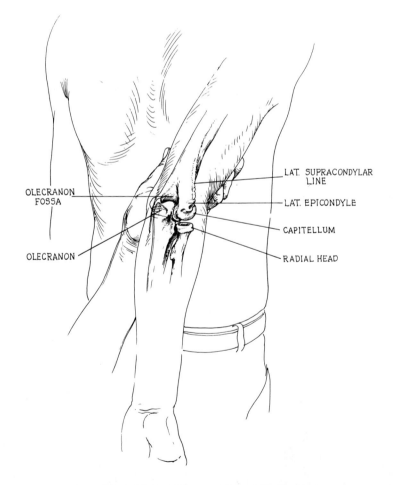

Fig. 13. Anatomy of the elbow (lateral view).

Olecranon Fossa. The olecranon fossa, which lies at the distal end of the posterior humerus, receives the olecranon during elbow extension (Fig. 12). It is filled with fat and covered by a portion of the triceps muscle and aponeurosis, and precise palpation is difficult. Partial extension of the elbow slackens the triceps muscle, bringing its insertion and origin closer together and exposing a portion of the fossa for palpation. If the elbow is extended too far, however, the olecranon process will fill the fossa and make palpation impossible.

Lateral Epicondyle. Located lateral to the olecranon process is the lateral epicondyle. It is prominent, but somewhat smaller and less defined than the medial epicondyle (Figs. 13, 14).

Lateral Supracondylar Line of the Humerus. This is better defined and longer than the medial supracondylar line, extending almost to the deltoid tuberosity. From the lateral epicondyle, palpate up the lateral supracondylar line and then back down to the lateral epicondyle (Fig. 15).

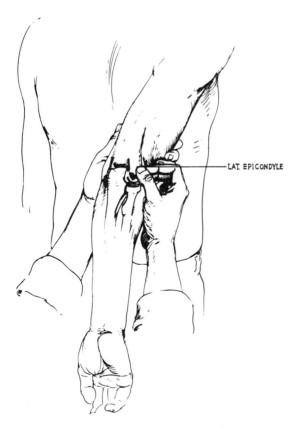

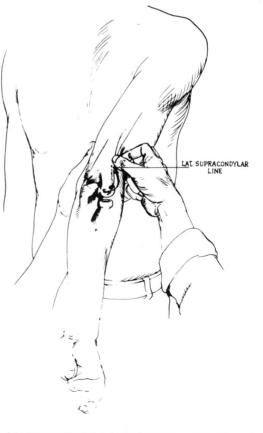

Fig. 14. The lateral epicondyle of the humerus.　　　**Fig. 15.** The lateral supracondylar line of the humerus.

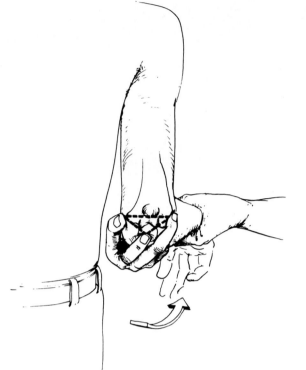

Fig. 16. When the elbow is flexed, the olecranon and the medial and lateral epicondyles form an isosceles triangle.

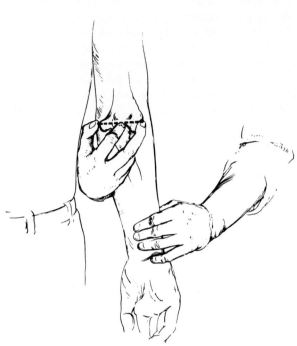

Fig. 17. When the elbow is extended, the points at the olecranon and the epicondyles lie in a straight line.

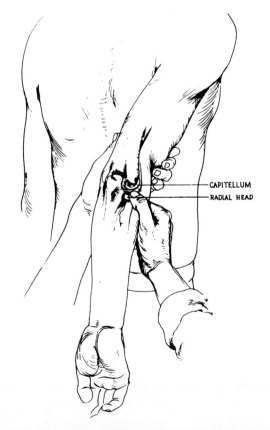

CAPITELLUM
RADIAL HEAD

Fig. 18. The radial head lies within a depression medial and posterior to the wrist extensor muscle group.

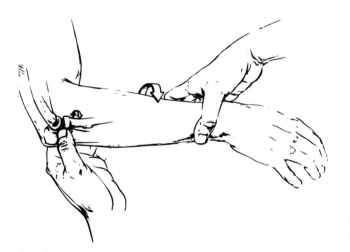

Fig. 19. Palpation of the radial head: Supination and pronation of the forearm rotate the radial head under your thumb.

The medial epicondyle, the olecranon process, and the lateral epicondyle have an interesting, almost geometric, alignment, which can be appreciated if you place your thumb upon the lateral epicondyle, your index finger upon the olecranon, and your middle finger upon the medial epicondyle. When the patient's elbow is flexed (90°), your fingers form an isosceles triangle (Fig. 16). When his elbow is extended, your fingers, moving with the bony prominences, form a relatively straight line (Fig. 17). Any appreciable deviation from this alignment may be indicative of some anatomic problem, and requires further investigation.

Radial Head. With the patient's arm abducted, ask him to maintain his elbow in a flexed position (90°). To orient yourself, relocate the lateral epicondyle, and move your fingers about one inch distally until you find a visible depression in the skin just medial and posterior to the wrist extensor muscle group (Fig. 18). The radial head lies deep within this depression, and is palpable through the thick muscle mass of the wrist extensors. Ask the patient to turn his forearm slowly, first in supination, then in pronation; the radial head will rotate under your thumb (Fig. 19). If the patient can perform supination and pronation fully, approximately three-quarters of the radial head is palpable. The radius articulates with the capitellum (condyle) of the humerus on its proximal end and with the ulnar radial notch on its distal end. Both the capitellum and the radial notch lie deep and are not palpable. Pain in and around the area of the radial head may indicate synovitis or osteoarthritis of the head itself. The radial head may be out of position and more easily palpable if it has been dislocated congenitally or traumatically.

SOFT TISSUE PALPATION

The examination of the elbow's soft tissues has been divided into four parts, or clinical zones: (1) the medial aspect, (2) the posterior aspect, (3) the lateral aspect, and (4) the anterior aspect. The bony structures of the elbow are palpated in a linear fashion. Since most of the soft tissues surrounding the elbow joint also run longitudinally, this linear fashion of examination should continue.

Zone I—Medial Aspect

With the patient's elbow in a flexed position (90°), extend and abduct his shoulder slightly so that the soft tissue structures of the medial aspect become more accessible. The elbow should remain in this position throughout soft tissue palpation.

Ulnar Nerve. The ulnar nerve is situated in the sulcus (groove) between the medial epicondyle and the olecranon process, and can be palpated as it is rolled gently under the index and middle fingers (Fig. 20). It feels soft, round, and tubular. Follow its course up the arm as far as possible, and return to the sulcus at the level of the medial epicondyle. As you do so, gently check to see if you can displace the nerve from its groove.

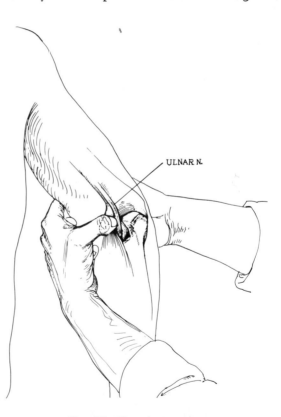

ULNAR N.

Fig. 20. The ulnar nerve.

A thickening in this region, usually due to a build-up of scar tissue, may cause nerve compression, which will lead to a tingling sensation in the patient's ring and little fingers (the ulnar distribution of the hand). The nerve must be palpated with a gentle touch or the patient will experience pinprick-like shocks down the forearm and into the ulnar distribution of his hand. The ulnar nerve is popularly known as the "funny bone" because of this tingling. As the nerve runs distally, it crosses the elbow joint and pierces the flexor carpi ulnaris muscle to gain entrance to the forearm. The ulnar nerve may be injured secondary to supracondylar or epicondylar fracture or by direct trauma. However, loss of continuity is rare.

Wrist Flexor–Pronator Muscle Group. This group is composed of four muscles: (1) the pronator teres, (2) the flexor carpi radialis, (3) the palmaris longus, and (4) the flexor carpi ulnaris. These four originate from the medial epicondyle as a common tendon, then split and continue in their individual courses down the forearm. You can easily remember their order and pattern if you place your hand over your forearm with your thenar eminence upon the medial epicondyle. With your fingers spread down the forearm, your thumb represents the pronator teres, your index finger the flexor carpi radialis, your middle finger the palmaris longus, and your ring finger the flexor carpi ulnaris (Fig. 21).

The wrist flexors should be palpated first as a unit and then individually. As you move from their origin at the medial epicondyle and supracondylar line down the forearm and toward the wrist, check for any tenderness that may be present (Fig. 22). The muscle mass and origin may become tender if they are strained by activities requiring wrist flexion pronation (tennis, golf, using a screwdriver, and so on). Note that the palmaris longus, the flexor carpi radialis, and the flexor carpi ulnaris are palpable to the wrist. The entire flexor pronator group can be surgically removed from its common origin and transferred proximally onto the humerus to substitute for a weak or absent biceps muscle.

Pronator Teres. This muscle is covered by other muscles and is not distinctly palpable.

Flexor Carpi Radialis. Ask the patient to make a tight fist, and then to radially deviate and flex his wrist. The flexor carpi radialis stands out

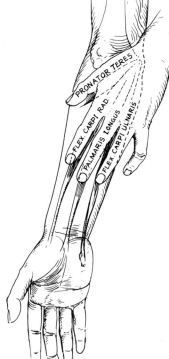

Fig. 21. The wrist flexor–pronators (Redrawn from Henry, AK: Extensile Exposure, 2nd ed. London, Churchill Livingston, 1957).

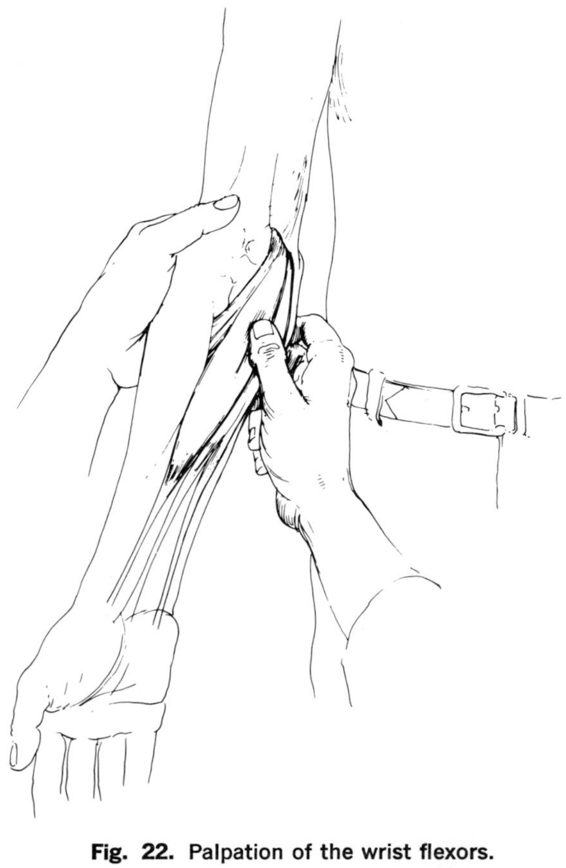

Fig. 22. Palpation of the wrist flexors.

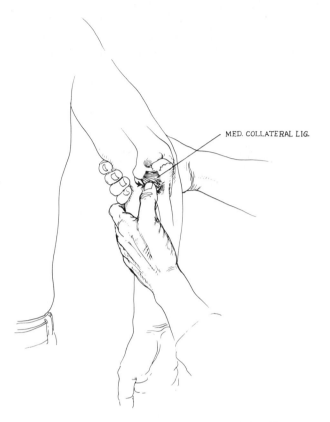

Fig. 23. The medial collateral ligament of the elbow.

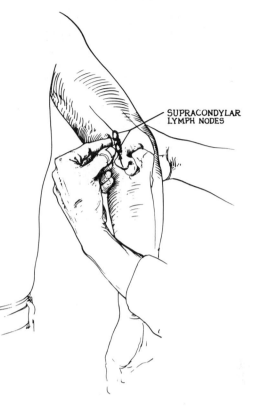

Fig. 24. Enlarged supracondylar lymph nodes.

radial to the palmaris longus and may be palpated proximally toward its origin at the medial epicondyle.

Palmaris Longus. See Wrist and Hand Chapter, page 82.

Flexor Carpi Ulnaris. Even if the patient makes a tight fist, this muscle will be less prominent than the palmaris longus or the flexor carpi radialis, but it does stand out slightly on the ulnar side of the palmaris longus proximal to the pisiform bone. Palpate along its length toward its origin at the medial epicondyle of the humerus.

Medial Collateral Ligament. The medial collateral ligament of the elbow is one of the basic stabilizers for the humeroulnar articulation. Fan-shaped and similar to the knee's medial collateral ligament, it rises from the medial epicondyle and extends to the medial margin of the ulna's trochlear notch (Fig. 23). While it cannot be palpated directly, the area in which it lies should be checked for tenderness which could result from a sprain caused by a sudden, forced valgus stress to the elbow. (A test for ligamentous stability is described in the special tests portion of this chapter.)

Supracondylar Lymph Nodes. At this time, check the medial supracondylar line for the presence of enlarged supracondylar (epicondylar) lymph nodes. If they are swollen, they will feel like slippery lumps under your fingers (Fig. 24). An enlarged node frequently implies an infection in the hand or forearm. As you gain experience, palpation of the nodes can be integrated into bony palpation of the medial supracondylar line.

Zone II—Posterior Aspect

Olecranon Bursa. The olecranon bursa covers the olecranon, and is not distinctly palpable. However, the area in which it lies should be palpated. If the bursa is inflamed (bursitis) or inspissate (thickened), the area will feel boggy and thick (Figs. 5, 25). As you palpate this area, explore along the posterior ulnar border and check for rheumatoid nodules, which are occasionally found in the region.

Triceps Muscle. As its name indicates, the triceps muscle has three heads: the long head, the lateral head, and the medial head. The long head crosses the glenohumeral joint of the shoulder and

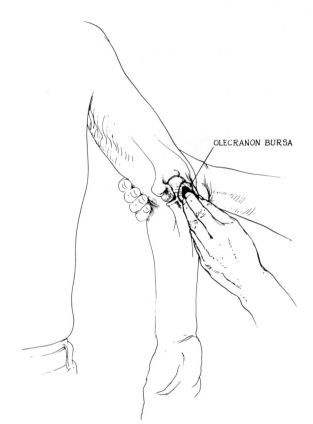

Fig. 25. The olecranon bursa.

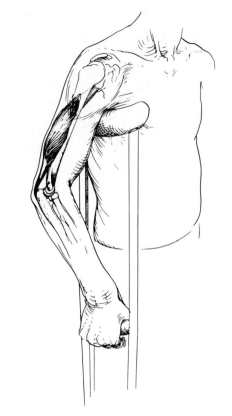

Fig. 26. The triceps muscle becomes prominent when weight is supported by a crutch. The triceps muscle is necessary for the use of a standard crutch.

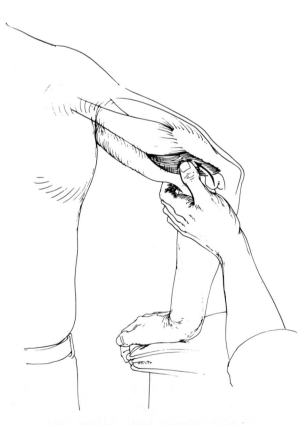

Fig. 27. The long head of the triceps.

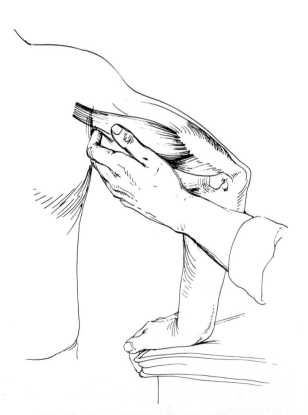

Fig. 28. The medial head of the triceps.

the elbow joint as well, making the triceps a two-joint muscle. To facilitate palpation, have the patient lean on a table or desk as if he were supporting his weight on a cane or crutch. Since the triceps muscle is integral to the act of walking with a standard crutch, it will stand out prominently on the posterior aspect of the arm (Fig. 26).

The long head of the triceps is subcutaneous and lies on the posteromedial portion of the arm. Palpate it by tracing its course up the arm toward its origin (Fig. 27), and then back down to the point where it forms a common muscle belly with the lateral head. The lateral head lies on the posterolateral aspect of the arm and may be palpated in the same manner as the long head. The medial, or deep, head lies deep under the long head, but is distinctly palpable on the medial aspect of the distal end of the humerus, to the point where it submerges beneath the long head (Fig. 28). The triceps aponeurosis, which expands distally, is broad and thin and palpable only to the proximal end of the olecranon process; however, its course should be checked for any tenderness or defects secondary to trauma.

Zone III—Lateral Aspect

Wrist Extensors. The wrist extensors originate from the lateral epicondyle and its supracondylar line and are commonly called "the mobile wad of three." This group is composed of three muscles: (1) the brachioradialis, (2) the extensor carpi radialis longus, and (3) the extensor carpi radialis brevis.

The mobile wad of three is an elongated muscle mass, and should initially be palpated as a unit. Notice that the muscles are tractable under the skin and are easily held and moved between the fingers (Fig. 29). The consistency of the muscle mass can best be assessed when the patient's forearm is in a neutral position (neither pronated nor supinated), and his wrist is at rest.

Brachioradialis. The brachioradialis originates from the lateral supracondylar ridge of the humerus. To make this muscle more prominent, have the patient close his fist, place it in a neutral position under the edge of a table, and then lift up against the weight of the table. The brachioradialis is easily identifiable on the anterolateral aspect of the arm (Fig. 30). Palpate it from its origin to its insertion at the radial styloid process, and note any tenderness elicited or defects felt along the way. The brachioradialis is the only muscle in the body that extends from the distal end of one bone to the distal end of another. Although it is considered a part of the wrist extensor muscle group, it actually functions as an elbow flexor.

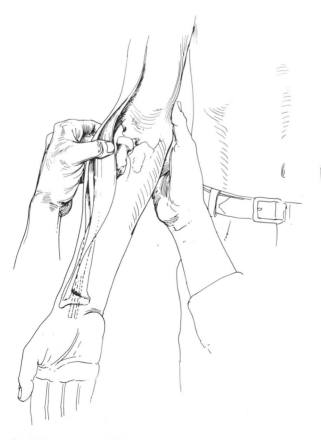

Fig. 29. The "mobile wad of three"—the wrist extensors.

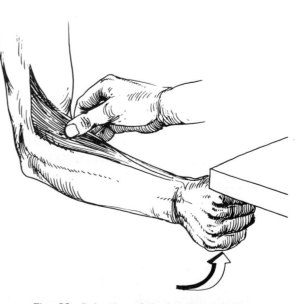

Fig. 30. Palpation of the brachioradialis.

Extensor Carpi Radialis Longus and Brevis. To make these muscles prominent, have the patient make a fist as you offer resistance to the dorsum of his hand. Wrist extension accentuates the contour of these two muscles at the wrist, just proximal to the second and third metacarpal. Palpate the muscles proximally, moving up the forearm to the lateral epicondyle. Notice that the muscle bellies do not run in straight lines from the lateral epicondyle of the humerus, but rather trace oblique paths from origin to insertion, as do most of the forearm muscles. It is a widely held belief that the muscles of the mobile wad of three (and the extensor carpi radialis brevis in particular) are involved in "tennis elbow," a condition in which the extensor muscles, strained by an unusual amount of stress, cause pain at the lateral epicondyle of the elbow and along the course of the muscles. In some cases, pain may even be referred as high as the shoulder (Fig. 50). A test for "tennis elbow" is described in the special test section of this chapter (Fig. 49).

Lateral Collateral Ligament. This ligament is a ropelike structure, similar to the knee's lateral collateral ligament. It extends from the lateral epicondyle to the side of the annular ligament, which encircles the radius. A sprain of this ligament, usually the result of a sudden varus stress, can make it tender to palpation.

Annular Ligament. This ligament is attached to the lateral collateral ligament and cups the radial head and neck, holding them in place as they articulate with the ulna (Fig. 31). Neither the lateral collateral or the annular ligament is directly palpable, but the area in which they lie should be probed for possible pathology involving either the ligaments themselves or the radial head. (A test for the stability of the lateral collateral ligament is described in the special tests section of this chapter.)

Zone IV—Anterior Aspect

Cubital Fossa. The cubital fossa is a triangular space, bordered laterally by the brachioradialis and medially by the pronator teres. The fossa's base is defined by an imaginary line drawn between the two epicondyles of the humerus (Fig. 32). From its lateral to medial borders, the structures passing through the cubital fossa are: (1) the biceps tendon, (2) the brachial artery, (3) the median nerve, and (4) the musculocutaneous nerve.

Biceps Tendon. The biceps tendon and its muscle belly become more accessible to palpation if the patient places his closed fist (in supination)

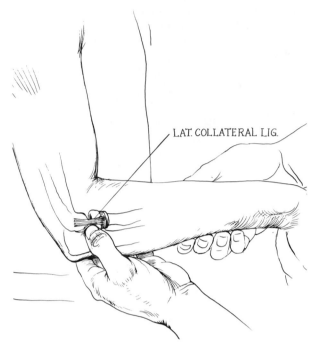

LAT. COLLATERAL LIG.

Fig. 31. The annular ligament.

under the edge of a table and tries to lift the table. The tendon, a long, taut structure, will then stand out medial to the brachioradialis muscle (Fig. 33). First, explore up the long muscle belly of the biceps. While neither its origins nor insertions are palpable, the muscle belly and the tendon are distinctly palpable. Pursue the biceps tendon distally, as far as you can, noting the medial expansion (lacertus fibrosus) which crosses the wrist flexor group and renders it immobile. A ruptured biceps tendon (at or near its insertion) usually occurs when the elbow has been flexed forcibly against strong resistance. The anticubital fossa then becomes tender, and the tendon is no longer palpable. A bulbous swelling forms in the upper arm as the muscle belly contracts, drawing the ruptured tendon upward.

Brachial Artery. The pulse of the brachial artery can be felt directly medial to the biceps tendon (Fig. 34).

Median Nerve. The median nerve is a round, tubular structure lying directly medial to the brachial artery. In its course, it leaves the elbow distally and pierces the pronator teres muscle as it enters the forearm on the way to the hand (Fig. 35).

Musculocutaneous Nerve. This nerve lies on the lateral side of the biceps tendon and provides sensation for the forearm. The nerve is not palpable, but for clinical purposes it is located deep

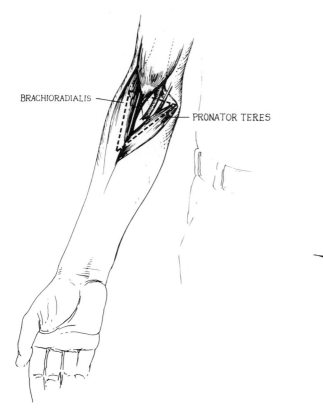

BRACHIORADIALIS

PRONATOR TERES

Fig. 32. The cubital fossa.

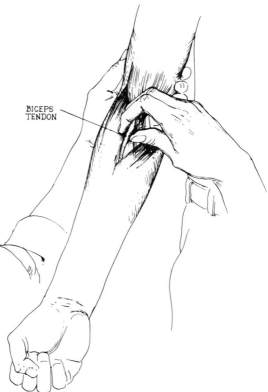

BICEPS
TENDON

Fig. 33. The biceps tendon.

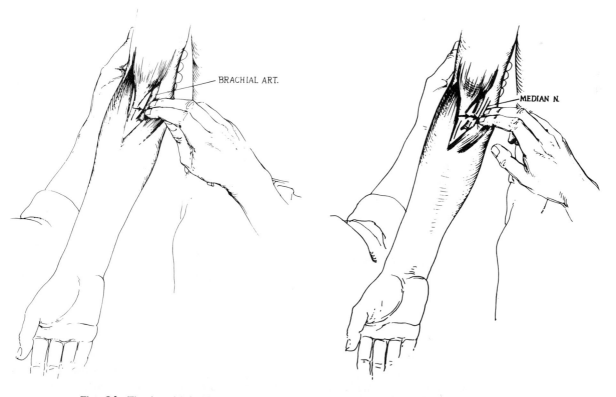

BRACHIAL ART.

Fig. 34. The brachial artery.

MEDIAN N.

Fig. 35. The median nerve.

under the brachiioradialis approximately one or two inches above the line of the elbow joint. As you palpate the cubital fossa, note any tenderness elicited over the joint capsule's attachment to the lower end of the humerus. Tenderness in this area can be caused by a hyperextension injury to the elbow, resulting in a sprain of the anterior joint capsule.

RANGE OF MOTION

A fairly wide range of motion in the upper extremity is desirable, for a severely limited range can prevent a patient from performing some of the necessary activities of daily living (such as feeding himself). Basically, the range of motion in the elbow joint involves four movements: (1) elbow flexion, (2) elbow extension, (3) forearm supination, and (4) forearm pronation. Flexion and extension originate primarily at the humeroulnar and humeroradial joints, while supination and pronation derive from the radioulnar articulations at the elbow and wrist. During supination and pronation, the radial head revolves at its articulation with the capitellum.

The patient may stand or sit during the active range of motion tests, while the examiner is either at his side or directly in front of him.

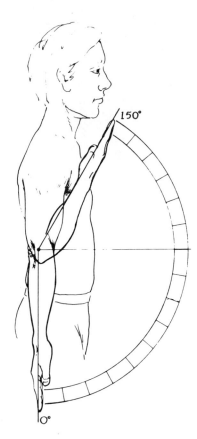

Fig. 36. The elbow range of motion in flexion and extension.

Active Range of Motion Tests

The tests which follow are termed "active" because they reveal the extent of a patient's ability to move his elbow without assistance. If a patient cannot perform the active tests, then passive testing should be conducted.

FLEXION—135°+. Instruct the patient to bend his elbow and to try to touch the front of his shoulder with his hand. Flexion is limited by the muscle mass of the anterior arm, but the patient should normally be able to touch his shoulder (Fig. 36).

EXTENSION—0°/−5°. Extension of the elbow joint is motored by the triceps muscle. Extension limits are defined by the point at which the olecranon strikes the olecranon fossa.

Ask the patient to straighten his elbow as far as he can. Most males can achieve the normal 0° extension; those who are unusually muscular may not be able to extend the elbow to 0° because of biceps muscle tension. Females are normally able to extend the arm to a minimum of 0° and many are able to hyperextend the elbow as much as 5°

beyond the straight position. Tests for flexion and extension may be performed in one continuous motion, and both elbows should be tested simultaneously (Fig. 36).

SUPINATION—90°. The limits of supination are defined by the degree to which the radius can rotate around the ulna. Pathology related to either the elbow or the wrist's radioulnar articulation may affect and limit such rotation.

To test active supination, instruct the patient to flex his elbow to 90° and then to hold the flexed elbow into his waist. This positioning will prevent him from substituting shoulder adduction and flexion for forearm supination. Then have him put his closed fist in front of him, palm downward, and rotate his fist until the palm faces upward. In a normal range of supination, the palm can turn until it faces directly upward.

Another method for testing supination is to have the patient hold a pencil in each hand, and then to move both forearms simultaneously into supination (Fig. 37). In normal supination, the pencils are parallel to the floor. Any asymmetry in their positions indicates restricted supination in the forearm.

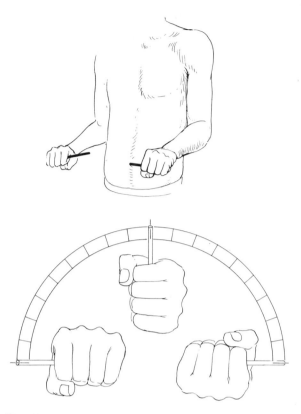

Fig. 37. The elbow range of motion in supination and pronation.

PRONATION—90°. As in supination, the limits of normal pronation are determined by the degree to which the radius can rotate around the ulna. Pronation can be limited by pathology at the elbows, at the wrist radioulnar articulations, or within the forearms.

In the active testing of pronation, the patient maintains the same position as in supination, with elbows flexed and at his waist, and fists holding the pencils. Ask the patient to rotate his fist from a fully supinated position until his palm faces downward (Fig. 37). In normal pronation, the palm will face the floor, and the pencils, having turned 180° from the position of supination, will again be parallel to the floor. Any dissimilarity in the position of the pencils implies a restricted range of pronation.

Supination and pronation should be performed as one test, since the two motions essentially describe a single arc of motion.

Passive Range of Motion Tests

These tests should be administered when a patient is unable to perform the active tests. Since

it is easier, as well as more effective, to test related motions as a unit, passive range of motion testing has been divided into two phases: (1) flexion and extension and (2) supination and pronation.

FLEXION AND EXTENSION. Ask the patient to tuck his elbow into his waist, and stabilize his arm in this position by cupping the olecranon process in your hand and holding his elbow against his body. Place your other hand just above the wrist to support it. Then flex and extend the forearm as far as the patient will permit. If you feel any blockage to motion within the elbow joint, or if you notice a splinting of the joint, move the forearm back to a neutral position. Determine if the blockage is abrupt in nature, as opposed to being rubbery or ill-defined. Then have the patient flex and extend his normal elbow, to provide a basis for comparison. Findings determining the type and potential cause of blockage and the degree of limitation should be recorded.

SUPINATION AND PRONATION. Hold the patient's elbow in the described stabilized position. With your other hand, grip his hand as if to shake it. Your grip should be firm enough to allow you to control the motion, but loose enough so as not to cause the patient discomfort. Supinate and pronate the forearm slowly to check whether or not a full range of motion can be achieved. Again, a loss or limitation of motion should be evaluated both in terms of the type of blockage and the degree of loss.

NEUROLOGIC EXAMINATION

The neurologic portion of the examination is comprised of tests designed to evaluate the strength of the elbow musculature as well as the integrity of the nerve supply to those muscles. Examination is conducted in three parts: (1) muscle testing, (2) reflex testing, and (3) sensation testing.

Muscle Testing

Essentially, the muscle tests for the elbow relate to the motions of flexion, extension, supination, and pronation. For the purpose of this discussion, these motions have been classified in distinct categories. In conducting the examination, however, it is much easier to continue the flow of testing and to move from one test to the next without interruption. The patient may either stand or sit during examination of the elbow, depending solely on his comfort.

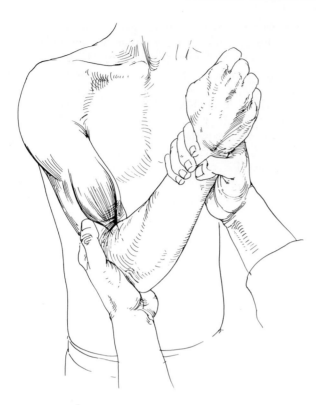

Fig. 38. Muscle test for flexion.

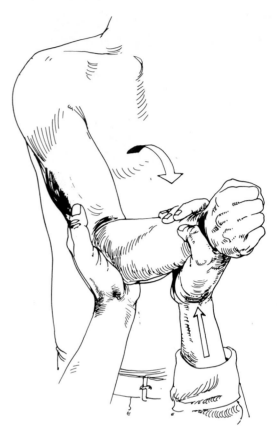

Fig. 39. Muscle test for extension.

FLEXION

Primary Flexors:
1) Brachialis
   musculocutaneous nerve, C5, C6
2) Biceps, when the forearm is supinated
   musculocutaneous nerve, C5, C6

Secondary Flexors:
1) Brachioradialis
2) Supinator

Stand in front of the patient and support and stabilize his arm by cupping your hand around the posterior portion of the elbow just proximal to the joint itself. Place your resisting hand on the forearm's palmar surface and wrap your fingers around its distal portion (Fig. 38).

Ask the patient to flex his arm slowly, and, as flexion approaches 45°, begin to apply resistance. After determining the maximum resistance he can overcome, test the opposite elbow in the same manner to provide a basis for comparison. Record

the muscle strength in accordance with the muscle grading chart (See Table 1, Shoulder Chapter, page 26).

EXTENSION

Primary Extensor:
1) Triceps
   radial nerve, C7

Secondary Extensor:
1) Anconeus

Remain in front of the patient and maintain the same hand positions as in the test for flexion.

Ask the patient to extend his arm slowly from the flexed position. Before he reaches a position of about 90°, increase your resistance until you determine the maximum resistance he can overcome. Resisting pressure should be constant and firm, for a jerky or pushing type of resistance is likely to result in an inaccurate evaluation (Fig. 39).

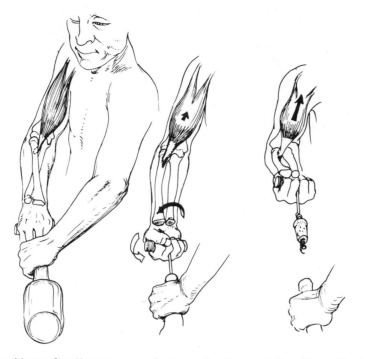

Fig. 40. The biceps functions as a supinator and a flexor of the elbow. Its function is illustrated by twisting a corkscrew into the bottle and then pulling the cork out.

SUPINATION

Primary Supinators:
1) Biceps
   musculocutaneous nerve, C5, C6
2) Supinator
   radial nerve, C6

Secondary Supinator:
1) Brachioradialis

In addition to its role in supination, the biceps also functions as an elbow flexor. Its total function is well illustrated in the act of twisting (supination) a corkscrew into the cork of a bottle and then pulling (flexion) the cork out of the bottle (Fig. 40).

Remain in position in front of the patient with your hand stabilizing and supporting his elbow at his side. This support will prevent the substitution of shoulder adduction and external rotation for forearm supination. Place the thenar eminence of your resisting hand upon the dorsal surface of the patient's radius (at the distal end), and wrap your fingers medially around the ulna (Fig. 41).

Instruct the patient to begin supination from a position of pronation, and, as he moves his forearm into supination, gradually increase your resist-

ing pressure against the radius until you determine the maximum resistance he can overcome.

PRONATION

Primary Pronators:
1) Pronator teres
   median nerve, C6
2) Pronator quadratus
   anterior interosseous branch of median nerve, C8, T1

Secondary Pronator:
1) Flexor carpi radialis

Stand in front of the patient and continue to stabilize the elbow just proximal to the joint to prevent the substitution of shoulder abduction and internal rotation for pure forearm pronation. Adjust your resisting hand so that the thenar eminence presses against the volar surface at the distal end of the radius. Wrap your fingers around the posterior border of the ulna (Fig. 42). This adjustment requires only that you turn your resisting hand from the dorsal to the volar surface of the wrist.

Ask the patient to begin forearm pronation from a position of supination. As he moves into pronation, increase resisting pressure against the radius until you ascertain the maximum resistance he can overcome.

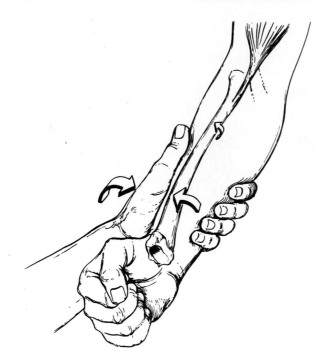

Fig. 41. Muscle test for supination.

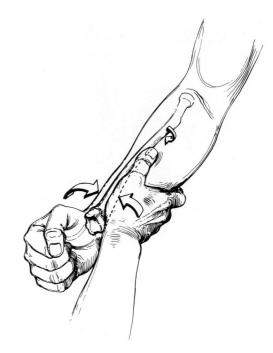

Fig. 42. Muscle test for pronation.

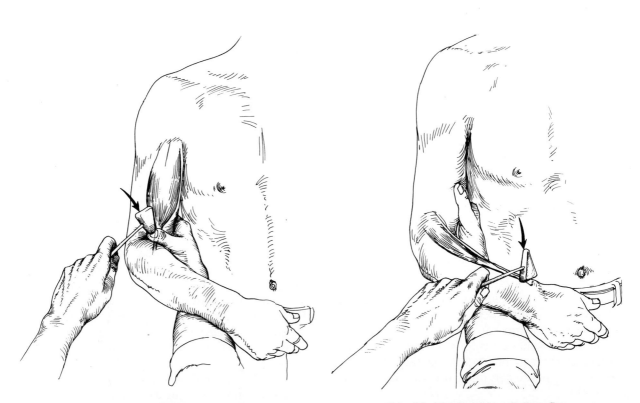

Fig. 43. Testing the biceps reflex.

Fig. 44. The brachioradialis reflex.

Reflex Testing

The three basic reflexes which evaluate the integrity of the nerve supply to the elbow are: (1) the biceps reflex, (2) the brachioradialis reflex, and (3) the triceps reflex. Each of these is a *deep tendon reflex*, a lower motor neuron reflex, transmitted to the cord as far as the anterior horn cell and returning to the muscle via the peripheral nerves.

BICEPS REFLEX—C5

Although the biceps is innervated by the musculocutaneous nerve at neurologic levels C5 and C6, its reflex action is largely a function of C5. Thus, in testing the biceps reflex, you are primarily assessing the integrity of neurologic level C5.

To test the reflex, place the patient's arm over your opposite arm, so that it rests upon your forearm. With your hand supporting the patient's arm under the elbow's medial side, place your thumb on the tendon of the biceps in the cubital fossa (Fig. 43). If the patient flexes his elbow slightly you will feel the tendon stand out under your thumb.

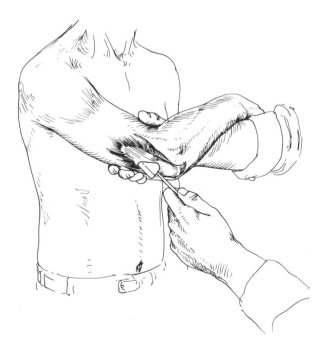

Fig. 45. The triceps reflex.

Have the patient rest his arm on your forearm and let it relax completely. When his arm is totally relaxed, tap your thumbnail with the narrow end of a reflex hammer. The biceps should jerk slightly. You will be able either to see or to feel its movement (Fig. 43).

If there is a slight response, you may consider the C5 neurologic level as normal in its innervation of the biceps muscle. If, after several attempts to elicit a reflex, there is no perceptible response, there may be a lesion at the C5 neurologic level anywhere from the root at C5 to the innervation of the biceps muscle. An excessive response may be the result of an upper motor neuron lesion, such as a cardiovascular attack (stroke), while a decreased response may be caused by a lower motor neuron lesion, such as a peripheral nerve injury secondary to a herniated cervical disc. (Note that the brain exerts an inhibitory, or regulatory, control over a lower motor neuron reflex and prevents it from excessive activity or briskness.) Test the reflexes on both sides; they should be equal. Reflexes are recorded as normal, increased, or decreased.

BRACHIORADIALIS REFLEX—C6

The brachioradialis muscle is innervated by the radial nerve via the C5 and C6 neurologic levels, but its reflex is largely a function of C6. To test the reflex, support the patient's arm in the same manner used to elicit the biceps reflex. Using the flat edge of the reflex hammer, tap the brachioradialis tendon at the distal end of the radius to elicit a radial jerk (Fig. 44). Then, test the opposite arm and compare and record the results.

TRICEPS REFLEX—C7

The triceps is innervated by the radial nerve. The reflex is largely a function of the C7 neurologic level.

Keep the patient's arm in the same position used for the two previous tests. Ask him to relax his arm completely. When you are certain it is relaxed (you can feel the lack of tension in the triceps muscle), tap the triceps tendon where it crosses the olecranon fossa with the narrower end of the reflex hammer (Fig. 45). You should be able to see the reflex or to feel it as a slight jerk on your supporting forearm.

Sensation Testing

Sensation around the elbow joint is controlled by four different nerve supplies:

1) C5—lateral arm
   sensory branches of the axillary nerve
2) C6—lateral forearm
   sensory branches of the musculocutaneous nerve
3) C8—medial forearm
   antibrachial cutaneous nerve
4) T1—medial arm
   brachial cutaneous nerve (Fig. 46).

SPECIAL TESTS

TEST FOR LIGAMENTOUS STABILITY.
This test is employed to assess the stability of the medial and lateral collateral ligaments of the elbow. To conduct this test, cup the posterior aspect of the patient's elbow in one hand and hold his wrist with the other. Your hand on the elbow will act as a fulcrum around which your other hand will force the forearm during the test. First, instruct the patient to flex his elbow a few degrees as you force his forearm laterally, producing a valgus stress on the joint's medial side (Fig. 47).

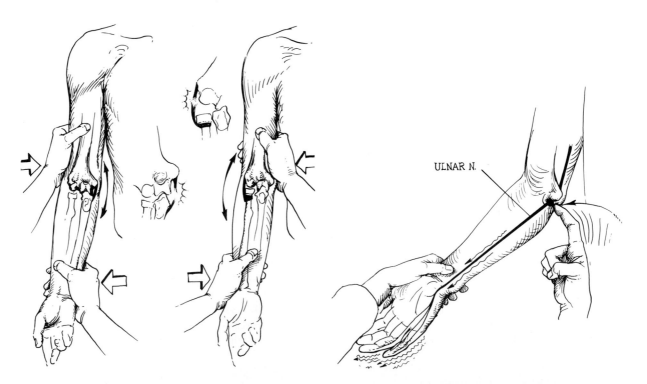

Fig. 46. Elbow sensation.

Fig. 47. Test for ligamentous stability.

Fig. 48. The Tinel sign.

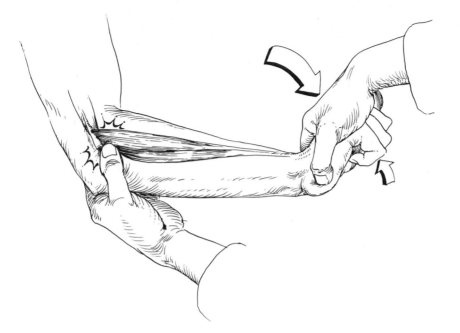

Fig. 49. The tennis elbow test.

Notice if there is any gapping on the medial side underneath your hand. Then reverse direction and push the forearm medially, producing a varus stress to the elbow's lateral side. Again, inspect for any gapping on the lateral side. Your hand, in its position on the elbow, acts not only as a stabilizer and a fulcrum but as a means for palpating the collateral ligament during the test.

TINEL SIGN. The Tinel sign is a test designed to elicit tenderness over a neuroma within a nerve. If there is a neuroma within the ulnar nerve, tapping the area of the nerve in the groove between the olecranon and the medial epicondyle will send a tingling sensation down the forearm to the ulnar distribution in the hand (Fig. 48).

TENNIS ELBOW TEST. This test is designed to reproduce the pain of tennis elbow. Stabilize the patient's forearm and instruct him to make a fist and to extend his wrist. When he has done so apply pressure with your other hand to the dorsum of his fist in an attempt to force his wrist into flexion (Fig. 49). If he has tennis elbow, the patient will experience a sudden severe pain at the site of the wrist extensors' common origin, the lateral epicondyle.

EXAMINATION OF RELATED AREAS

A herniated cervical disc and osteoarthritis are causes of pain referred to the elbow. Occasionally,

wrist pathology such as rheumatoid arthritis will refer symptoms to the elbow joint, since the wrist flexors and extensors are two-joint muscles which cross both the wrist and the elbow. In the same way, shoulder pathology may refer symptoms (Fig. 50). Pain is not as frequently referred to the elbow as it is to the shoulder.

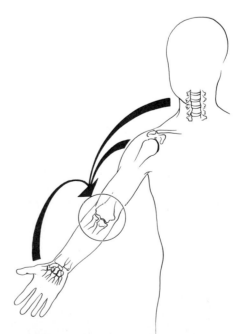

Fig. 50. Pathology of the wrist, the shoulder, and the cervical spine can refer symptoms to the elbow.

3

Physical Examination of the Wrist and Hand

INSPECTION
   The Palmar Surface
   The Dorsal Surface

SKIN PALPATION

BONY PALPATION
   Radial Styloid Process
   Anatomic Snuffbox
   Navicular
   Trapezium
   Tubercle of the Radius (Lister's Tubercle)
   Capitate
   Lunate
   Ulnar Styloid Process
   Triquetrium
   Pisiform
   Hook of Hamate
   Metacarpals
   First Metacarpal
   Metacarpophalangeal Joints
   Phalanges

SOFT TISSUE PALPATION
   Wrist: Zone I   — Radial Styloid Process
   Wrist: Zone II — Tubercle of the Radius
                    (Lister's Tubercle)
   Wrist: Zone III — Ulnar Styloid Process
   Wrist: Zone IV — Pisiform (Palmar Aspect)
   Wrist: Zone V — Palmaris Longus and
                    Carpal Tunnel
   Hand: Zone I   — Thenar Eminence
   Hand: Zone II — Hypothenar Eminence
   Hand: Zone III — Palm
   Hand: Zone IV — Dorsum
   Hand: Zone V — Phalanges
   Hand: Zone VI — Tufts of the Fingers

RANGE OF MOTION
   Active Range of Motion
   Passive Range of Motion
   Wrist:
      Flexion   — 80°
      Extension — 70°

Wrist:
   Ulnar Deviation — 30°
   Radial Deviation — 20°
Fingers: Flexion and Extension at the
         Metacarpophalangeal Joints
   Flexion   — 90°
   Extension — 30°–45°
Fingers:
   Abduction — 20°
   Adduction — 0°
Fingers: Thumb
   Abduction — 70° (Palmar Abduction)
   Adduction — 0° (Dorsal Adduction)
Fingers: Opposition

NEUROLOGIC EXAMINATION
   Muscle Testing
      Wrist Extension — C6
      Wrist   Flexion   — C7
      Finger Extension — C7
      Finger   Flexion   — C8
      Finger Abduction — T1
      Finger Adduction — T1
      Thumb Extension
      Thumb Flexion (Transpalmar Abduction)
      Thumb Abduction (Palmar Abduction)
      Thumb Adduction
      Pinch Mechanism (Thumb and Index Finger)
      Opposition of Thumb and Little Finger
   Sensation Testing
      Peripheral Nerve Innervation
      Sensation in the Hand by Neurologic Levels
        (Dermatomes)

SPECIAL TESTS
   Long Finger Flexor Tests
      Flexor Digitorum Superficialis Test
      Flexor Digitorum Profundus Test
   Bunnel-Littler Test
   Retinacular Test
   Allen Test

EXAMINATION OF RELATED AREAS

The wrist and hand are constructed of a series of complex, delicately balanced joints whose function is integral to almost every act of daily living (Fig. 1).

While the hand is the most active portion of the upper extremity, it is, at the same time, the least protected; thus it is extremely vulnerable, and the incidence of injury is high. Considering the frequency with which the physician is called upon to treat the hand, his examination should be accurate and should include a methodical search for both intrinsic and extrinsic pathology.

As discussed in previous chapters, bilateral comparison is a fast way to discover the presence of pathologic signs; it is particularly useful in the examination of the wrist and hand.

INSPECTION

Initially, observe the patient's hands in function to ascertain if they are being used easily and spontaneously, rather than being guarded or protected. When the patient first enters the room, notice whether or not his upper extremities move normally and symmetrically, for pathology of the hand occasionally affects the swinging motion of the upper extremity. In most instances, a patient holds an injured hand splinted across his chest or positioned stiffly at his side.

Because of the possibility of symptom referral from other areas of the body, examination of the hand requires that the entire upper extremity be exposed, including the cervical spine. Therefore, ask the patient to undress to the waist, and observe his hand movements as he does so. Normal hand motion appears smooth and natural, with the fingers moving in a synchronous manner, while abnormal movement looks stiff or jerky. Occasionally, altered shoulder or elbow movements can compensate for pathology in the hand.

After observing the hands in function, appraise their overall structure. It may seem grossly elementary, but it is important that the fingers be counted to make certain that there are the necessary five on each hand. The loss of a finger is not always evident at a glance, if, for example, one

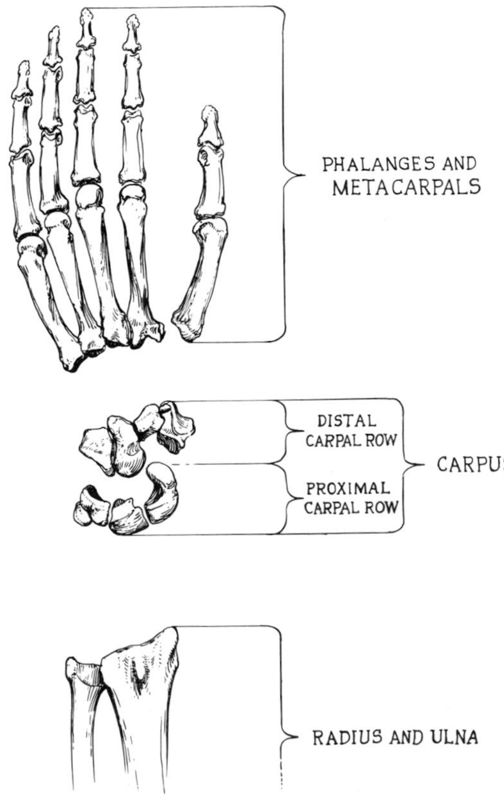

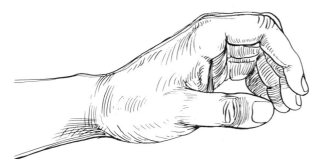

Fig. 2. The "attitude" of the hand.

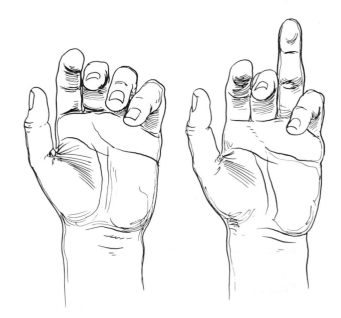

Fig. 1. The bony anatomy of the wrist and hand.

PHALANGES AND METACARPALS

DISTAL CARPAL ROW

PROXIMAL CARPAL ROW

CARPUS

RADIUS AND ULNA

Fig. 3. If one finger is held extended while others are flexed, its flexor tendon has been damaged or cut.

finger has been amputated and another surgically moved into the gap. It is particularly important to count the fingers of the newborn, since a congenital absence or excess of digits is sometimes less than obvious.

The attitude of the hand is another factor to be considered in inspection. At rest, both the metacarpophalangeal and the interphalangeal joints normally hold a position of slight flexion, with the fingers lining up almost parallel to each other (Fig. 2). If one finger, in comparison to the others, is extended, its flexor tendon may have been damaged or cut (Fig. 3).

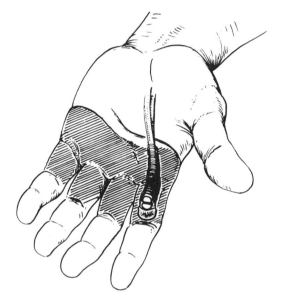

Fig. 4. The shaded area represents surgical no man's land.

The Palmar Surface

The palmar surface of the wrist and hand contains numerous creases, situated where the fascia attaches to the skin. Those creases of importance are:

1) *The distal palmar crease*, which roughly describes the palmar site of the metacarpophalangeal joints (knuckles) and marks the proximal border of surgical "no man's land" (where the two flexor tendons begin to run in one sheath) (Fig. 4).

2) *The proximal palmar crease*, which lies at the base of the fingers (within no man's land) and marks the location of the proximal pulley.

3) *The proximal interphalangeal crease*, which crosses the fingers at the proximal interphalangeal joints and defines the distal border of no man's land.

4) *The thenar crease*, which outlines the thenar eminence (Fig. 5).

Often, a patient's dominant hand can be identified merely by examining the palmar creases, since the musculature in a dominant hand is more developed and its creases are deeper than those of the weaker hand. In addition, the dominant hand usually looks somewhat larger than the nondominant hand, with more prominent callosities.

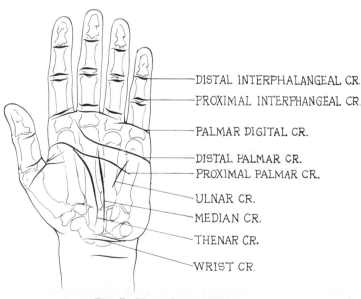

DISTAL INTERPHALANGEAL CR.
PROXIMAL INTERPHANGEAL CR.
PALMAR DIGITAL CR.
DISTAL PALMAR CR.
PROXIMAL PALMAR CR.
ULNAR CR.
MEDIAN CR.
THENAR CR.
WRIST CR.

Fig. 5. The palmar creases.

In respect to the contour of the palmar surface, the thenar and hypothenar eminences are significant because they represent the muscle bellies which motor the thumb and little fingers, respectively. In appearance, the eminences bulge slightly, lending an indented, cuplike shape to the center of the palm (Figs. 6, 72). This shape is actually created by three arches (Fig. 7), two of which run across the palm (one at the carpal level and one at the metacarpal head and neck level), the third longitudinally down its center. The arch framework is supported by the hand's intrinsic muscles, which, when absent or atrophic, cause the palm to lose its normal contour and to appear flat, without concavity (Figs. 8, 9). The strategic location of these arches enhances the volar projection of the thumb, and promotes an efficient pinch unit between the thumb and the index and middle fingers (Fig. 10).

On the palmar surface of the hand, the metacarpophalangeal joint area is characterized by "hills and valleys." The fleshy mounds, or hills, are composed of neurovascular bundles which supply the fingers and lumbrical muscles, while the valleys designate the paths of the flexor tendons at the point where they cross the joints (Fig. 6).

Normally, a slight webbing is noticeable between the fingers, with a more substantial web space between the thumb and index finger. An abnormal distal extension of the web space between the fingers (syndactyly) limits hand function by restricting the range of finger abduction (Fig. 11).

The Dorsal Surface

On the dorsal aspect, the metacarpophalangeal joints and the soft tissue valleys between them should appear bilaterally symmetrical. Generally, the valleys are approximately the same depth on both hands, although a unilateral swelling around

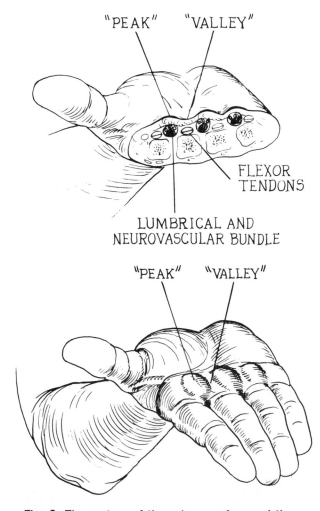

Fig. 6. The contour of the palmar surface and the underlying anatomy.

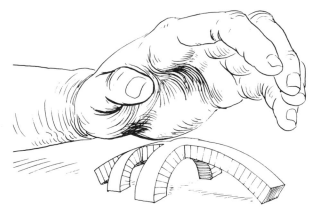

Fig. 7. The arched framework of the hand is supported by the hand's intrinsic muscles.

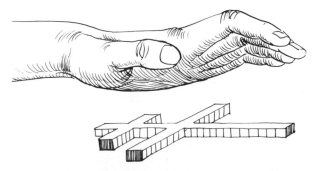

Fig. 8. If the intrinsic muscles of the hand are absent or atrophied, the palmar surface will lose its contour.

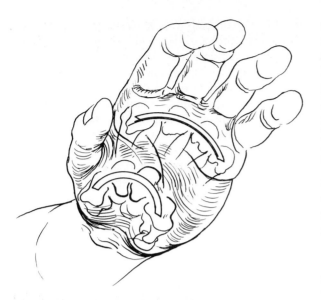

Fig. 9. The two transverse arches of the hand and wrist.

a knuckle can diminish the depth of the valleys on either side, and, in the case of extreme swelling, can fill the valleys completely. The knuckles should be inspected when the patient's fist is clenched, and should be compared to those of the opposite hand (Fig. 12). The knuckle of the middle finger is usually the most prominent. Variations in the length of the individual metacarpals cause corresponding differences in size of the metacarpal heads, but an obvious difference seen between the corresponding knuckles on each hand may be an indication of disease or trauma. In addition to the metacarpophalangeal joints, the proximal and distal interphalangeal joints should be inspected and compared with those of the opposite hand.

The general condition and color of the fingernails can sometimes indicate serious pathologic problems and should not be overlooked during inspection. Normal nails are pink in color, while pale

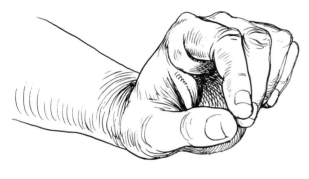

Fig. 10. The pinch unit.

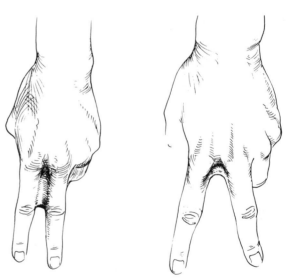

Fig. 11. Left—abnormal web space between fingers (syndactyly). **Right**—normal webbing between fingers.

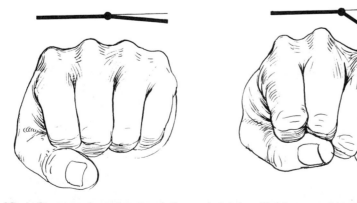

Fig. 12. Left—normal metacarpophalangeal joints. **Right**—normal metacarpophalangeal joint contour with a clenched fist.

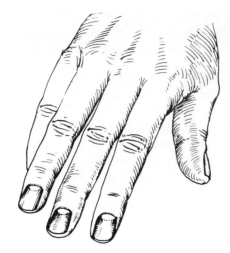

Fig. 13. Good general condition of the hand and nails.

or whitish nail beds can be a sign of anemia or circulatory problems. The nails should be in good condition, neither pitted nor split, and the lunula (the small crescent-shaped area at the nailbase) should be white (Fig. 13). In abnormal circumstances, fingernails may become spoon-shaped or clubbed. Spoon nails are weakly structured, appearing concave or dug out, and are usually the result of a severe fungus infection (Fig. 14A). Clubbed nails are domed, and are much broader and larger than normal (Fig. 14B). They are most often due to hypertrophy of the underlying soft tissues, but may also indicate respiratory or congenital heart problems.

SKIN PALPATION

Normally, the skin is palpated in conjunction with the bony prominences underneath it. However, in this chapter, the skin will be palpated as a separate entity since it is frequently involved in trauma.

The skin of both the palm and the palmar surface of the fingers is much thicker than that of the dorsal surface because it must protect the delicate underlying structures. The palmar skin is fixed by fascia, which binds it to the structures beneath at the palmar creases. This fixation allows for objects to be held securely in the hand, whereas the looser

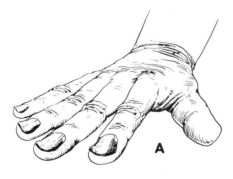

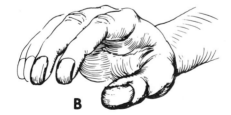

Fig. 14. A. Spoon nails. **B.** Clubbed nails.

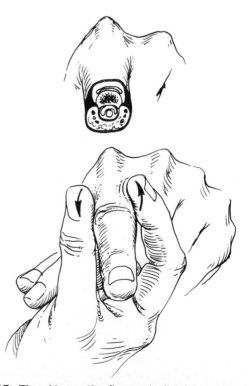

Fig. 15. The skin on the fingers is fixed by septa and small ligaments running from skin to bone.

skin on the hand's dorsal surface permits the extreme metacarpophalangeal joint flexion necessary for making a fist. Occasionally, swelling secondary to an infection which may have originated in the palmar surface is transported by the lymphatics and manifests itself in the larger, more accommodating area of the dorsum.

The skin on the fingers is fixed to bone by septa and small ligaments running from skin to bone along the lateral and medial sides of the fingers (Cleland's and Grayson's Ligaments). Thus, there is very little rotary movement of the skin around the fingers. It would be extremely difficult to hold anything in the hand without this relative fixation since the skin would roll around the fingers (Fig. 15).

As you palpate the wrist and hand, check the skin for any unusually warm or dry areas. An excessive localized warmth of the skin may be a sign of infection, while an unnaturally dry condition (anhydrosis) may indicate nerve damage. Particular attention should be given to any lesions, swellings, or scars observed during inspection: They should be palpated carefully. An immobile scar (one that seems fixed to the underlying soft tissues or bone) or any tenderness elicited within scar tissue should be noted.

BONY PALPATION

To begin palpation of the wrist and hand, place your thumb upon the patient's radial styloid process (proximal to his thumb) and your index and middle fingers upon the ulnar styloid process (proximal to his little finger). These two bony prominences are the basic reference points of the carpal region (Fig. 17). From these points, palpation will proceed in a linear fashion through the bony and soft tissue structures of the hand.

Bones of the Wrist. The wrist is composed of eight carpal bones situated in two rows: The proximal carpal row and the distal carpal row. The proximal carpal row from radial to ulnar contains the navicular, the lunate, the triquetrium, and the pisiform (anterior to the triquetrium). The distal carpal row from radial to ulnar is composed of the trapezium, the trapezoid, the capitate, and the hamate bones (Fig. 16).

Radial Styloid Process. The radial styloid process is truly lateral when the hand is in the anatomic position (palm facing anteriorly) (Fig. 17). As you palpate its distal tip, note the small but distinct groove that can be felt along the lateral

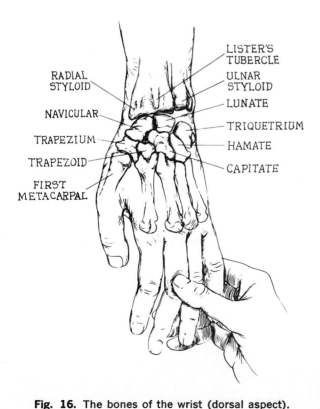

Fig. 16. The bones of the wrist (dorsal aspect).

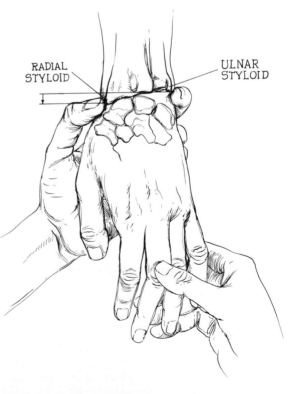

Fig. 17. The basic reference points in palpation of the wrist. The radial styloid process is more distal than the ulnar.

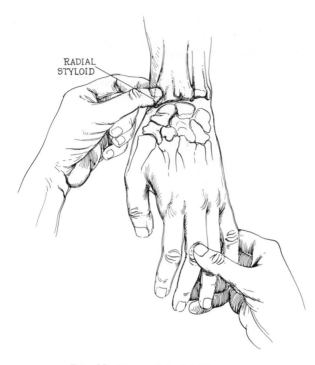

Fig. 18. The radial styloid process.

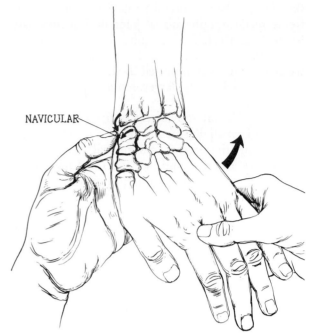

Fig. 19. Ulnar deviation facilitates palpation of the navicular.

edge (Fig. 18). From there, palpate up the length of the styloid process, and continue up the radial shaft until it becomes obscured by overlying soft tissues about halfway up the forearm. Then return to the most prominent point of the radial styloid process, just proximal to the carpal joint.

Anatomic Snuffbox. The anatomic snuffbox is a small depression located immediately distal and slightly dorsal to the radial styloid process. It becomes outlined and is palpable when the patient extends his thumb laterally away from his fingers (Fig. 43).

Navicular. The navicular, also known as the scaphoid bone, is situated on the radial side of the carpus. It represents the floor of the snuffbox. The navicular is the largest bone in the proximal carpal row. Of all the carpal bones, it is the most commonly fractured. Ulnar deviation causes the navicular to slide out from under the radial styloid process so that it becomes palpable (Fig. 19).

Trapezium. The trapezium is located on the radial side of the carpus where it articulates with the first metacarpal (Fig. 20). Move distal to the snuffbox to palpate the trapezium/first metacarpal articulation. The articulation is saddlelike and lies immediately proximal to the thenar eminence (Figs. 21, 22). It is more easily palpable if you instruct the patient to flex and extend his thumb.

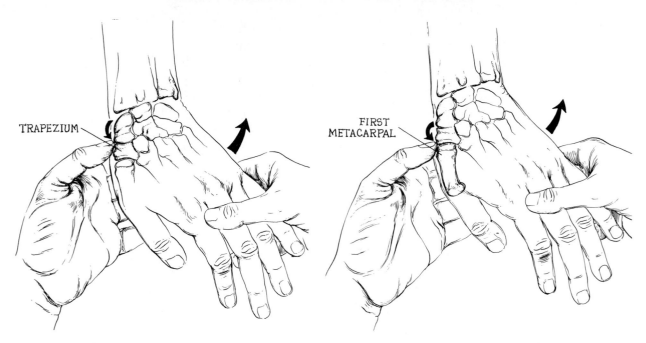

Fig. 20. Palpation of the trapezium.

Fig. 21. The trapezium/first metacarpal articulation.

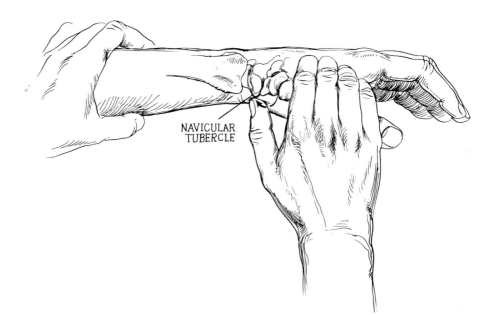

Fig. 22. The trapezium/first metacarpal is palpated radially. The navicular tubercle is palpated proximally.

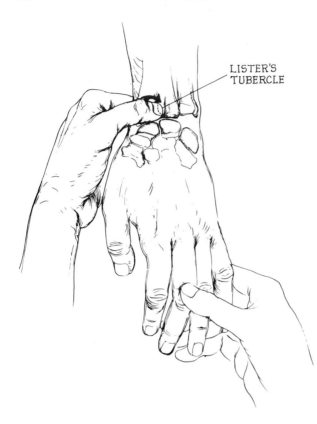

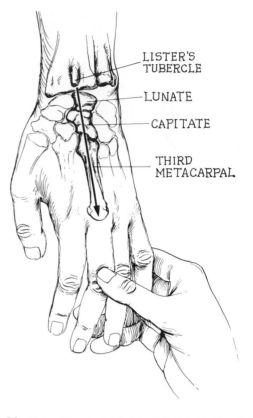

Fig. 23. Palpation of the tubercle of the radius (Lister's tubercle).

Fig. 24. The alignment of the radial tubercle, the lunate, the capitate, and the third metacarpal.

Tubercle of the Radius. (Lister's Tubercle) Lister's tubercle lies about one-third of the way across the dorsum of the wrist from the radial styloid process. It feels like a small, longitudinal bony prominence or nodule (Fig. 23).

Capitate. As you move distally from Lister's tubercle, you will encounter the base of the third metacarpal bone, the largest and most prominent of the metacarpal bases (Fig. 25). The capitate lies in the distal carpal row between the third metacarpal base and the tubercle of the radius. It is the largest of all the carpal bones and is palpable immediately proximal to the base of the third metacarpal (Fig. 24). When the wrist is in a neutral position, you will find a small depression in the area of the capitate, a depression which is actually a curve in the capitate itself (Fig. 26). When

the wrist is flexed this depression rolls distally, and the capitate slides out from under the lunate to create a fullness where the depression has been.

Lunate. The lunate, just proximal to the capitate, has the distinction of being the most frequently dislocated as well as the second most often fractured bone in the wrist. It lies in the proximal carpal row and articulates proximally with the radius and distally with the capitate. It is palpable just distal to the radial tubercle. As you palpate, ask the patient to flex and extend his wrist so that the motion at the lunate/capitate articulation can be felt (Fig. 27). The lunate, capitate, and the base of the third metacarpal are in line with each other and are covered by the extensor carpi radialis brevis tendon which inserts into the base of the third metacarpal (Fig. 25).

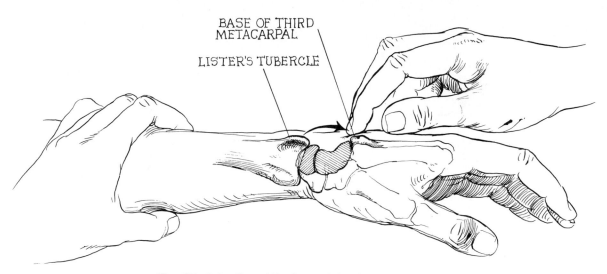

Fig. 25. Palpation of the base of the third metacarpal.

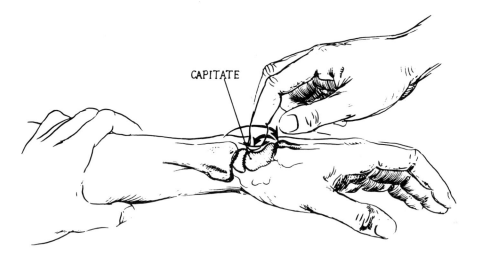

Fig. 26. There is a slight palpable depression in the dorsum of the capitate.

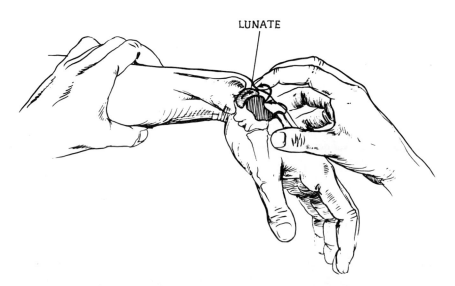

Fig. 27. Flexion of the wrist facilitates palpation of the lunate.

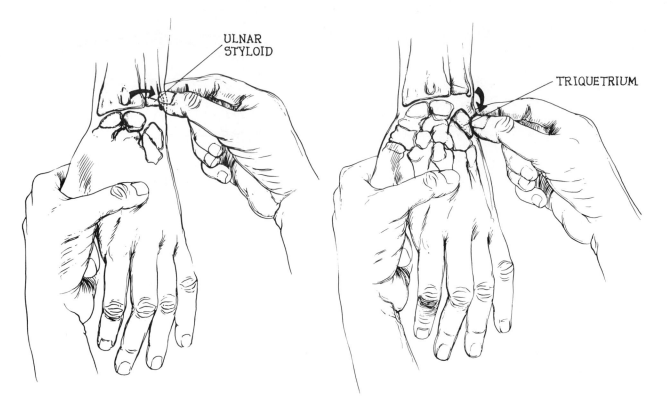

Fig. 28. The ulnar styloid process.

Fig. 29. Radial deviation of the hand facilitates palpation of the triquetrium.

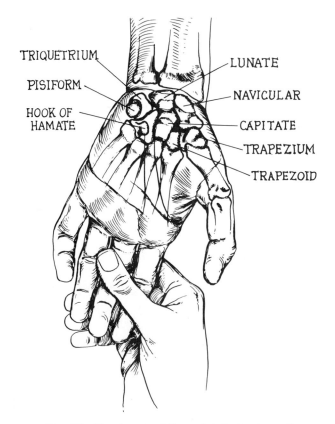

Fig. 30. The bones of the wrist (volar aspect).

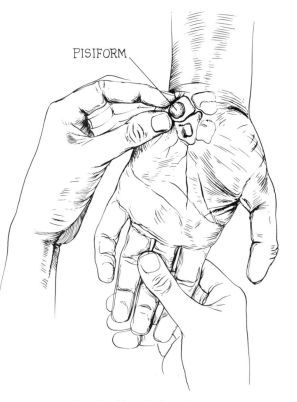

Fig. 31. The pisiform bone.

Ulnar Styloid Process. Return to the basic position with your fingers on the ulnar and radial styloid processes. Note first that the ulnar styloid process does not extend as far distally as does the radial process (Fig. 17), and that it is more prominent and thicker than its radial counterpart (Fig. 28). In the anatomic position, the ulnar styloid process does not lie directly along the side of the wrist but rather is both medially and posteriorly located. The ulna and its styloid process actually take no part in wrist articulation; only the radius articulates with the proximal carpal row. Palpate up the sharp, subcutaneous ulnar border to the olecranon process of the elbow and return to the ulnar process via the same route. On the distal tip of the ulnar styloid process, you should feel a small, shallow dorsal groove running longitudinally (Fig. 59). The extensor carpi ulnaris tendon runs through this groove. It is most easily palpated when the hand is radially deviated and the tendon is contracted.

Triquetrium. The triquetrium lies just distal to the ulnar styloid process, in the proximal carpal row. To facilitate its palpation, the hand must be radially deviated so that the triquetrium moves out from under the ulnar styloid process (Fig. 29).

Even then the triquetrium may be difficult to find, since it also lies under the pisiform. The triquetrium is vulnerable to injury, ranking third highest of all the carpal bones in incidence of fracture.

Pisiform. As you probe the anterolateral region of the triquetrium, you will feel a small sesamoid bone, the pisiform, which is formed within the flexor carpi ulnaris tendon (Figs. 30, 31).

Hook of the Hamate. The hook of the hamate is situated slightly distal and radial to the pisiform. To locate it, place the interphalangeal joint of your thumb upon the pisiform, pointing the tip of your thumb toward the web space between the patient's thumb and index fingers (Fig. 32) and rest the tip of your thumb upon his palm. The hook of the hamate lies directly under your thumb tip, but, since it is buried deep under layers of soft tissue, you must press firmly to find its rather shallow contour (Fig. 33). The hook is of clinical importance because it forms the lateral (radial) border of the tunnel of Guyon, which transports the ulnar nerve and artery to the hand (Fig. 63). The medial border of the tunnel of Guyon is formed by the pisiform bone.

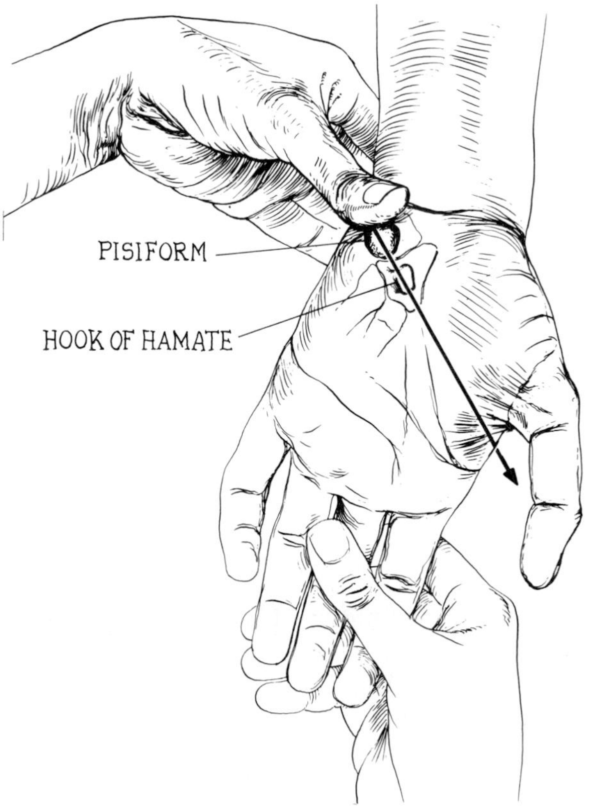

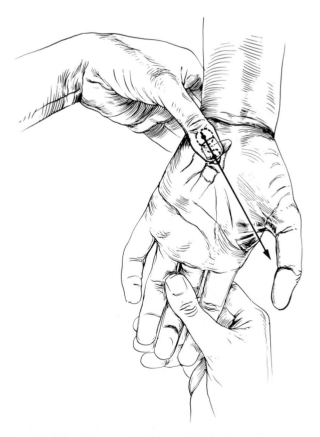

PISIFORM

HOOK OF HAMATE

Fig. 32. The hook of the hamate lies in a direct line between the pisiform bone and the web space of the thumb and index finger.

Fig. 33. Palpation of the hook of the hamate.

Metacarpals. The metacarpals may be palpated in order, moving from the index to the little finger. Keep your thumb on the patient's palm and locate the base of the second metacarpal with your index and middle fingers, and palpate its full length. The dorsal and radial aspects are almost subcutaneous and are easily palpable (Fig. 34). Interruptions or excrescences of bone along the dorsal aspect or unusual tenderness suggest a possible fracture. The third, fourth, and fifth metacarpals should be palpated in the same manner.

The second and third metacarpals are anchored firmly to the carpus and are consequently immobile, providing for the index and middle fingers the stability necessary to perform pinch movement and fine motion. In contrast, the fourth and fifth metacarpals are mobile. As such, they furnish a greater range of motion for the ring and little fingers and allow the palm to close on the ulnar side of the hand, preventing objects from slipping out (Figs. 35, 36, 37).

First Metacarpal. The first metacarpal should be palpated for continuity in bone structure from the anatomic snuffbox to the metacarpophalangeal joint. Note that it is shorter and broader than the other metacarpals. Tenderness elicited in the joints at either end should be noted (Fig. 38).

Metacarpophalangeal Joints. Move distally from the metacarpals and palpate the fusiform joints (knuckles) while they are flexed so that their articulations are exposed, the condyles at the ends of the metacarpal bones accessible, and the joint lines more evident (Figs. 39, 40). A slight indentation is palpable on the dorsal aspect of the joint.

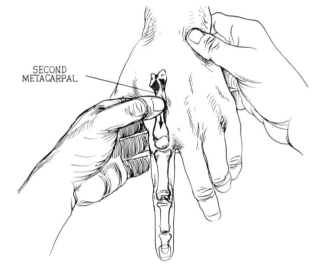

Fig. 34. Palpation of the second metacarpal.

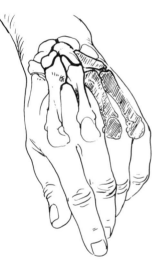

Fig. 35. The second and third metacarpals are almost subcutaneous and are easily palpated.

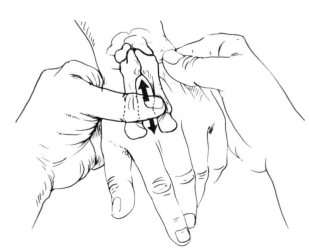

Fig. 36. The second and third metacarpals are immobile (stable).

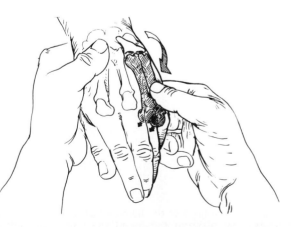

Fig. 37. The fourth and fifth metacarpals are mobile.

Through it passes the extensor tendon on its way to the finger. Fracture of the metacarpals occurs most often at the neck where the shaft meets the head. The incidence of fracture is greatest in the fifth metacarpal. Note again that the distal palmar crease is directly over the anterior aspect of the knuckles (Fig. 5).

Phalanges. There are fourteen phalanges on each hand, since the thumb has two and the other fingers three each. The proximal and middle phalanges articulate at the *proximal interphalangeal joints,* and the distal and middle phalanges at the *distal interphalangeal joints* (Fig. 41). Occasionally, you may find one finger palpably different from the others of the same hand as well as from

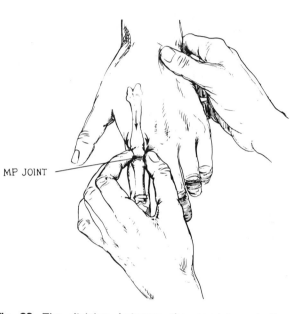

Fig. 39. The division between the condyles at the metacarpophalangeal joint is palpable.

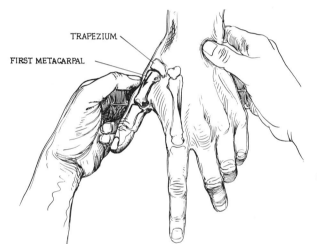

Fig. 38. Palpation of the first metacarpal.

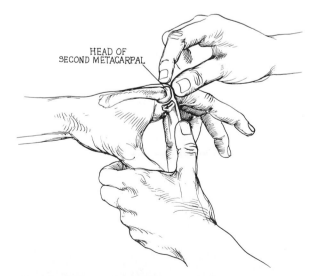

Fig. 40. Flexion of the metacarpophalangeal joint facilitates palpation of its bony structures.

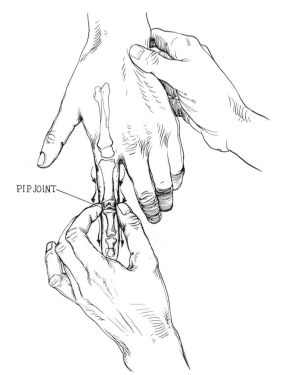

Fig. 41. Palpation of the phalanges.

its counterpart on the opposite hand. For example, a fractured finger, healing in a poor position, can lose its smooth linear continuity along one of its phalangeal rays and develop a callosity over the point of fracture. The interphalangeal joints should be palpated for swelling, tenderness, and symmetry, and should be compared to the opposite hand.

SOFT TISSUE PALPATION

The soft tissue portion of the wrist and hand examination has been divided into clinical zones to present a more clinical picture. Although each zone shall be discussed as a separate entity, in actuality the zones have no such clearcut distinction and are vitally related both clinically and anatomically.

Within the wrist, there are six dorsal passageways, or tunnels (Fig. 47), which transport the extensor tendons, and two palmar tunnels which transport the nerves, arteries, and flexor tendons to the hand. These tunnels (and the structures within

them) are palpable, and each will be discussed in detail under its respective clinical zone.

Wrist: Zone I—Radial Styloid Process

Anatomic Snuffbox. This lies just dorsal and distal to the radial styloid process. The tendons bordering it become more prominent when the thumb is extended (Fig. 45). The radial border of the snuffbox is composed of the abductor pollicis longus and the extensor pollicis brevis tendons which pass over the radial styloid process and etch a small groove on its lateral aspect (Fig. 44). The ulnar border of the snuffbox is the extensor pollicis longus tendon and the floor the navicular bone (Fig. 43). Any tenderness elicited on the floor of the snuffbox suggests a fracture. Occasionally, the deep branch of the radial artery is palpable where it crosses the navicular bone (Fig. 46). The terminal branches of the superficial radial nerve are also palpable where they cross the extensor pollicis longus tendon (Fig. 42).

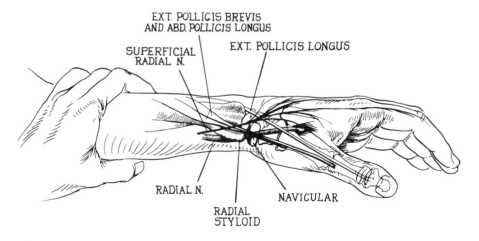

Fig. 42. Bony and soft tissue landmarks around the anatomic snuffbox.

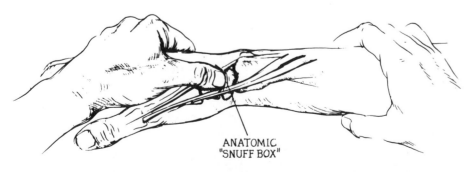

Fig. 43. The anatomic snuffbox.

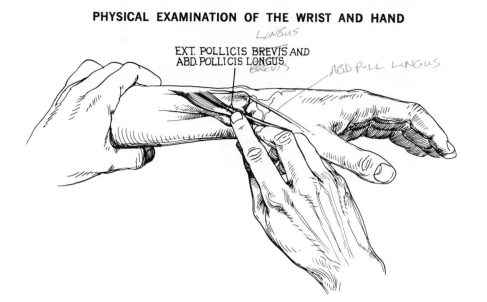

EXT. POLLICIS BREVIS AND
ABD. POLLICIS LONGUS

Fig. 44. The radial border of the snuffbox is defined by the abductor pollicis longus and the extensor pollicis brevis tendons.

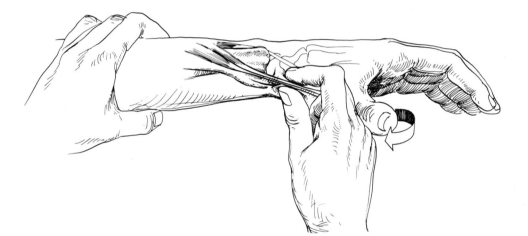

Fig. 45. The tendons of the abductor pollicis longus and brevis are made more prominent for palpation when the thumb is extended.

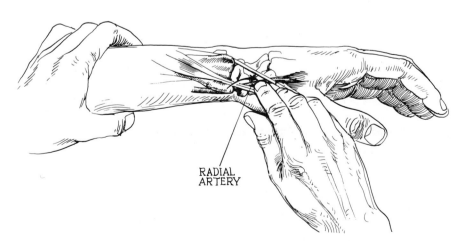

RADIAL
ARTERY

Fig. 46. Palpation of the radial artery.

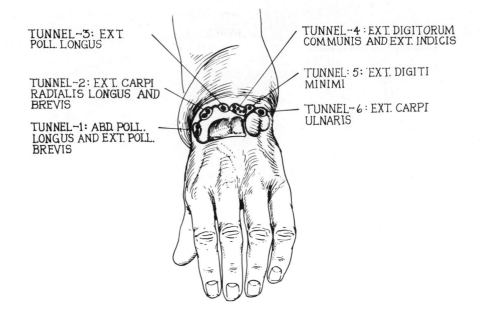

TUNNEL~3: EXT. POLL. LONGUS

TUNNEL~2: EXT. CARPI RADIALIS LONGUS AND BREVIS

TUNNEL~1: ABD. POLL. LONGUS AND EXT. POLL. BREVIS

TUNNEL~4: EXT. DIGITORUM COMMUNIS AND EXT. INDICIS

TUNNEL: 5: EXT. DIGITI MINIMI

TUNNEL~6: EXT. CARPI ULNARIS

Fig. 47. The tunnels on the dorsum of the wrist which transport extensor tendons to the hand.

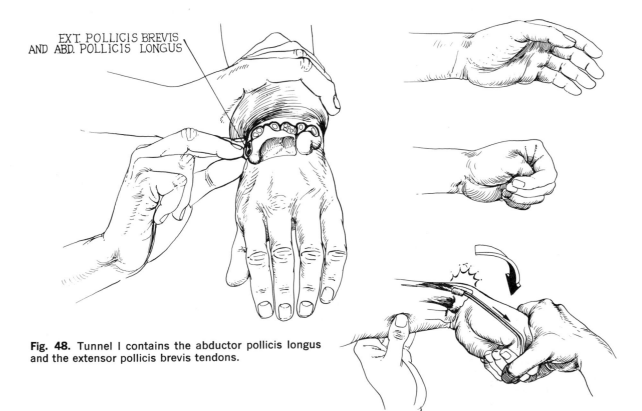

EXT. POLLICIS BREVIS AND ABD. POLLICIS LONGUS

Fig. 48. Tunnel I contains the abductor pollicis longus and the extensor pollicis brevis tendons.

Fig. 49. Finkelstein Test.

Tunnel I. Tunnel I, which lies in Zone I of the wrist, transports the *abductor pollicis longus* and the *extensor pollicis brevis* tendons (Fig. 48). As stated previously, these tendons represent the radial border of the anatomic snuffbox. When the patient's thumb is extended, you can distinguish between the tendons as they exit the tunnel. Near the insertions of the tendons, distal to the tunnel, the extensor pollicis brevis lies on the ulnar side of the abductor pollicis longus. Tunnel I is of clinical significance because it is a site for stenosing tenosynovitis (De Quervain's disease), in which inflammation of the synovial lining of the tunnel narrows the tunnel opening and results in pain when the tendons move. Tenderness elicited in the area during palpation may be an indication of this pathology.

To test specifically for stenosing tenosynovitis of the tendons in Tunnel I, instruct the patient to make a fist, with his thumb tucked inside of his other fingers. Then, as you stabilize his forearm with one hand, deviate his wrist to the ulnar side with the other. If he feels a sharp pain in the area of the tunnel, there is strong evidence of stenosing tenosynovitis (Finkelstein Test) (Fig. 49).

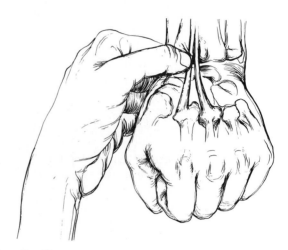

Fig. 51. The extensor carpi radialis longus and brevis tendons become palpable when the fist is clenched.

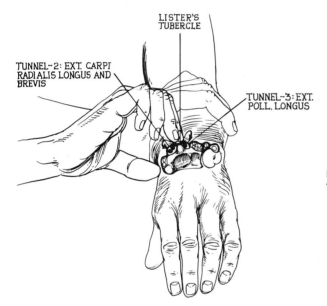

Fig. 50. Tunnel II contains the extensor carpi radialis longus and brevis tendons.

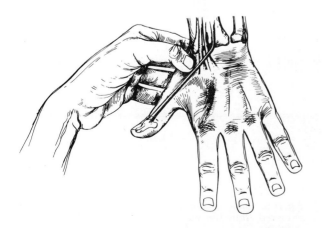

Fig. 52. The extensor carpi radialis longus and brevis tendons are situated on the radial side of the tubercle of the radius.

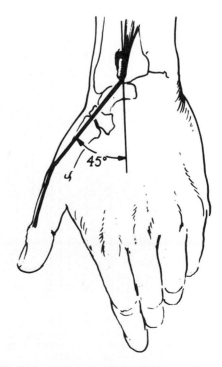

Fig. 53. The course of the extensor pollicis longus tendon.

Wrist: Zone II—Tubercle of the Radius (Lister's Tubercle)

Tunnel II.   Tunnel II, on the radial side of the radial tubercle, contains the *extensor carpi radialis longus* and the *extensor carpi radialis brevis* tendons (Fig. 50). To palpate them, ask your patient to clench his fist. The tendons then stand out slightly on the radial side of the dorsal radial tubercle (Fig. 51). Clinically, either the extensor carpi radialis longus or the brevis may be used for tendon transplants (Fig. 52).

Tunnel III.   Tunnel III on the ulnar side of the radial tubercle contains the *extensor pollicis longus*, which defines the ulnar border of the anatomic snuffbox (Figs. 44, 50). At the point where the extensor pollicis longus passes the dorsal radial tubercle, the tendon takes a 45° turn around the tubercle. Then, after passing over the extensor carpi radialis longus and brevis tendons of tunnel II, it continues along its course to the thumb (Fig. 53). As you palpate along the length of this tendon, look for any signs of rupture. If the dorsal radial tubercle has been disturbed by a Colles' fracture (producing an irregularity of the process), the extensor pollicis longus tendon may rupture due to the added friction imposed upon it as it turns around the roughened tubercle. It is not uncommon to find this tendon ruptured in conjunction with rheumatoid arthritis, since synovitis secondary to that disease increases the friction at the tubercle and causes tendon attrition.

Tunnel IV.   Tunnel IV, just ulnar to tunnel III and just radial to the radioulnar articulation, transports the *extensor digitorum communis* and the independent *extensor indicis* to the hand (Fig. 54).

Although the tendons of the extensor digitorum communis are palpable when the fingers are extended, they are not as distinctly palpable as the tendons in Tunnels I, II, and III. Each of the extensor tendons of the hand should be palpated between the carpus and the metacarpophalangeal joints (Fig. 55). After you palpate the extensor digitorum communis, ask the patient to move his index finger into flexion and extension and observe the independent motion of the extensor indicis tendon. The extensor indicis should be palpated along its course to the index finger. Note that it is not distinctly palpable at the level of the tunnel. All the extensor tendons of the wrist and fingers are subject to rheumatoid arthritis, which may cause them to be tender to palpation. The extensor indicis is sometimes transferred surgically to replace a torn extensor pollicis longus tendon.

On occasion, a cystic, pea-sized swelling (ganglion) with a jellylike consistency may develop on the dorsal or volar aspect of the wrist. Such ganglia are not usually fixed to the connective tissues, nor are they tender to palpation (Fig. 56).

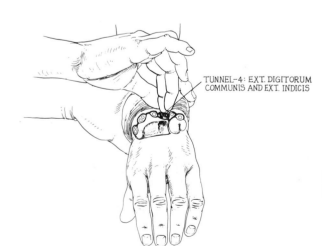

TUNNEL-4: EXT. DIGITORUM COMMUNIS AND EXT. INDICIS

Fig. 54. Tunnel IV contains the extensor digiti communis and the extensor indicis tendons.

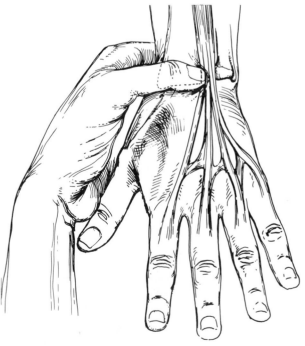

Fig. 55. Each of the tendons in the hand should be palpated from the carpus to the metacarpophalangeal joint.

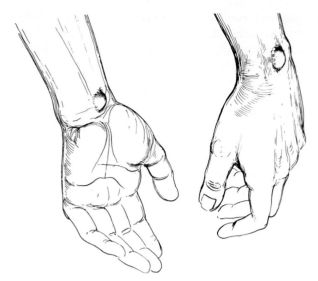

Fig. 56. Ganglia may be found on the wrist's dorsal or volar surfaces.

Wrist: Zone III—Ulnar Styloid Process

Tenderness in the area of the ulnar styloid process may be due either to pathology within the process itself or to a Colles' fracture with an associated fracture of the distal end of the ulnar styloid process. If the ulnar styloid process is eroded due to rheumatoid arthritis, localized pain, swelling, and possible deformity will develop.

Tunnel V. Tunnel V, which overlies the distal ends of the radioulnar articulation on the dorsum of the wrist, contains the *extensor digiti minimi* tendon. The tunnel is palpable as a slight indentation just lateral to the ulnar styloid process. To palpate the extensor digiti minimi, have the patient rest his palm upon a table or desk and ask him to raise his little finger. The movement of the extensor digiti minimi can be felt in the depression radial to the ulnar styloid process (Fig. 57). Like the extensor indicis, the extensor digiti minimi can move independently. This independent movement is demonstrable by having the patient extend both his index and little fingers while keeping the other fingers in flexion (in the familiar "hex" sign) (Fig. 58).

The extensor digiti minimi lies over the radioulnar articulation and may become involved in

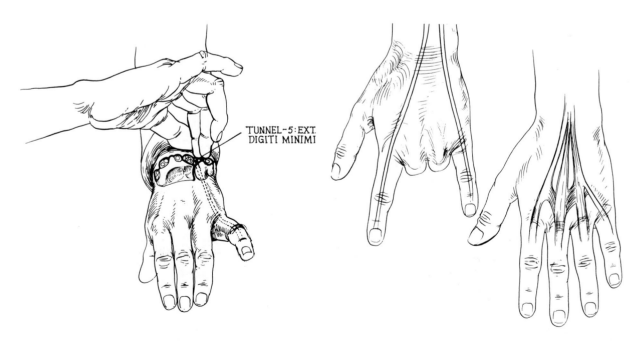

Fig. 57. Tunnel V contains the extensor digiti minimi.

Fig. 58. The extensor indicis and the extensor digiti minimi tendons are capable of independent action.

rheumatoid arthritis of the joint. It may also be subject to attrition, either from friction due to dorsal dislocation of the ulnar head or from synovitis.

Tunnel VI. Tunnel VI, in the groove between the apex of the ulnar styloid process and the ulnar head, contains the *extensor carpi ulnaris* tendon, which is palpable from where it passes over the ulnar styloid process to its insertion into the side of the fifth metacarpal base (Fig. 59). The extensor carpi ulnaris is more palpable when the patient's wrist is extended and ulnarly deviated (Fig. 60). In a Colles' fracture with an associated fracture of the distal end of the ulnar styloid process, the dorsal carpal ligament of tunnel VI may tear. As a consequence, the extensor tendon may dislocate over the styloid process during pronation. In this instance, there is a perceptible, audible snap which may cause some attendant pain. In rheumatoid arthritis, the tendon may displace in an ulnar direction or rupture.

Wrist: Zone IV—Pisiform (Palmar Aspect)

Flexor Carpi Ulnaris. The pisiform bone is situated over the anterior surface of the triquetrium, and is enclosed by the flexor carpi ulnaris. The flexor carpi ulnaris stands out proximal to the pisiform bone on the ulnar side of the palmaris longus when the wrist is flexed against resistance (Fig. 61). Palpate the tendon proximally, moving up the forearm, then returning to the level of the wrist. Calcific deposits, which occasionally form at the site of the insertion of the tendon, can cause severe pain. The flexor carpi ulnaris tendon is sometimes surgically transferred to other sections of the wrist and hand to substitute for a variety of pathologically involved musculotendinous units.

Tunnel of Guyon. The depression between the pisiform and the hook of the hamate (Figs. 32, 33) is converted into a fibro-osseous tunnel, the tunnel of Guyon, by the pisohamate ligament. The tunnel of Guyon is clinically significant because it contains the ulnar nerve and artery and is a site for compression injuries. Although neither the nerve nor the artery is distinctly palpable under the thick layer of soft tissue covering the tunnel, the area is unusually tender if there is pathology present (Figs. 62, 63). Some tenderness is to be expected in the palpation of any nerve. Therefore, it is important to note the degree of tenderness elicited and to compare it to that of the opposite side.

Ulnar Artery. The pulse of the ulnar artery is palpable proximal to the pisiform bone just before the artery crosses the wrist on the anterior aspect of the ulna. The pulse can be felt if you press the artery against the ulna (Fig. 64).

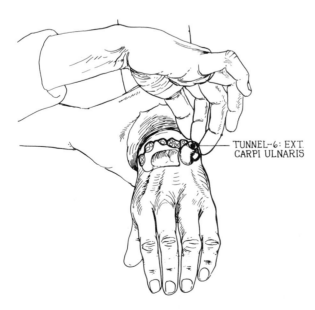

Fig. 59. Tunnel VI contains the extensor carpi ulnaris tendon.

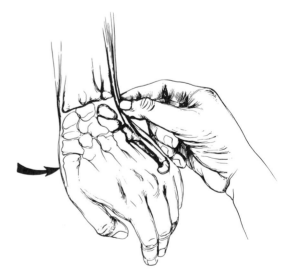

Fig. 60. Ulnar deviation facilitates palpation of the extensor carpi ulnaris tendon.

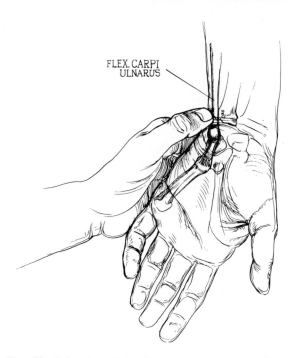

FLEX. CARPI ULNARUS

Fig. 61. Palpation of the flexor carpi ulnaris tendon.

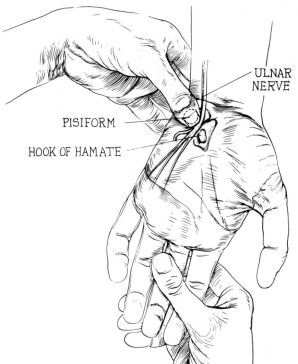

ULNAR NERVE

PISIFORM

HOOK OF HAMATE

Fig. 62. The Tunnel of Guyon contains the ulnar nerve and artery.

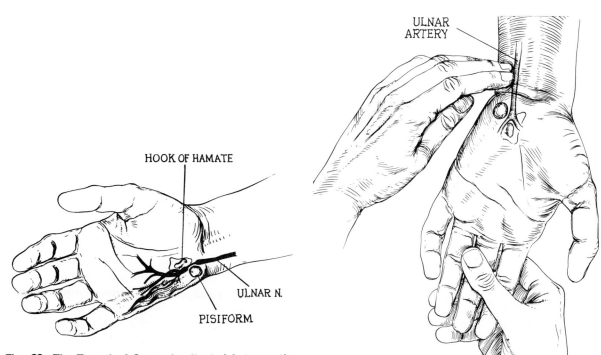

HOOK OF HAMATE

ULNAR N.

PISIFORM

Fig. 63. The Tunnel of Guyon is situated between the hook of the hamate and the pisiform bone. The ulnar nerve may be compressed in the tunnel.

ULNAR ARTERY

Fig. 64. Palpation of the ulnar artery.

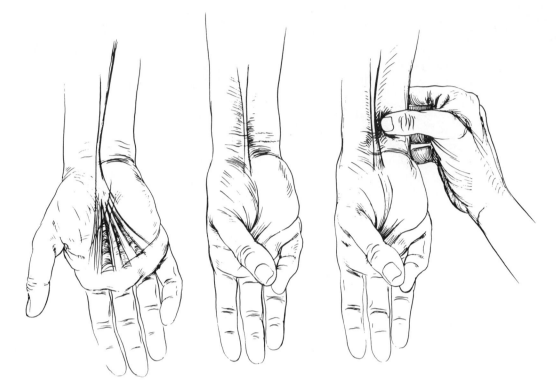

Fig. 65. Opposition of the thumb and little finger facilitates the palpation of the palmaris longus.

Wrist: Zone V—*Palmaris Longus and Carpal Tunnel*

Palmaris Longus.   The palmaris longus bisects the anterior aspect of the wrist. Its distal end marks the anterior surface of the carpal tunnel. To facilitate palpation of this tendon, have the patient flex his wrist and touch the tips of his thumb and little finger together in opposition (Fig. 65); the palmaris longus becomes prominent along the midline of the anterior aspect of the wrist. Palpate it in linear fashion, first up the forearm, then back down to the wrist.

In approximately 7 percent of the population, the palmaris longus is absent. Such absence, however, is not a problem since the condition does not hinder hand function. The tendon is of major clinical importance in that it is frequently used as a tendon graft to replace severely traumatized flexor tendons of the fingers.

Carpal Tunnel.   The carpal tunnel lies deep to the palmaris longus and is defined by four palpable bony prominences: proximally, by the pisiform and the tubercle of the navicular; distally, by the hook of the hamate and the tubercle of the trapezium (Fig. 66). The transverse carpal ligament, a portion of the volar carpal ligament, runs between these four prominences and forms a

fibrous sheath which contains the carpal tunnel anteriorly within a fibro-osseous tunnel. Posteriorly, the tunnel is bordered by the carpal bones. This tunnel transports the median nerve and the finger flexor tendons from the forearm to the hand.

The carpal tunnel is clinically significant not only because of the importance of the structures within it, but also because of the frequent incidence of carpal tunnel syndrome (narrowing of the carpal tunnel) and its resulting clinical problems. In this syndrome, compression of the median nerve can restrict motor function as well as sensation along the median nerve distribution of the hand. Less frequently, constriction of the tunnel traps the tendons running through it, and restricts, and may even prevent, flexion in the fingers. Compression of the carpal tunnel can stem from a variety of factors, such as anterior dislocation of the lunate bone, swelling secondary to Colles' fracture of the distal end of the radius, synovitis secondary to rheumatoid arthritis, or anything causing swelling secondary to other general trauma affecting the wrist, such as sprains and a host of systemic diseases, such as myxedema and Paget's disease.

To confirm a diagnosis of carpal tunnel syndrome, you can elicit or reproduce pain in the distribution of the median nerve by tapping over the volar carpal ligament (Tinel sign) (Fig. 67).

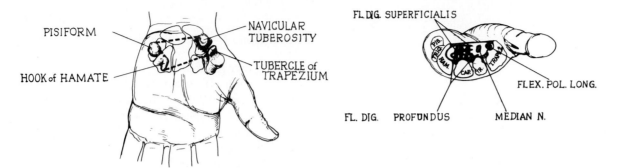

PISIFORM

NAVICULAR
TUBEROSITY

HOOK of HAMATE

TUBERCLE of
TRAPEZIUM

FL. DIG. SUPERFICIALIS

FLEX. POL. LONG.

FL. DIG.   PROFUNDUS   MEDIAN N.

Fig. 66. The Carpal Tunnel. It contains the median nerve and the finger flexor tendons, and is defined proximally by the pisiform and navicular bones, and distally by the hook of the hamate and the trapezium.

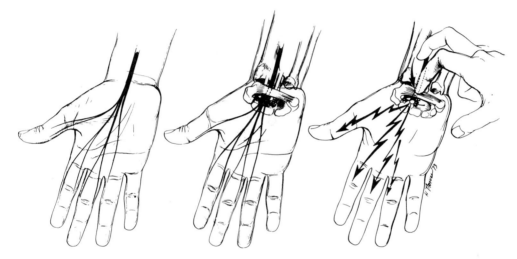

Fig. 67. Carpal Tunnel Syndrome (left and middle). Tinel sign (right).

Symptoms common to the syndrome such as tingling of the fingers may also be reproduced by flexing the patient's wrist to its maximum degree and holding it in that position for at least a minute (Phalen's Test) (Fig. 68). Although the anatomic structures within the carpal tunnel are not palpable, the examiner should be aware of their location, since their function is vital to the normal function of the hand.

Flexor Carpi Radialis. The flexor carpi radialis lies radial to the palmaris longus at the level of the wrist. This tendon crosses the navicular before inserting into the base of the second metacarpal and stands out more prominently at the wrist level than does the flexor carpi ulnaris. When the patient flexes his wrist and radially deviates his hand, the tendon becomes prominent next to the palmaris longus (Fig. 69). Palpate it proximally until it becomes indistinct beneath the fascia covering the wrist flexor–pronator group.

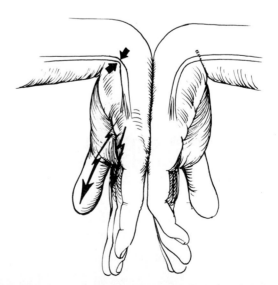

Fig. 68. Phalen's Test to reproduce symptoms of carpal tunnel syndrome.

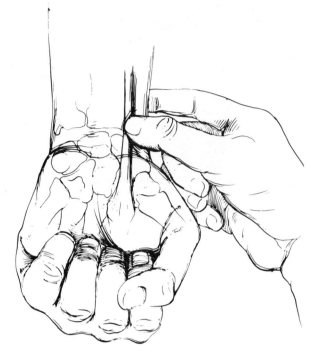

Fig. 69. Palpation of the flexor carpi radialis tendon.

Hand: Zone I—Thenar Eminence

The thenar eminence is situated at the base of the thumb. It is composed of three muscles which activate thumb motion: the abductor pollicis brevis (superficial layer), the opponens pollicis (middle layer), and the flexor pollicis brevis (deep layer). It feels fleshy to the touch and is mobile since it is not bound by any fascial covering (Fig. 70). The thenar eminence on the dominant hand may look and feel somewhat more developed than its counterpart on the opposite hand. It should be examined for hypertrophy or atrophy and compared to the other hand for visible or palpable differences in size, shape, and consistency.

Compression of the median nerve within the carpal tunnel can cause the thenar eminence to atrophy, since its muscles are supplied by the recurrent branch of the median nerve. If carpal tunnel syndrome is a possible pathology, look for an atrophic thenar eminence and a more readily palpable first metacarpal as concomitant signs of its existence. At the onset of atrophy, the thenar muscles appear somewhat flat. Later, the effects of the pathology become more obvious, and a hollow develops in this normally prominent muscle mound (Fig. 73).

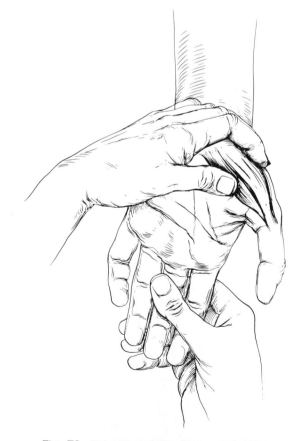

Fig. 70. Palpation of the thenar eminence.

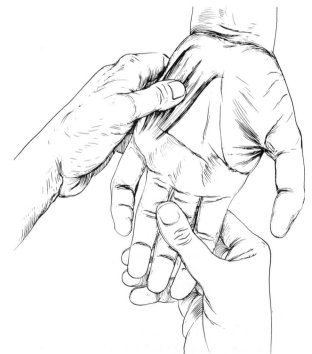

Fig. 71. Palpation of the hypothenar eminence.

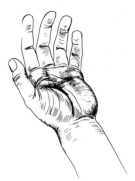

Fig. 72. Normally developed thenar and hypothenar eminences.

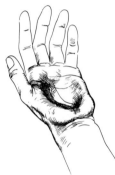

Fig. 73. Atrophy of the thenar and hypothenar eminences.

Hand: Zone II—Hypothenar Eminence

The hypothenar eminence lies just proximal to the little finger and extends longitudinally to the pisiform. This eminence, too, is composed of three mobile muscles: the abductor digiti quinti, the opponens digiti, and the flexor digiti quinti. These three muscles are indistinguishable from each other since they lie in layers (Fig. 71).

The hypothenar eminence should be checked for hypertrophy or atrophy. Since the eminence is supplied by the ulnar nerve, atrophy may result from ulnar nerve compression taking place either in the tunnel of Guyon or, more proximally, in the extremity (Figs. 72, 73). Compression also alters sensation within the ulnar nerve distribution of the hand.

Hand: Zone III—Palm

The structures within the palm are not distinctly palpable because of the thick muscular padding (thenar and hypothenar eminences) and palmar fascia which obscure them. The flexor tendons are barely palpable deep to the palmar fascia; the nerves and vessels within the palm cannot be palpated at all.

Palmar Aponeurosis. The palmar aponeurosis consists of four broad, divergent bands that extend to the base of the fingers (Fig. 74). The

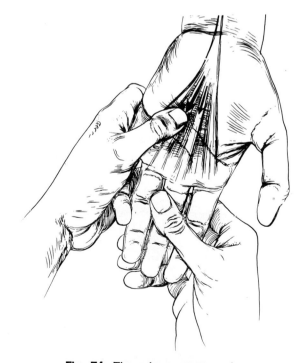

Fig. 74. The palmar aponeurosis.

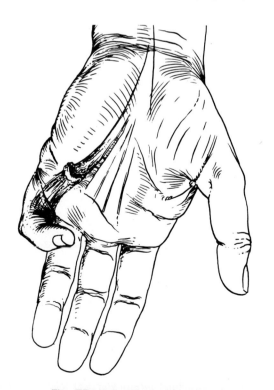

Fig. 75. Dupuytren's contracture.

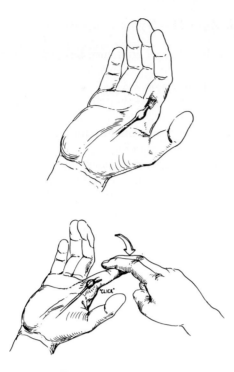

palmar fascia should be probed for palpable thickened areas in the form of discrete nodules which are found, for the most part, on the ulnar side proximal to the ring and little fingers. These discrete nodules can cause a flexion deformity of the fingers (Dupuytren's Contracture) (Fig. 75).

Finger Flexor Tendons. The finger flexor tendons run in a common sheath deep to the bands of the fascia and may be palpable, although as a general rule they are not. If they are, any tenderness elicited should be noted, for it may be the result of a direct trauma to the flexor tendons.

To palpate the tendons, ask the patient to flex and extend his fingers. A sudden palpable and audible snapping occurring upon movement of one of the fingers indicates "trigger finger." The snapping is most often caused by a nodule in the flexor tendon that catches on a narrower annular sheath or pulley opposite the metacarpal head (Fig. 76 A and B). It may take place either in flexion or in extension. A similar sound upon motion of the thumb indicating "trigger thumb" is a common finding.

Fig. 76. A. and B. Trigger finger.

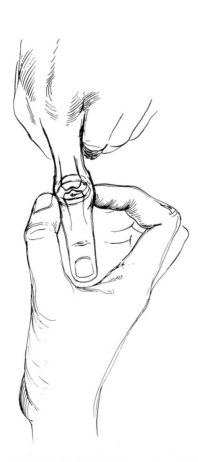

Fig. 77. The proximal interphalangeal joint is covered by a thick joint capsule and the collateral ligaments.

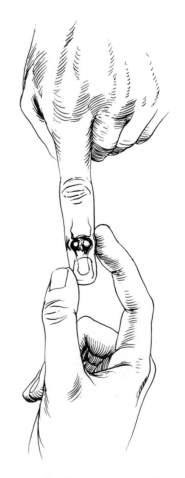

Fig. 78. Heberden's nodes.

Hand: Zone IV—Dorsum

Extensor Tendons. The extensor tendons run along the dorsum of the hand. They become palpable when the patient extends his fingers while his wrist is slightly extended. When extension is resisted by pressure upon the dorsum of the fingers, the extensor tendons stand out, especially where they cross the metacarpophalangeal joints.

Each tendon should be palpated individually, proximal and distal to the joint. Any tenderness elicited may be the result of a strained or ruptured tendon. In rheumatoid arthritis, the extensor tendons can become displaced to the ulnar side of the metacarpophalangeal joints and cause an ulnar drift of the fingers.

Hand: Zone V—Phalanges

The fingers contain no muscle bellies and are motored only by their flexor and extensor tendons.

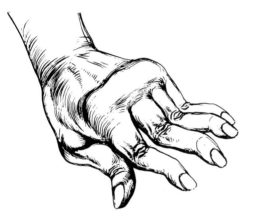

Fig. 79. Swan-neck deformity.

First palpate the soft tissues surrounding the proximal interphalangeal joints. The dorsal and palmar surfaces of the proximal interphalangeal joints feel smooth because the flexor and extensor tendons of the fingers cross them. The joint's lateral surfaces feel fusiform, since they are covered by a thick joint capsule and the collateral ligaments (Fig. 77). Enlarged joints should be gently palpated for they may be sensitive. An abnormal fusiform enlargement can indicate synovitis secondary to rheumatoid arthritis (Bouchard's nodes). Occasionally, rheumatoid arthritis can cause a so-called swan neck deformity, which occurs when the proximal interphalangeal joint is hyperextended and the distal interphalangeal joint is flexed (Fig. 79).

If the central slip of the extensor digitorum communis tendon is avulsed from its insertion into the base of the middle phalanx, the proximal interphalangeal joint becomes markedly flexed and the distal interphalangeal joint extended. In this condition, called a "boutonniere" deformity, the middle phalanx is sensitive to palpation (Fig. 80).

The distal interphalangeal joint, like the proximal interphalangeal joint, should feel smooth on its dorsal and palmar surfaces and fusiform on its lateral surfaces. Any unilateral swelling or tenderness that palpation might elicit should be noted. Discrete but palpable bony nodules (Heberden's nodes) found on the dorsal and lateral surfaces of the distal interphalangeal joint (Fig. 78) may indicate osteoarthritis.

If the distal insertion of the extensor digitorum communis has been torn away from the distal phalanx with an attendant avulsion of a bone fragment, a bony excrescence becomes palpable on the dorsal surface of the distal interphalangeal joint. The joint may be tender to the touch and the patient may be unable to extend it fully. This deformity is known as "mallet finger" (Fig. 81).

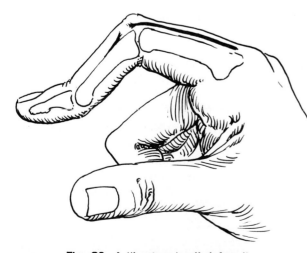

Fig. 80. A "boutonniere" deformity.

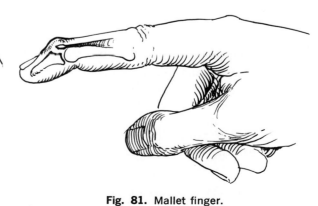

Fig. 81. Mallet finger.

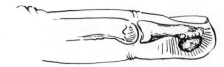

Fig. 82. An infection (a felon) of the finger tufts.

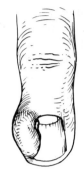

Fig. 83. Paronychia

Hand: Zone VI—Tufts of the Fingers

The finger tufts contain most of the hand's sensory nerve endings and are instrumental in almost every movement and task that the hand undertakes. Pathology involving the tufts of the fingers is considered a serious matter inasmuch as it affects the vital functioning of the hand.

The distal ends of the fingers are particularly susceptible to infection. A localized infection (a felon) of the finger tufts has no way of decompressing itself because it becomes trapped between the septa that attach the skin to the bone (Fig. 82). In such an infection, pressure increases proportionate to the amount of pus, and the site becomes very painful.

Since infection in the fingers can travel proximally, the dorsum of the hand should be checked for swelling and red streaks. If swelling is present, the supracondylar and axillary lymph nodes also should be probed for enlargement, because drainage from an infection follows the course of the lymphatics.

An infection, originating in the finger tufts, may also travel along the tendon sheaths, producing the four cardinal signs of Kanavel: (1) fingers held in flexion, (2) uniform swelling of the finger, (3) intense pain upon passive extension of the finger, and (4) sensitivity upon palpation along the course of the tendon sheaths.

A runaround, or "hangnail" infection (paronychia), usually starts at the side of the nail but does not localize, since it has room to spread around the nail base (Fig. 83).

RANGE OF MOTION

The wrist and the fingers will be assessed separately. Those movements pertaining to wrist function are:

1) flexion
2) extension
3) radial deviation
4) ulnar deviation
5) supination (of the forearm)
6) pronation (of the forearm)

Movements to be tested in the fingers are:

1) finger flexion and extension at the metacarpophalangeal joints
2) finger flexion and extension at the interphalangeal joints
3) finger abduction and adduction at the metacarpophalangeal joints
4) thumb flexion and extension at the metacarpophalangeal joint and the interphalangeal joint (transpalmar abduction and radial abduction)
5) thumb abduction and adduction at the carpometacarpal joint (palmar abduction)
6) opposition

Active Range of Motion

In evaluating the range of motion of the wrist and hand, bilateral comparison is most useful in determining the degrees of restriction in any given situation. A patient should be able to complete the quick active tests without any strain or symptoms of pain. If, however, he has any difficulty or is unable to complete the active range of motion satisfactorily, passive range of motion tests should be conducted.

WRIST FLEXION AND EXTENSION. Instruct the patient to flex and extend his wrist. Normal flexion allows him to move his wrist to about 80° from the neutral or straight position (0°). The normal limit for extension is approximately 70° (Fig. 84).

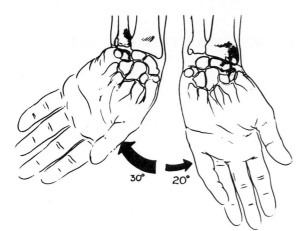

Fig. 84. Ulnar and radial deviation of the wrist.

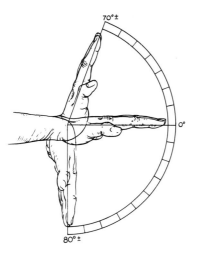

Fig. 85. Wrist flexion and extension range of motion.

WRIST ULNAR AND RADIAL DEVIATION. Ask the patient to move his wrist from side to side into ulnar and radial deviation. Ulnar deviation is the greater of the two, since the ulna does not extend distally as far as the radius and does not articulate directly with the carpus. Ulnar deviation has a range of approximately 30°, while the range of radial deviation is about 20° (Fig. 85).

SUPINATION AND PRONATION. Tests are given in the Elbow Chapter, pages 50 and 51.

FINGER FLEXION AND EXTENSION. To test flexion and extension of the fingers (metacarpophalangeal, proximal, and distal interphalangeal joints), ask the patient first to make a tight fist and then to extend his fingers, observing whether or not he is able to do so with all fingers working in unison. In normal flexion, the fingers close together in an even motion, touching the palm approximately along the distal palmar crease (Figs. 86–88). In normal extension, the fingers move in unison and extend to, or beyond, the straight position. Extension is not within normal limits if the patient has difficulty bringing one or more fingers out of the palm, if his fingers show an incomplete extension, or if they do not move at all. Watch for a sudden mass movement that would tend to mask the restricted movement of any one digit.

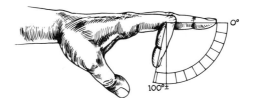

Fig. 87. Proximal interphalangeal joint range of motion: flexion–extension.

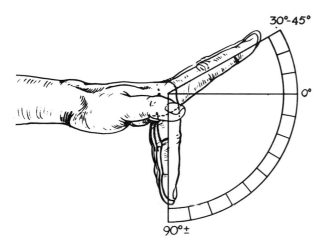

Fig. 86. Metacarpophalangeal joint range of motion: flexion–extension.

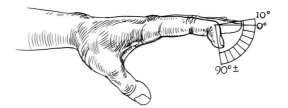

Fig. 88. Distal interphalangeal joint range of motion: flexion–extension.

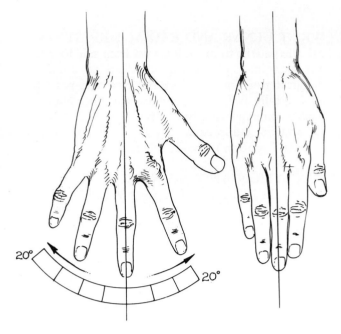

Fig. 89. Finger abduction and adduction.

FINGER ABDUCTION AND ADDUCTION.

Ask the patient to spread his fingers apart and back together again (Fig. 89). Clinically, abduction and adduction are measured from the axial line of the hand which runs longitudinally down the middle finger. In abduction, the fingers should separate in equal amounts of approximately 20°; in adduction, they should come together and touch each other.

THUMB FLEXION.

Have the patient move his thumb across his palm and touch the pad at the base of the little finger (Figs. 90–92). This motion, transpalmar abduction, tests active flexion of the metacarpophalangeal as well as the interphalangeal joints of the thumb.

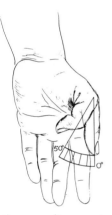

Fig. 91. Thumb flexion and extension: metacarpophalangeal joint.

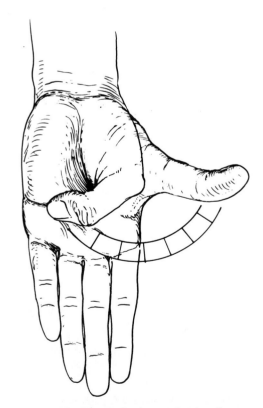

Fig. 90. Thumb flexion and extension.

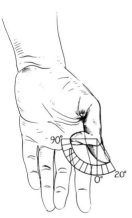

Fig. 92. Thumb flexion and extension: interphalangeal joint.

THUMB EXTENSION (radial abduction). Ask the patient to move his thumb laterally away from his fingers. There should be an angle of approximately 50° between the index finger and thumb.

PALMAR ABDUCTION/ADDUCTION OF THE THUMB. Instruct the patient to spread his thumb anteriorly away from his palm and then to return it to the palm. Normally, the thumb and index finger form an angle of about 70° when the thumb is in full abduction (Fig. 93). Bringing the thumb back to the palm demonstrates full adduction.

OPPOSITION. Normally, the patient should be able to touch the tip of his thumb to each of the other fingertips (Fig. 94).

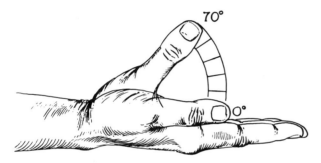

Fig. 93. Palmar abduction/adduction of the thumb.

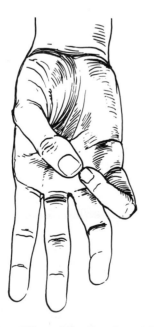

Fig. 94. Opposition of the thumb and fingertips.

Passive Range of Motion

WRIST:
FLEXION —80°
EXTENSION—70°

In preparation for the wrist flexion and extension test, isolate the wrist by placing your stabilizing hand at the distal end of the patient's forearm and holding his hand with your other hand. Then move the wrist into flexion and from flexion into extension (Fig. 84). A limited range of wrist motion may be due to ankylosis of the joint secondary to infection or to a poorly reduced Colles' fracture of the radius.

WRIST:
ULNAR DEVIATION—30°
RADIAL DEVIATION—20°

Keep your hands in the same positions used for the flexion and extension tests and move the patient's wrist into radial and ulnar deviation (Fig. 85). Restricted ulnar deviation of the wrist may be due to a comminuted Colles' fracture.

FINGERS: FLEXION AND EXTENSION AT THE METACARPOPHALANGEAL JOINTS
FLEXION —90°
EXTENSION—30°–45°

To fully test flexion and extension at the metacarpophalangeal joints, test the fingers both individually and together. To prepare for the test, place your stabilizing hand around the ulnar border of the patient's hand so that your thumb lies in his palm and your fingers spread across the dorsum of his hand. Your other hand should be positioned with your thumb on the palmar surface of his proximal phalanges and your fingers spread over the dorsum of his fingers to isolate the metacarpophalangeal joints of the four fingers. Now move the metacarpophalangeal joints into flexion and extension. Normally, the fingers can hyperextend beyond their active range of extension (Fig. 86).

To test the fingers individually, keep your stabilizing hand in its position around the hand and grasp the proximal phalanx of the index fingers. Then flex and extend the metacarpophalangeal joint of the index finger slowly. You should be able to move the index finger (and the other fingers as well) into approximately 90° of flexion and nearly 45° of hyperextension. Since the finger flexor tendons influence each others' actions, you may be unable to move a normal finger to the maximum

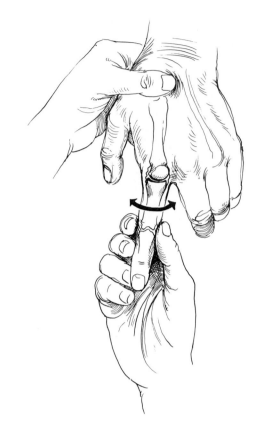

Fig. 95. The metacarpophalangeal joints can be moved laterally a few degrees when extended.

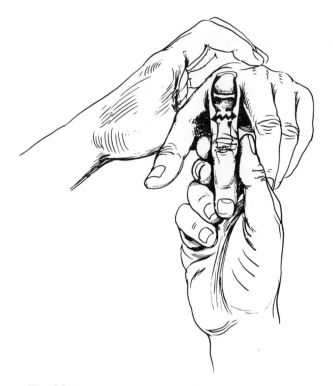

Fig. 96. There is no motion in the metacarpophalangeal joints when they are flexed.

limits because of problems with another finger. The metacarpophalangeal joints of the hand have a few degrees of lateral motion in extension, but none in flexion (Figs. 95, 96) because the collateral ligaments of the metacarpal joints are slack in extension and tight in flexion (Fig. 97). When the hand is placed in a cast, the metacarpal joint must be flexed; otherwise, in time, the slack collateral ligament will shorten, and the joint will not flex properly when the cast is removed.

FINGERS

	Flexion	Extension
Proximal interphalangeal joint	100°	0°
Distal interphalangeal joint	90°	20°

To conduct the passive range of motion tests for the interphalangeal joints, isolate each individual joint. This can be done by stabilizing the phalanges proximal and distal to the joint being tested and by moving the joint into flexion and extension with your more distally placed hand.

The interphalangeal joints are equally stable in flexion and extension because of the bony configuration of the joint surfaces.

FINGERS:
ABDUCTION—20°
ADDUCTION— 0°

Finger abduction and adduction are functions of the metacarpophalangeal joints. Before conducting the test, isolate the joint by stabilizing the metacarpal and the proximal phalanx of the finger being tested. Now move the finger into abduction and adduction. While they are being tested, the metacarpophalangeal joints must be fully extended to zero degrees.

FINGERS: THUMB

	Flexion	Extension
Metacarpophalangeal joint	50°	0°
Interphalangeal joint	90°	20°

Thumb flexion and extension should be tested at both the metacarpophalangeal and the interphalangeal joints. The joint should be isolated and the thumb moved slowly from flexion to extension.

To check flexion and extension of the thumb's interphalangeal joint, hold the proximal phalanx and the distal phalanx, and move the joint into flexion and extension. Both joints of the thumb

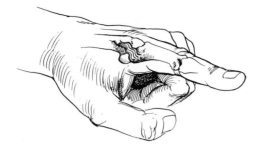

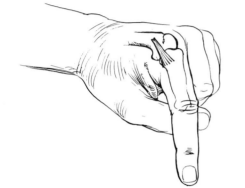

Fig. 97. Above. The collateral ligament of the metacarpophalangeal joint is slack in extension. **Below.** The ligament becomes tight in flexion.

may be tested for flexion and extension at the same time.

FINGERS: THUMB
ABDUCTION—70°.   (Palmar Abduction)
ADDUCTION— 0°.   (Dorsal Adduction)

Thumb abduction and adduction are functions of the carpometacarpal joint, which can be isolated if you place your stabilizing hand just proximal to the thumb at the level of the snuffbox and the radial styloid process and your active hand on the first metacarpal. To test palmar abduction, move the thumb slowly away from the palm. To test dorsal adduction, return it to the palm.

FINGERS: OPPOSITION

For the most part, opposition takes place at the carpometacarpal joint of the thumb. To test opposition, hold the metacarpal bone of the thumb at the metacarpophalangeal joint, then slowly move the thumb toward the palmar surface to the tips of each of the other fingers. Normally, the thumb touches the fingertips with relative ease. However, in abnormal circumstances, the motion

may be difficult or painful for the patient. Note that the opponens digiti muscle is also involved in opposition.

NEUROLOGIC EXAMINATION

Ordinarily, the neurologic examination includes tests that establish the integrity of the nerves relative to muscular strength, sensation, and reflex action. However, since there are no clearly distinguished reflexes in the wrist and hand, this discussion concerns only muscular assessment and sensation testing.

Muscle Testing

Wrist:
1) extension
2) flexion
3) supination
4) pronation

Fingers:
1) extension
2) flexion
3) abduction
4) adduction
5) thumb extension (radial abduction)
6) thumb flexion (transpalmar abduction)
7) thumb abduction (palmar abduction)
8) thumb adduction
9) pinch mechanism (thumb and index finger
10) opposition (thumb and little finger)

WRIST EXTENSION—C6

Primary Extensors:
1) Extensor carpi radialis longus
   radial nerve, C6, (C7)
2) Extensor carpi radialis brevis
   radial nerve, C6, (C7)
3) Extensor carpi ulnaris
   radial nerve, C7

To test wrist extension, stabilize the patient's forearm by placing your palm on the dorsum of his wrist and wrapping your fingers around it. Then instruct the patient to cock his wrist up. When it is fully extended, place the palm of your resisting hand upon the dorsum of his hand, and try to force his wrist out of its extended position (Fig. 98). Normally it is not possible to move the patient's wrist out of its position. The opposite side

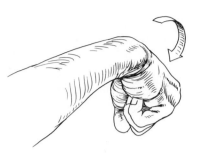

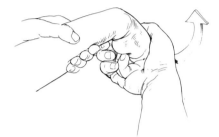

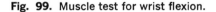

Fig. 99. Muscle test for wrist flexion.

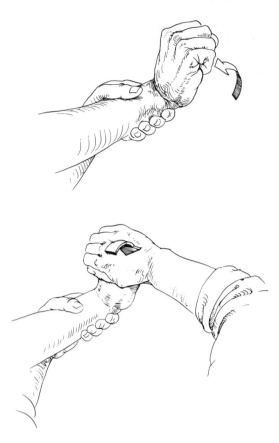

Fig. 98. Muscle test for wrist extension.

should be tested for comparison, and your findings should be evaluated in accordance with the muscle grading chart (Table 1, Shoulder Chapter).

WRIST FLEXION—C7

Primary Flexors:
1) Flexor carpi radialis
   median nerve, C7
2) Flexor carpi ulnaris
   ulnar nerve, C8 (T1)

The flexor carpi radialis is the more effective of the two flexors, although the flexor carpi ulnaris is important in that it provides an axis for motion and guides the wrist into ulnar deviation during flexion.

To test wrist flexion, instruct the patient to make a fist since, in some instances, the finger flexors can act as wrist flexors. By having the patient make a fist, you eliminate the finger flexors as active factors in wrist flexion. Then, stabilize the wrist and ask the patient to flex his closed fist at the wrist. When the wrist is in flexion, place your resisting hand over the patient's flexed fingers, and try to pull the wrist out of flexion (Fig. 99).

WRIST SUPINATION—(See page 53 Elbow Chapter)
WRIST PRONATION—(See page 53 Elbow Chapter)

FINGER EXTENSION—C7

Primary Extensors:
1) Extensor digitorum communis
   radial nerve, C7
2) Extensor indicis
   radial nerve, C7
3) Extensor digiti minimi
   radial nerve, C7

In testing finger extension, the wrist should first be stabilized in a neutral position. Ask the patient to extend his metacarpophalangeal joints, while he flexes his proximal interphalangeal joints. Flexion of the interphalangeal joints prevents him from using the intrinsic muscles of the hand in substitution for the long finger extensors. Then place your hand on the dorsum of the proximal phalanges and try to force them into flexion (Fig. 100).

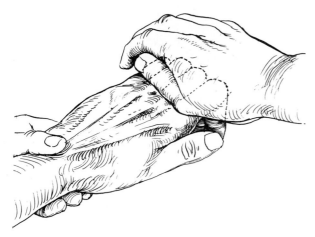

Fig. 100. Muscle test for finger extension.

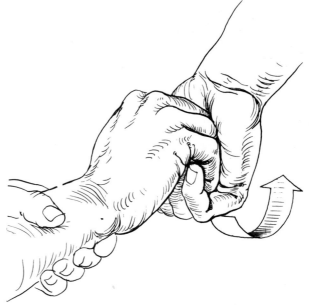

Fig. 101. Muscle test for finger flexion.

FINGER FLEXION—C8

Primary Flexor, Distal Interphalangeal Joint:
1) Flexor digitorum profundis
   ulnar nerve, C8, T1
   anterior interosseous branch of median
   nerve

Primary Flexor, Proximal Interphalangeal Joint:
1) Flexor digitorum superficialis
   median nerve, C7, C8, T1

Flexors, Metacarpophalangeal Joint:
1) Lumbricals
   Medial two lumbricals:
      ulnar nerve, C8
   Lateral two lumbricals:
      median nerve, C7

To check finger flexion, ask the patient to flex his fingers at all the phalangeal joints. Then curl and lock your fingers into his and try to pull his fingers out of flexion (Fig. 101). Normally, all joints should remain flexed. In your evaluation of the test results, note those joints that failed to hold flexion against your pull. (See page **100** in the special tests section of this chapter to differentiate between the flexor digitorium profundus and the flexor digitorum superficialis.)

FINGER ABDUCTION—T1

Primary Abductors:
1) Dorsal interossi
   ulnar nerve, C8, T1
2) Abductor digiti minimi
   ulnar nerve, C8, T1

To test finger abduction, have the patient abduct his extended fingers away from the axial midline of the hand, and try to force each pair together; pinch the index to the middle, ring, and little fingers; the middle finger to the ring and little fingers; and the ring finger to the little finger (Figs. 102, 103).

FINGER ADDUCTION—T1

Primary Adductor:
1) Palmar interossei
   ulnar nerve, C8, T1

To test finger adduction, have the patient try to keep his extended fingers together while you attempt to pull them apart. Test in pairs as follows: the index and middle fingers, the middle and ring fingers, and the ring and little fingers.

Finger adduction can also be checked if you place a piece of paper between two of the patient's extended fingers, and, as he tries to maintain his hold on the paper, pull it out from in between. The strength of his grasp should be compared to that of the opposite hand (Fig. 104).

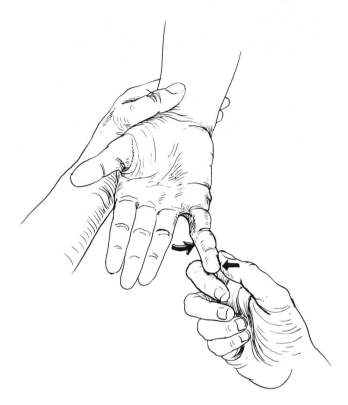

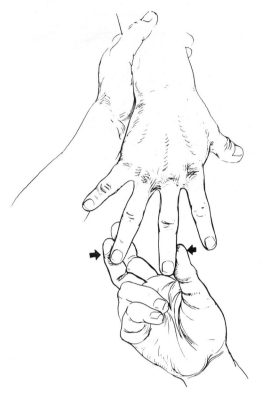

Fig. 102. Muscle test for finger abduction.

Fig. 103. Muscle test for finger abduction.

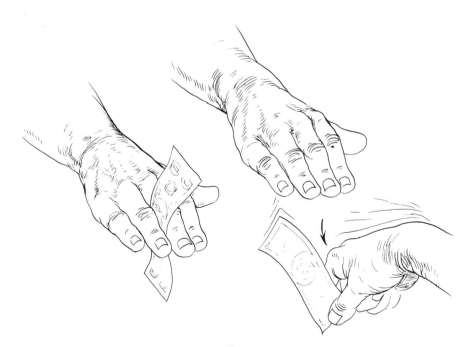

Fig. 104. An alternate method of testing finger adduction.

THUMB EXTENSION

Primary Extensor, Metacarpophalangeal Joint:
1) Extensor pollicis brevis
   radial nerve, C7

Primary Extensor, Interphalangeal Joint:
1) Extensor pollicis longus
   radial nerve, C7

First, have the patient extend his thumb. Then press upon the distal phalanx to push the thumb into flexion. Notice if either joint flexes without taking much pressure. If the thumb extensors are weak or nonfunctional, the patient may substitute the thumb abductors to perform extension at the metacarpophalangeal joint.

THUMB FLEXION (Transpalmar Abduction)

Primary Flexor, Metacarpophalangeal Joint:
1) Flexor pollicis brevis
   medial portion: ulnar nerve, C8
   lateral portion: median nerve, C6, C7

Primary Flexor, Metacarpophalangeal Joint:
1) Flexor pollicis longus
   median nerve, C8, T1

To test thumb flexion, have the patient touch his hypothenar eminence with his thumb. When his thumb is fully flexed, hook your thumb into his, and try to pull his thumb out of flexion.

THUMB ABDUCTION (Palmar Abduction)

Primary Abductors:
1) Abductor pollicis longus
   radial nerve, C7
2) Abductor pollicis brevis
   median nerve, C6, C7

In preparation for this test, first stabilize the patient's metacarpals by wrapping your hand around the ulnar side of his hand. Then instruct him to abduct his thumb fully as you attempt to push his thumb back toward the palm. If the thumb abductors are weak or nonfunctional, the patient may substitute thumb extensors to accomplish abduction (Fig. 105).

THUMB ADDUCTION

Primary Adductor
1) Adductor pollicis (obliquus and transversus)
   ulnar nerve, C8

The patient's hand should first be stabilized along its ulnar border as it was in the test for abduction. Then, while you hold his thumb, instruct him to adduct it, and apply resistance gradually until you determine the maximum resistance he can overcome.

PINCH MECHANISM
(Thumb and Index Finger)

The pinch motion is a complicated movement that involves several muscles. The long flexors and extensors stabilize the interphalangeal, metacarpophalangeal, and carpometacarpal joints and provide a good arch for the thumb and index fingers. This arch creates an effective "O" type pinch. The lumbricals and the interossei must be functional to provide the finger pinch motion.

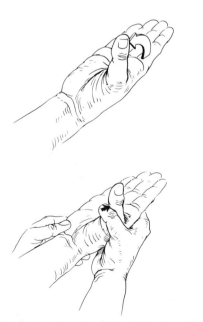

Fig. 105. A muscle test for thumb abduction.

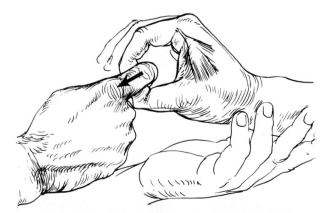

Fig. 106. Muscle test for the pinch mechanism.

To test the pinch mechanism, instruct the patient to touch the tips of his thumb and index finger together. Then hook or curl your index finger in the circle created by the two fingers and try to pull the fingers apart by pulling at their point of union (Fig. 106). Normally, with a moderate to strong pull there should be no collapse or change in the "O," and you will not be able to pull the fingers apart.

OPPOSITION OF THUMB AND LITTLE FINGER

Primary Opposers:
1) Opponens pollicis
    median nerve, C6, C7
2) Opponens digiti minimi
    ulnar nerve, C8

To test opposition, instruct the patient to touch the tips of his thumb and little finger together. Then take hold of the patient's thenar eminence with one hand and his hypothenar eminence with your other, and try to pull his fingers apart by forcing the metacarpals underlying the eminences away from the midline of the hand.

Sensation Testing

Sensation in the wrist and hand should be evaluated in two ways:

1) testing the major peripheral nerves that innervate the hand
2) testing each neurologic level involved in the hand.

PERIPHERAL NERVE INNERVATION. The hand is supplied by three major peripheral nerves (See Table 2, Cervical Spine Chapter, page 125.): (1) the radial nerve, (2) the median nerve, and (3) the ulnar nerve.

The Radial Nerve. The radial nerve supplies the dorsum of the hand on the radial side of the third metacarpal, as well as the dorsal surfaces of the thumb, index, and middle fingers as far as the distal interphalangeal joints. The web space (dorsal surface) between the thumb and index fingers is almost wholly supplied by the radial nerve (Fig. 107).

The Median Nerve. The median nerve supplies the radial portion of the palm and the palmar surfaces of the thumb, index, and middle fingers; it may also supply the dorsum of the terminal phalanges of these fingers. Its innervation is purest on the palmar skin of the tip of the index finger (Fig. 108).

The Ulnar Nerve. The ulnar nerve supplies the ulnar side of the hand (both dorsal and palmar surfaces) and the ring and little fingers. Its purest area for sensation is on the volar surface of the tip of the little finger (Fig. 108).

SENSATION IN THE HAND BY NEUROLOGIC LEVELS (Dermatomes). The sensation in the hand is supplied by three neurologic levels (See Table 1, Cervical Spine Chapter, page 125.):

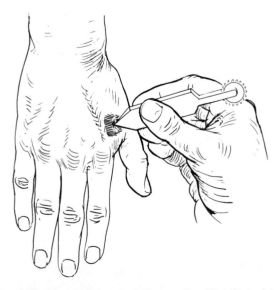

Fig. 107. The web space between the thumb and index fingers is almost autonomous for the radial nerve.

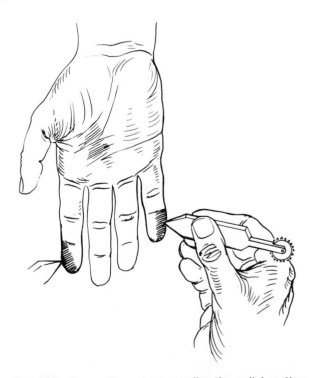

Fig. 108. The median nerve supplies the radial portion of the palm. The ulnar nerve supplies the ulnar side of the hand.

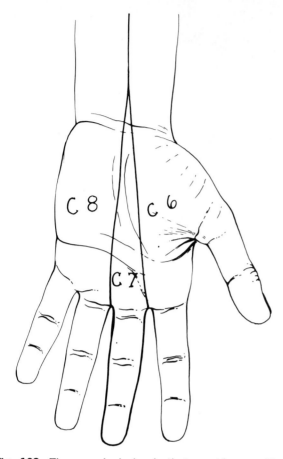

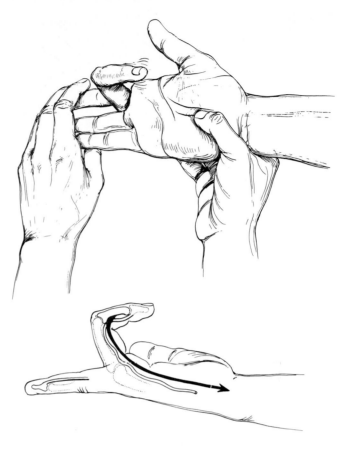

Fig. 109. The neurologic levels that provide sensation to the hand.

Fig. 110. A test for the flexor digitorum superficialis tendon.

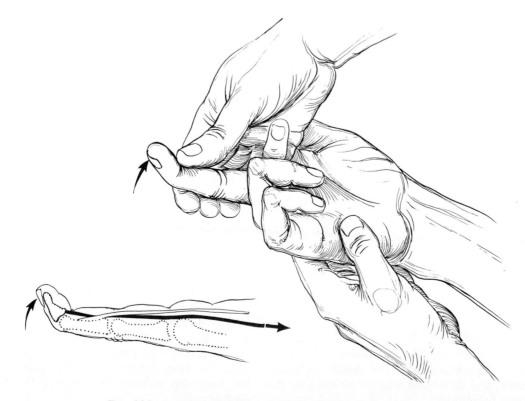

Fig. 111. A test for the flexor digitorum profoundus tendon.

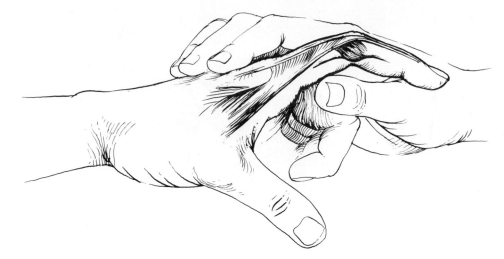

Fig. 112. The Bunnel-Littler test for tightness of the hand intrinsics.

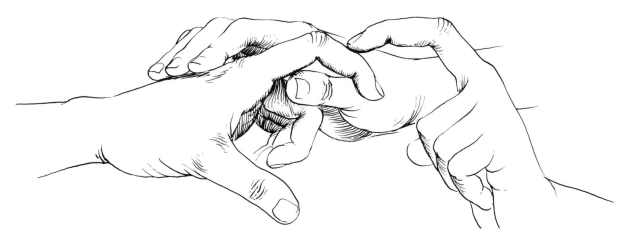

Fig. 113. The Bunnel-Littler Test: with the metacarpophalangeal joint held in a few **degrees** of extension, attempt to flex the proximal interphalangeal joint. If the joint **cannot** be flexed, either the intrinsics are tight or there is a joint capsule contracture.

C6. C6 supplies sensation to the thumb, the index, and half of the middle finger. The pinch unit, which is so necessary to effective function of the hand, receives sensory innervation from C6 via the median nerve.

C7. C7 supplies the middle finger, with contributions from C6 and C8.

C8. C8 supplies the ring and little fingers (Fig. 109).

SPECIAL TESTS

LONG FINGER FLEXOR TESTS. The two tests which follow establish the status of the flexor digitorum superficialis and the flexor digitorum profundus, and determine whether or not they are intact and functioning.

Flexor Digitorum Superficialis Test. To perform this test, hold the patient's fingers in extension, except for the finger being tested. This isolates the flexor digitorum superficialis tendon. Then instruct him to flex the finger in question at the proximal interphalangeal joint (Fig. 110). If he can flex his finger at the specified joint, the flexor digitorum superficialis tendon is intact. If he cannot, the superficialis tendon is either cut or absent. Since this tendon can act independently because of the position of the finger, it is the only functioning tendon at the proximal interphalangeal joint. This can be proved if you wiggle the distal interphalangeal joint of the finger being tested. The distal interphalangeal joint, motored by the flexor digitorum profundus has no power of flexion when the other fingers are held in extension, and the finger tip is loose and beyond the patient's control.

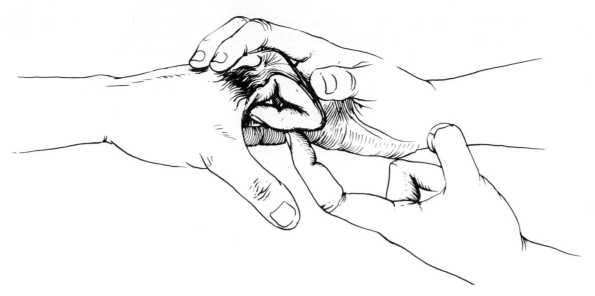

Fig. 114. Place the metacarpophalangeal joint in a few degrees of flexion to relax the intrinsic muscles. If the joint can now flex fully, the intrinsics are tight.

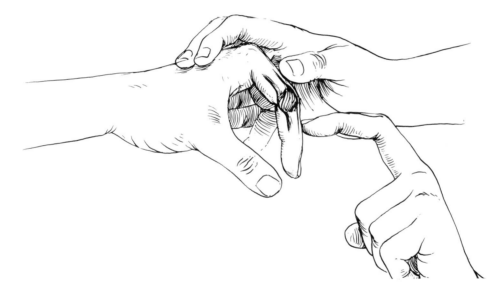

Fig. 115. If, with the intrinsic muscles relaxed, you still cannot flex the proximal interphalangeal joint, a joint capsule contracture is limiting flexion of the joint.

Flexor Digitorum Profundus Test. The flexor digitorum profundus tendons work only in unison. By limiting three of them, you also limit the fourth. This phenomenon is demonstrable if you ask the patient to try to flex his finger at any given distal interphalangeal joint. Because these tendons work only in unison, the patient is unable to accomplish such individual flexion.

To test the flexor digitorum profundus, isolate the distal interphalangeal joint (which is motored only by that tendon) by stabilizing the metacarpophalangeal and interphalangeal joints in extension. Then ask the patient to flex his finger at the distal interphalangeal joint (Fig. 111). If he is able to do so, the tendon is functional. If he cannot, the tendon may be cut or the muscle denervated.

BUNNEL-LITTLER TEST. This test evaluates the tightness of the intrinsic muscles of the hand (the lumbricals and interossei). The test may also be used to determine whether flexion limitation in the proximal interphalangeal joint is due to tightness of the intrinsics or to joint capsule contractures, a condition which prevents the finger from curling into the palm.

To test the tightness of the intrinsic muscles, hold the metacarpophalangeal joint in a few degrees of extension (Fig. 112), and try to move the proximal interphalangeal joint into flexion (Fig. 113). If, in this position, the proximal interphalangeal joint can be flexed, the intrinsics are not tight and are not limiting flexion. If, however, the proximal interphalangeal joint cannot be flexed, either the intrinsics are tight, or there are joint capsule contractures.

You can distinguish between intrinsic muscle tightness and joint capsule contractures by letting the involved finger flex a few degrees at the metacarpophalangeal joint (thereby relaxing the intrinsics) and moving the proximal interphalangeal joint into flexion. If the joint is now capable of full flexion, the intrinsics are probably tight (Fig. 114). If the joint still does not flex completely, the limitation is probably due to proximal interphalangeal joint capsule contractures (Fig. 115).

RETINACULAR TEST. This test verifies the tightness of the retinacular ligaments. The test may be used to determine whether flexion limitation in the distal interphalangeal joints is due to tightness of retinacular ligaments or to joint capsule contractures. To conduct the test, hold the proximal interphalangeal joint in a neutral position

and try to move the distal interphalangeal joint into flexion (Fig. 116). If the joint does not flex, limitation is due either to joint capsule contraction or to retinacular tightness. To distinguish between these two, flex the proximal interphalangeal joint slightly to relax the retinaculum. If the distal interphalangeal joint then flexes, the retinacular ligaments are tight. If however, the joint still does not flex, the distal interphalangeal joint capsule is probably contracted (Fig. 117).

ALLEN TEST. This test makes it possible to determine whether or not the radial and ulnar arteries are supplying the hand to their full capacities.

To perform the test, instruct the patient to open and close his fist quickly several times, and then to squeeze his fist tightly so that the venous blood is forced out of the palm. Place your thumb over the radial artery and your index and middle fingers over the ulnar artery, and press them against the underlying bones to occlude them (Fig. 118). With the vessels still occluded, instruct the patient to open his hand. The palm of the hand should be pale. Then release one of the arteries at

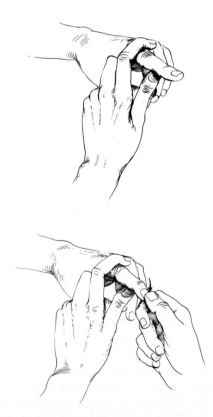

Fig. 116. Test for tightness of the retinacular ligaments.

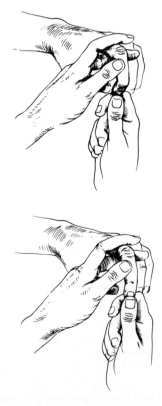

Fig. 117. Above. Flexion of the proximal interphalangeal joint relaxes the retinaculum. If the distal interphalangeal joint now flexes, the retinacular ligaments are tight. **Below.** Nonflexion at the distal interphalangeal joint indicates joint capsule contracture.

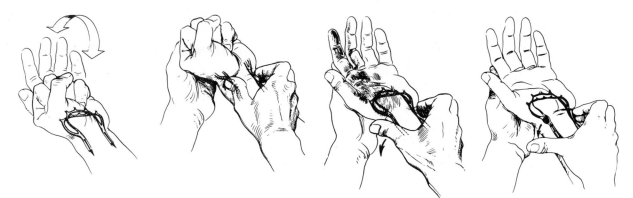

Fig. 118. The Allen test evaluates blood supply to the hand. **Left.** The patient first opens and closes his fist several times. **Right.** With the patient's fist closed, pressure is applied to the radial and ulnar arteries to occlude them.

Fig. 119. Left. When the patient opens his hand, pressure is released from one of the arteries, and the hand should flush immediately. **Right.** If the hand does not flush or reacts slowly, the artery is either completely or partially occluded.

the wrist, while maintaining the pressure upon the other one. Normally, the hand flushes immediately. It does not react, or if it flushes very slowly the released artery is partially or completely occluded (Fig. 119). The other artery should be tested similarly, and the opposite hand checked for comparison.

A modified version of the Allen test permits the evaluation of the patency of the digital arteries. Instruct the patient to open and close his fist quickly, several times, and then to hold it tightly closed to force the venous blood from the palmar aspect of the fingers. With the hand still in a fist, place your thumb and index finger on the sides of the base of the involved finger, pressing them to the bone to occlude the digital arteries. When the patient opens his hand, the test finger should be paler than the others. The finger normally flushes when pressure is released from one of the arteries (Fig. 120). If it does not, the patency of that digital vessel is in question (Fig. 121). The other digital artery should be tested in the same way and the corresponding finger on the opposite hand checked for comparison.

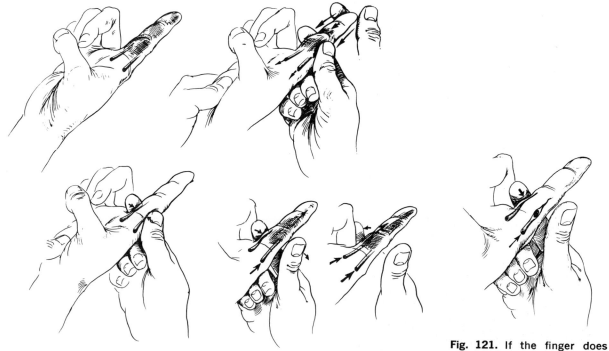

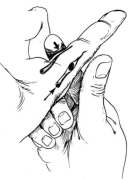

Fig. 120. A modified version of the Allen Test checks the patency of the digital arteries.

Fig. 121. If the finger does not flush upon removal of pressure from one of its arteries, the patency of the digital vessel is in question.

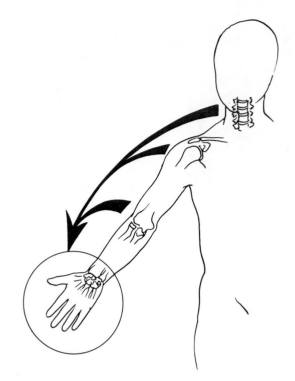

EXAMINATION OF RELATED AREAS

Symptoms can be referred to the hand from the elbow, the shoulder, and the cervical spine. The causes of referred pain to the wrist and hand include: Herniated cervical discs, osteoarthritis, brachial plexus outlet syndromes, and elbow and shoulder entrapment syndrome. In the interest of establishing the true etiology of the symptoms presented in the wrist and hand, the related clinical areas should be investigated thoroughly (Fig. 122).

Fig. 122. Related Areas. Symptoms can be referred to the wrist and hand from the elbow, the shoulder, and the cervical spine.

4
Physical Examination of the Cervical Spine
and Temporomandibular Joint

The cervical spine has three functions: (1) it furnishes support and stability for the head, (2) its articulating vertebral facets allow for the head's range of motion, and (3) it provides housing and transport for the spinal cord and the vertebral artery.

In this chapter, emphasis will be placed upon the neurologic examination, since cervical spine pathology, while of concern in itself, may be reflected to the upper extremity to show up as muscle weakness, altered reflexes or sensation, or pain. Since these symptoms may be the result of interference with the peripheral nerves at the C5–T1 (brachial plexus) level of the cervical spine, an expanded neurologic examination provides a more comprehensive interpretation of the integrity of the brachial plexus, and of pathologic signs and symptoms in the upper extremity as well.

INSPECTION

Inspection begins as the patient enters the examining room. As he enters, note the attitude and posture of his head. Normally, the head is held erect, perpendicular to the floor; it moves in smooth coordination with the body motion. Because of the possibility of reflected pathology, a complete examination of the neck requires that the patient undress to the waist, exposing the neck area as well as the entire upper extremity. As the patient disrobes, his head should move naturally with his body movements. If he holds his head stiffly to one side to protect or splint an area of pain, there may be a pathologic reason for such a posture.

The neck region should then be inspected for normal characteristics as well as for abnormalities, such as blisters, scars, and discoloration.

Surgical scars on the anterior portion of the neck most often indicate previous thyroid surgery, while irregular, pitted scars in the anterior triangle are likely evidence of previous tuberculous adenitis.

BONY PALPATION

The neck should be palpated while the patient is supine, since muscles overlying the deeper prominences of the neck are relaxed in that position and the bony structures become more sharply defined.

Anterior Aspect

To palpate the anterior bony structures of the neck, stand at the patient's side and support the back of his neck with one hand, leaving the other free for palpation. Firm support at the base of the neck allows the patient to feel more secure and to relax more thoroughly.

Hyoid Bone. The hyoid bone, a horseshoe-shaped structure, is situated above the thyroid cartilage. On a horizontal plane, it is opposite the C3 vertebral body. To palpate the hyoid, cup your hand around the anterior portion of the patient's neck, just above the thyroid cartilage. Probe with a pincerlike action of your finger and thumb to palpate its two stems. These long, thin processes originate in the midline of the neck, then proceed laterally and posteriorly (Fig. 1). Ask the patient to swallow; when he does so, the movement of the hyoid bone becomes palpable.

Thyroid Cartilage. Move inferiorly in the midline until your fingers come in contact with the thyroid cartilage and its small, identifiable superior notch. From there, palpate the bulging upper portion of the cartilage (Fig. 2). The top portion of the cartilage, commonly known as the "Adam's Apple," marks the level of the C4 vertebral body, while the lower portion designates the C5 level. Although the thyroid cartilage is not as broad as the hyoid bone, it is longer in a cephalad–caudad direction.

First Cricoid Ring. The first cricoid ring is situated immediately inferior to the sharp lower border of the thyroid cartilage, opposite C6. It is the only complete ring of the cricoid series (which is an integral part of the trachea) and is immediately above the site for an emergency tracheostomy. The ring should be palpated gently, for too much pressure may cause the patient to gag. Ask the patient to swallow; when he does so, the movement of the first cricoid ring becomes palpable, although it is not as pronounced as that of the thyroid cartilage (Fig. 3).

Carotid Tubercle. As you move laterally about one inch from the first cricoid ring, you will come across the carotid tubercle, the anterior tubercle of the C6 transverse process. The carotid tubercle is small and lies away from the midline, deep under the overlying muscles, but it is definitely palpable. It can be felt if you press posteriorly from the lateral position of your fingers (Fig.

4). The carotid tubercles of C6 should be palpated separately, since simultaneous palpation can restrict the flow of both carotid arteries, which run adjacent to the tubercles, and cause a carotid reflex. The carotid tubercle is frequently used as an anatomic landmark for an anterior surgical approach to C5–C6 and as a site for injection of the stellate cervical ganglion.

While exploring the anterior portion of the neck, locate the small, hard bump of the C1 transverse process, which lies between the angle of the jaw and the skull's styloid process, just behind the ear. As the broadest transverse process in the cervical spine, it is readily palpable, and, although it has little clinical significance, it serves as an easily identifiable point of orientation.

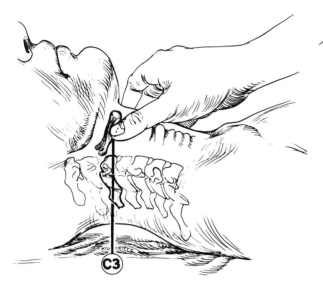

Fig. 1. The hyoid bone.

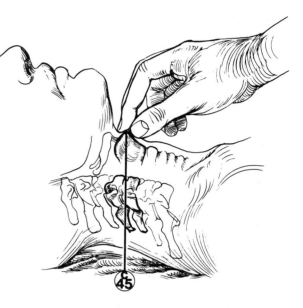

Fig. 2. The thyroid cartilage.

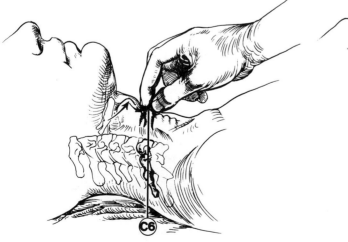

Fig. 3. The first cricoid ring.

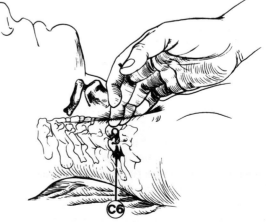

Fig. 4. The carotid tubercle.

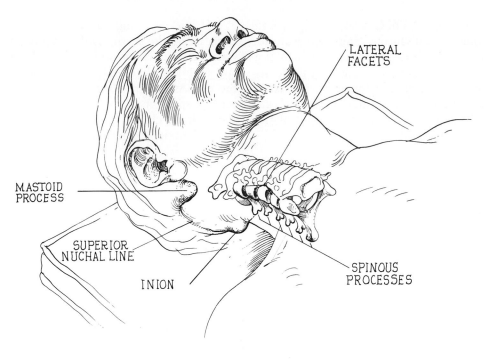

Fig. 5. The anatomy of the neck (posterior aspect).

Posterior Aspect

The posterior landmarks of the neck (Fig. 5) are more accessible to palpation if you stand behind the patient's head and cup your hands under his neck so that your fingertips meet at the midline. Since tensed muscles measurably inhibit the palpation of the deeper posterior bony prominences, hold the patient's head so that he need not use his neck muscles for support and encourage him to relax.

Occiput. Palpation of the posterior aspect begins at the occiput, the posterior portion of the skull.

Inion. The inion, a dome-shaped bump (bump of knowledge), lies in the occipital region on the midline and marks the center of the superior nuchal line (Fig. 6).

Superior Nuchal Line. Move laterally from the inion to palpate the superior nuchal line, which is a small, transverse ridge extending out on both sides of the inion.

Mastoid Processes. As you palpate laterally from the lateral edge of the superior nuchal line, you will feel the rounded mastoid processes of the skull (Fig. 7).

Spinous Processes of the Cervical Vertebrae. The spinous processes lie along the posterior midline of the cervical spine. To palpate them, cup one hand around the side of the neck and probe the midline with your fingertips. Since no muscle crosses the midline, it is indented. The lateral soft

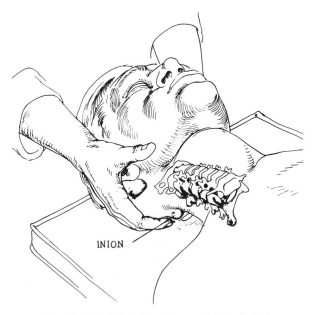

Fig. 6. The inion (the bump of knowledge).

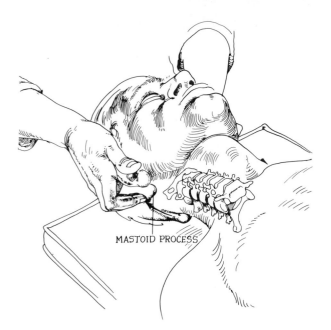

Fig. 7. The mastoid process.

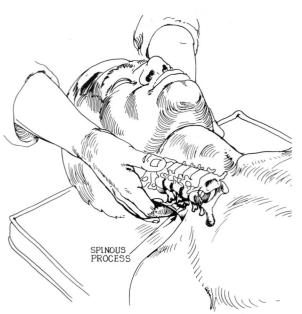

Fig. 8. Palpation of the cervical spinous processes.

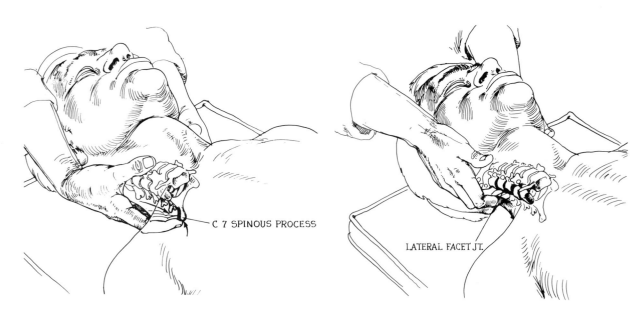

Fig. 9. The C7 spinous process is larger than those above it.

Fig. 10. Palpation of the facet joints.

tissue bulges outlining the indentation are composed of the deep paraspinal muscles and the superficial trapezius. Begin at the base of the skull; the C2 spinous process is the first one that is palpable (the C1 spinous process is a small tubercle and lies deep). As you palpate the spinous processes from C2 to T1, note the normal lordosis of the cervical spine (Fig. 8). On some patients, you may find bifid C3–C5 spinous processes (divided, and consisting of two small excrescences of bone). The C7 and T1 spinous processes are larger than those above them (Fig. 9). The processes are normally in line with each other; a shift in their normal alignment may be due to a unilateral facet dislocation or to a fracture of the spinous process following trauma (Fig. 11).

Facet Joints. From the spinous processes of C2, move each hand laterally about one inch and begin to palpate the joints of the vertebral facets that lie between the cervical vertebrae. These joints often cause symptoms of pain in the neck region. The joints feel like very small domes and lie deep beneath the trapezius muscle. They are not always clearly palpable, and the patient must be completely relaxed for you to feel them. Take note of any tenderness elicited, and palpate the joints bilaterally at each articulation until you reach the articulation between C7 and T1 (Fig. 10). The facet joints between C5 and C6 are most often involved in pathology (osteoarthritis) and are therefore most often tender (and possibly slightly enlarged). If the vertebral level of any one joint is uncertain, its level can be determined by lining up the vertebra in question with the anterior structures of the neck; the hyoid bone at C3, the thyroid cartilage at C4 and C5, and the first cricoid ring at C6 (Fig. 12).

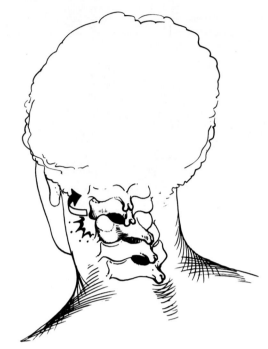

Fig. 11. Unilateral facet dislocation.

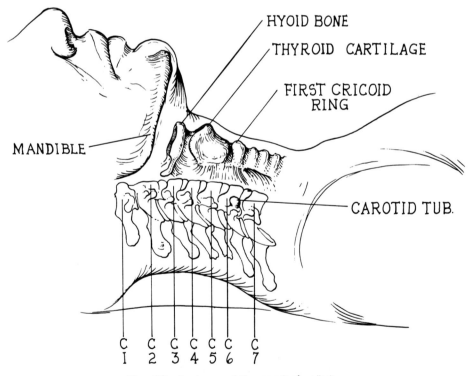

HYOID BONE

THYROID CARTILAGE

FIRST CRICOID RING

MANDIBLE

CAROTID TUB.

C C C C C C C
1 2 3 4 5 6 7

Fig. 12. Anatomy of the cervical spine.

SOFT TISSUE PALPATION

Palpation of the soft tissues of the neck is divided into two clinical zones: (1) the anterior aspect (anterior triangle) and (2) the posterior aspect. The important bony landmarks located in previous exploration may serve as useful guides in this portion of your examination.

Zone I—Anterior Aspect

The anterior zone is defined laterally by the two sternocleidomastoid muscles, superiorly by the mandible, and inferiorly by the suprasternal notch (forming a rough triangle). It is easier to palpate the anterior triangle of the neck when the patient is supine, because his muscles are more relaxed.

Sternocleidomastoid Muscle. This muscle, which extends from the sternoclavicular joint to the mastoid process, is frequently stretched in hyperextension injuries of the neck during automobile accidents (Fig. 13). To expedite palpation of the sternocleidomastoid, ask the patient to turn his head to that side opposite the muscle to be examined. When he does so, the muscle will stand out sharply near its tendinous origin. The sternocleidomastoid is long and tubular, and is palpable from origin to insertion (Fig. 14). The opposite sternocleidomastoid should also be examined for any discrepancies in size, shape, or tone. Palpable, localized swellings within the muscle may be due to hematoma and may cause the head to turn abnormally to one side (torticollis). Tenderness elicited during palpation may be associated with hyperextension injuries of the neck.

Lymph Node Chain. The lymph node chain is situated along the medial border of the sternocleidomastoid muscle. When they are normal, the lymph nodes are usually not palpable; if, however, they become enlarged, they may be palpable as small lumps which are often tender to the touch (Fig. 15). Enlarged lymph nodes in the region of the sternocleidomastoid muscle usually indicate an infection in the upper respiratory tract. They, too, may cause torticollis.

Thyroid Gland. The thyroid cartillage lies in a central position along the anterior midline of the neck, anterior to the C4–C5 vertebrae. The thyroid gland overlies the cartilage in an "H" pattern, with two extensive bodies located laterally and a thinner isthmus between. The normal thyroid gland feels smooth and indistinct, whereas the abnormal gland may contain unusual local enlargements due to cysts or nodules and is often tender to palpation. With practice, the gland can be palpated in conjunction with the thyroid cartilage (Fig. 17).

Carotid Pulse. The carotid artery is situated next to the carotid tubercle (C6). The carotid pulse is palpable if you press at this point with the tips of your index and middle fingers (Fig. 16). Palpate only one side at a time, for simultaneous palpation of the carotid pulses can provoke a carotid reflex. The pulses on each side of the neck should be approximately equal; both should be checked to determine their relative strengths.

Parotid Gland. The parotid gland partially covers the sharp angle of the mandible. The gland itself is not distinctly palpable, but if it is normal, the angle of the mandible feels sharp and bony to the touch (Fig. 18). If the gland is swollen (as in cases of mumps) the angle of the mandible is covered by a boggy, soft gland and no longer feels sharp.

Supraclavicular Fossa. The supraclavicular fossa lies superior to the clavicle and lateral to the suprasternal notch. It should be palpated for any unusual swellings or lumps. The platysma muscle crosses the fossa but does not fill out its contours. Therefore, the fossa normally describes a smooth indentation, with the subcutaneous clavicle further accentuating its depth. Swelling within the fossa may be caused by edema secondary to trauma, such as a clavicular fracture, and small lumps may be due to an enlargement of the lymph glands in the fossa. While it is not palpable, the cupola (dome) of the lung extends into the fossa and is sometimes injured by puncture wounds, a fracture of the clavicle, or the biopsy of an enlarged lymph node. If a cervical rib is present, it may be palpable in the fossa.

Note that a cervical rib can cause vascular or neurologic symptoms in the upper extremity.

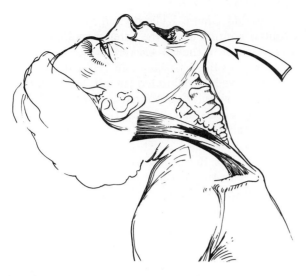

Fig. 13. Hyperextension injury of the sternocleidomastoid muscles.

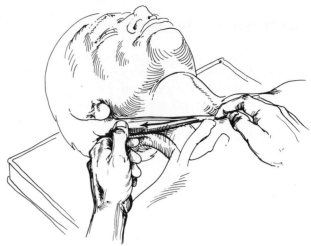

Fig. 14. The sternocleidomastoid is palpable from origin to insertion.

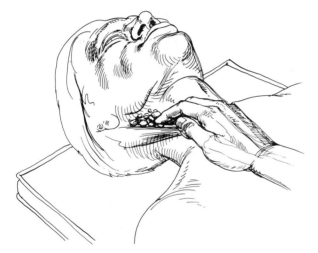

Fig. 15. The lymph node chain along the medial border of the sternocleidomastoid muscle.

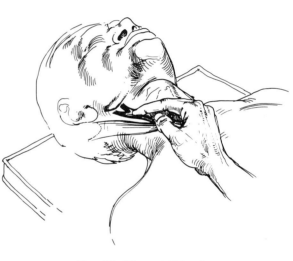

Fig. 16. The carotid pulse.

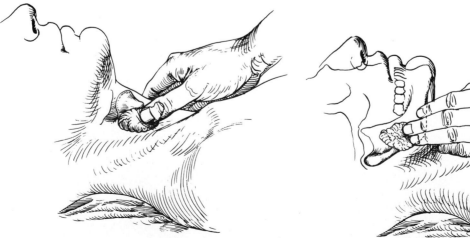

Fig. 17. The normal thyroid gland is smooth and indistinct.

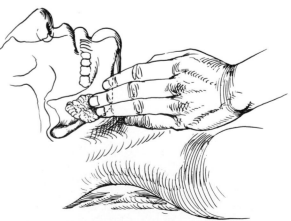

Fig. 18. Palpation of the parotid gland.

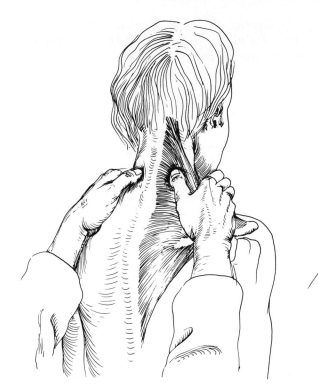

Fig. 19. Palpation of the trapezius muscles—from origin to insertion.

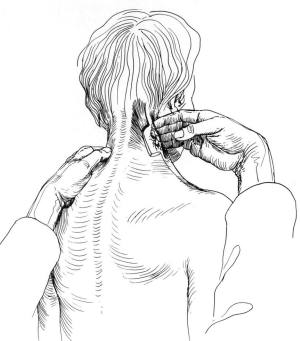

Fig. 20. Lymph nodes on the anterolateral aspect of the trapezius muscle.

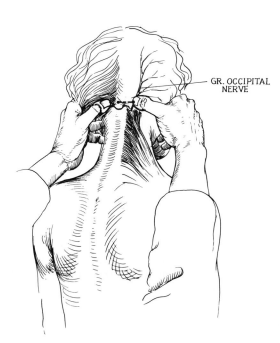

Fig. 21. Palpation of the greater occipital nerves.

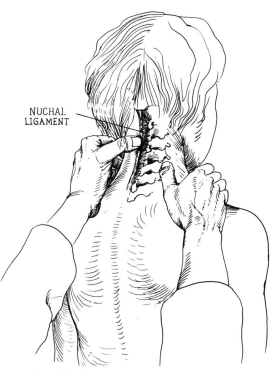

Fig. 22. The superior nuchal ligament.

Zone II—Posterior Aspect

In preparation for palpation of the posterior aspect of the neck, stand behind the seated patient. When the patient is seated, the posterior soft tissues of the neck become more accessible. If sitting is painful for the patient, however, he may remain supine.

Trapezius Muscle. The broad origin of this muscle extends from the inion to T12. It then inserts laterally in a continuous arc into the clavicle, the acromion, and the spine of the scapula. Palpate the trapezius from origin to insertion, beginning with its prominent superior portions at the side of the neck and moving towards the acromion. The superior portion of the trapezius is frequently stretched in flexion injuries of the cervical spine, such as may occur in automobile accidents. When your fingertips reach the dorsal surface of the acromion, follow its course until you reach the spine of the scapula. Although the trapezius' insertion is not distinctly palpable, you may encounter unusual tenderness in the area, a symptom usually due to defects or to hematoma secondary to a flexion/extension injury of the neck. Then move your fingertips up the longitudinal bulges of the trapezius muscle, on both sides of the spinous processes, to the origin at the superior nuchal line. The trapezius muscle is best palpated bilaterally to provide instant comparison. Any discrepancy in the size or shape of either side and any tenderness, unilateral or bilateral, should be noted. Tenderness most often presents in the superior lateral portion (Fig. 19).

The trapezius and the sternocleidomastoid muscles share a continuous attachment along the base of the skull to the mastoid process where they split, with each muscle then having a different and noncontinuous attachment along the clavicle. Embryologically, the trapezius and sternocleidomastoid muscles form as one muscle, but split into two during later development. Because of their common origin, these muscles share the same nerve supply, the spinal accessory nerve or cranial nerve number IX.

Lymph Nodes. The lymph nodes on the anterolateral aspect of the trapezius muscle are not normally palpable, but pathologic conditions such as infection may cause them to become tender and enlarged. As your experience increases, palpation of the lymph node chains can be incorporated into palpation of the trapezius muscle (Fig. 20).

Greater Occipital Nerves. Move from the trapezius muscle to the base of the skull and probe both sides of the inion for the greater occipital nerves. If they are inflamed (usually as a result of trauma sustained in whiplash injury), the nerves are distinctly palpable. Inflammation of the greater occipital nerves commonly results in headache (Fig. 21).

Superior Nuchal Ligament. This ligament rises from the inion at the base of the skull, and extends to the C7 spinous process. It overlays and attaches itself by fibers to each spinous process of the cervical vertebrae and lies directly under your fingertips during palpation of the spinous processes. Although it is not a distinctly palpable structure, the area in which it lies should be palpated to elicit tenderness. Tenderness might indicate either a stretched ligament as a result of a neck flexion injury, or perhaps a defect within the ligament itself (Fig. 22).

RANGE OF MOTION

The normal range of neck motion provides the patient not only with a wide scope of vision but with an acute sense of balance as well. Range of motion in the neck region involves the following basic movements: (1) flexion, (2) extension, (3) lateral rotation to the left and right, and (4) lateral bending to the left and right. These specific motions are also used in combination, giving the head and neck a capacity for widely diversified motion. Although the entire cervical spine is involved in head and neck motion, the greatest amount of motion is concentrated: Approximately 50 percent of flexion and extension occurs between the occiput and C1, with the remaining 50 percent distributed relatively evenly among the other cervical vertebrae (with a slight increase between C5 and C6) (according to William Fielding). Approximately 50 percent of rotation takes place between C1 (atlas) and C2 (axis). These two cervical vertebrae have a specialized shape to allow for this greater range of rotary motion (Fig. 23). The remaining 50 percent of rotation is then relatively evenly distributed among the other five cervical vertebrae. Although lateral bending is a function of all the cervical vertebrae, it does not occur as a pure motion, but rather functions in conjunction with elements of rotation. A significant restriction in a specific motion may be caused by blockage in the articulation that provides the greatest amount of motion as, for example, in Klippel-Feil Deformity, where the bodies of two or more vertebrae are fused.

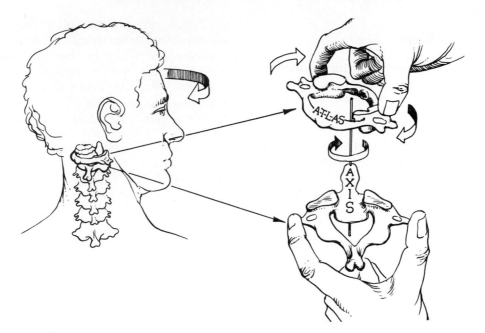

Fig. 23. The specialization of the C1 (Atlas) and the C2 (Axis) vertebrae allow for rotary motion.

Active Range of Motion Tests

FLEXION AND EXTENSION. To test active flexion and extension of the neck, instruct the patient to nod his head forward in a "yes" movement. He should be able to touch his chin to his chest (normal range of flexion) and to look directly at the ceiling above him (normal range of extension) (Fig. 24). As he moves his head, watch to see if the arc of motion is smooth, rather than halting. An auto accident, which may cause soft tissue trauma around the cervical spine, may result in a limitation in the range of motion and a disruption in the normal, smooth arc.

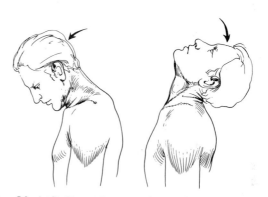

Fig. 24. Left. Normal range of neck flexion. **Right.** Normal range of neck extension.

ROTATION. Ask the patient to shake his head from side to side. He should be able to move his head far enough to both sides so that his chin is almost in line with his shoulder (Fig. 25). Again, observe the motion to determine whether or not the head is rotating fully and with ease in a smooth arc. Torticollis is one frequent limiter of neck motion.

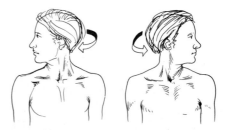

Fig. 25. Normal range of neck rotation.

LATERAL BENDING. To test active lateral bending (with its elements of rotation), have the patient try to touch his ear to his shoulder, making certain that he does not compensate for limited motion by lifting his shoulder to his ear. Normally, he should be able to tilt his head approximately 45° toward each shoulder (Fig. 26). Enlarged cervical lymph nodes may limit motion, especially in lateral bending.

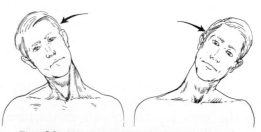

Fig. 26. Normal range of lateral bending.

Passive Range of Motion Tests

Since muscles can act to restrict motion, the patient must feel secure throughout the passive range of motion tests so that his muscles remain relaxed.

FLEXION AND EXTENSION. To conduct the passive tests for neck flexion and extension, place your hands on either side of the patient's cranium and bend his head forward. A normal range of flexion will allow you to push the chin forward to the chest. Then, lift the patient's head and tilt it backward. If his range of extension is normal, he will be able to see the ceiling directly above him. Note that the head cannot normally extend to touch the spinous processes of the cervical vertebrae.

ROTATION. To test rotation, return the head to a neutral position and move it from side to side in a "no" motion. Normally the head should turn far enough so that the chin is nearly in line with the shoulder, almost touching it. The degree of rotation achieved on each side should be compared.

LATERAL BENDING. Start from a neutral position and bend the head laterally toward the shoulder. A normal range of lateral bending permits the head to be tilted approximately 45° toward the shoulder. Results of the lateral bending tests should be compared, and any sign of restricted motion should be noted.

A note of caution! If you suspect that the patient has an unstable spine (for example, from trauma), do not put the spine through a passive range of motion. You may cause neurologic damage.

NEUROLOGIC EXAMINATION

The neurologic examination of the cervical spine has been divided into two phases: (1) muscle testing of the intrinsic muscles of the cervical spine, and (2) neurologic examination of the entire upper extremity by neurologic levels.

The first phase of the neurologic examination concerns testing the intrinsic muscles in the neck and cervical spine in functional groups. In this respect, muscle testing will indicate the presence of any motor weakness which might affect the motion of the neck, and, in addition, will demonstrate the integrity of the nerve supply.

The second phase of the examination will follow a different format. In previous chapters, functional groups of muscles, reflexes, and areas of sensation have been tested as they related only to a specific joint. However, since the upper extremity is innervated by nerves originating in the cervical spine, we will, in the second phase, trace the neurologic problems found anywhere in the upper extremity to their possible primary source in the cervical spine.

Phase I—Muscle Testing of the Intrinsic Muscles

Muscle tests are conducted with the patient seated, unless he is unable to hold his head erect, in which case he may lie down. If the patient is lying down during testing, gravity is eliminated as a variable.

FLEXION

Primary Flexors:
    1) Sternocleidomastoids (in conjunction) spinal accessory, or cranial XI nerve

Secondary Flexors:
    1) Scalenus muscles
    2) Prevertebral muscles

To test neck flexion, stabilize the patient's upper thorax (sternum) with one hand to prevent the substitution of flexion of the thorax for neck flexion. Place the palm of your resisting hand against the patient's forehead and cup his forehead in your palm to establish a firm and broad base of support (Fig. 27). Then ask the patient to flex his neck slowly. As he does so, steadily increase the pressure of resistance against his head until you determine the maximum resistance he can overcome. Record your findings in accordance with the muscle grading chart located in the Shoulder Chapter, page 26.

EXTENSION

Primary Extensors:
    1) Paravertebral extensor mass (splenius, semispinalis, capitis)
    2) Trapezius Spinal accessory or cranial XI nerve

Secondary Extensors:
    1) Various small intrinsic neck muscles

Prior to testing neck extension, place your stabilizing hand over the midline of the patient's upper posterior thorax and scapulae. This stabilization prevents him from substituting trunk extension for pure neck extension, or from leaning back to produce the illusion of neck extension. Cup the palm of your resisting hand over the occipital region of the skull to provide a firm base of support (Fig. 28).

Ask the patient to extend his neck. As he does so, slowly and steadily increase pressure of resistance until you determine the maximum resistance he can overcome. To evaluate the tone of the trapezius muscle as it contracts, palpate it with your stabilizing hand (Fig. 19).

LATERAL ROTATION

Primary Rotator:
1) Sternocleidomastoid
      spinal accessory, or cranial XI nerve
Secondary Rotators:
1) Small intrinsic neck muscles

One sternocleidomastoid, functioning alone, provides the primary pull for rotation to the side being tested. To test the muscle for right lateral rotation of the neck, stand in front of the patient and place your stabilizing hand on his left shoulder, preventing the substitution of thoracolumbar spine rotation for rotation within the cervical spine. Place the open palm of your resisting hand along the right side of the mandible (Fig. 29).

Instruct the patient to rotate his head in a "no" motion toward the open palm of your resisting hand, and increase the pressure until you can gauge the maximum resistance he can overcome. To evaluate the right sternocleidomastoid, change your hand positions to the opposite shoulder and mandible. Then compare your findings.

LATERAL BENDING

Primary Lateral Benders:
1) Scalenus anticus, medius, and posticus
      anterior primary divisions of lower cervical nerves
Secondary Lateral Benders:
1) Small intrinsic muscles of the neck

Test the muscles which power right lateral bending by placing your stabilizing hand on the right shoulder to prevent substitution of shoulder elevation. Then place the open palm of your resisting hand on the right side of the patient's head. To provide a firm base for resistance, your palm should lie on the temple, with fingers extending posteriorly.

Instruct the patient to bend his head laterally toward your palm, or to try to bring his ear to his shoulder. As he bends his head, gradually increase resistance until you determine the maximum resistance he can overcome (Fig. 30).

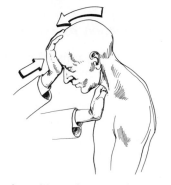

Fig. 27. Hand positions for neck flexion muscle test.

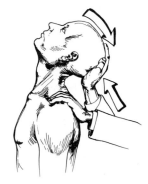

Fig. 28. Hand positions for neck extension muscle test.

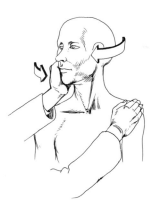

Fig. 29. Hand positions for testing the sternocleidomastoid muscles for lateral rotation.

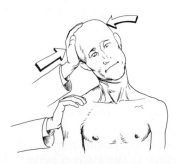

Fig. 30. Muscle test for lateral bending of the neck.

Phase II—Examination by Neurologic Levels

This phase of the examination is based upon the fact that pathology in the cervical spine, such as a herniated disc, is frequently reflected to the upper extremity via the brachial plexus (C5–T1), the innervation for the entire extremity.

The following diagnostic tests will help determine whether there is a relationship between upper extremity neurologic problems and a primary source in the neck. Motor power, reflexes, and areas of sensation will be tested by cord neurologic levels.

NEUROLOGIC ANATOMY.

While there are eight nerves that exit the cervical spine, there are only seven cervical vertebrae. The first through the seventh cervical nerves exit above the cervical vertebra with the corresponding number, while the eighth cervical nerve exits below the seventh cervical vertebra and above the first thoracic vertebra. The first thoracic nerve then exits below the first thoracic vertebra (Fig. 31).

The brachial plexus is composed of nerves emanating from the first thoracic and the lower four cervical levels (C5 to T1). Shortly after they exit the vertebral bodies and pass between the scalenus anticus and medius muscles, the nerve roots of C5 and C6 join to form the *upper trunk*. The nerve roots of C8 and T1 join to form the *lower trunk*. C7 does not join with any other nerve root; it alone makes up the *middle trunk*. As the trunks pass beneath the clavicle, they then divide to form cords. The upper trunk (C5 and C6) and the lower trunk (C8 and T1) contribute to the middle trunk (C7), to form the *posterior cord*. The middle trunk, in turn, sends a contribution to form, with C5 and C6, the *lateral cord*. The remainder of C8 and T1 forms the *medial cord*. These cords are called "posterior," "lateral," and "medial" in terms of their relation to the second part of the axillary artery.

The *branches* (or the named peripheral nerves) emanate from the cords. The lateral cord sends one branch to become the *musculocutaneous nerve*. The other branch of the lateral cord joins with a branch from the medial cord to form a *median nerve*. The second branch of the medial cord becomes the *ulnar nerve* and the posterior cord divides into two branches: the *axillary nerve* and the *radial nerve*. The branches from the cords may be summarized as follows:

From the lateral cord:
1) musculocutaneous nerve
2) branch to the median nerve

From the medial cord:
1) ulnar nerve
2) branch to the median nerve
From the posterior cord:
1) axillary nerve
2) radial nerve

The nerves included in the outline provide most of the innervation to the upper extremity. When relevant, the other peripheral nerves which emanate from the brachial plexus shall be discussed.

SENSORY DISTRIBUTION.

From C5 to T1, each neurologic level supplies sensation to a portion of the extremity in a succession of dermatomes around the extremity. The following outline lists the primary nerves involved in the sensory distribution of the brachial plexus:

C5—lateral arm
        axillary nerve
C6—lateral forearm, thumb, index, and half of middle finger
        sensory branches of the musculocutaneous nerve
C7—middle finger
C8—ring and little fingers, medial forearm
        medial antebrachial-cutaneous nerve (from posterior cord)
T1—medial arm
        medial brachial cutaneous nerve (from posterior cord) (Fig. 32)

With the above outline in mind, proceed to examine the upper extremity by neurologic levels.

NEUROLOGIC LEVEL C5 (Fig. 33)

Muscle Testing

The deltoid and the biceps are two muscles with C5 innervation that are easily tested. While the deltoid is innervated almost entirely by C5, the biceps has a dual innervation, from both C5 and C6. Therefore, evaluation of the C5 neurologic level through biceps testing alone becomes less accurate.

Deltoid: C5 Axillary Nerve

The deltoid is a three-part muscle: (1) the anterior deltoid flexes, (2) the middle deltoid abducts, and (3) the posterior deltoid extends the shoulder. To test deltoid strength, resist the motions of shoulder flexion, abduction, and extension, as described on pages 25 through 27 (Figs. 57 to 59, Shoulder Chapter).

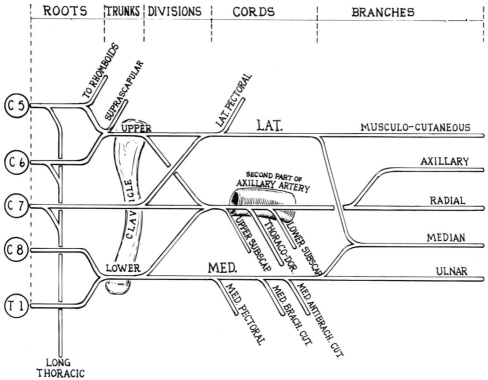

Fig. 31. The brachial plexus.

SENSATION

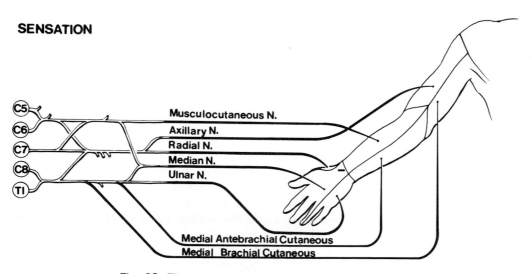

Fig. 32. The sensory distribution of the brachial plexus.

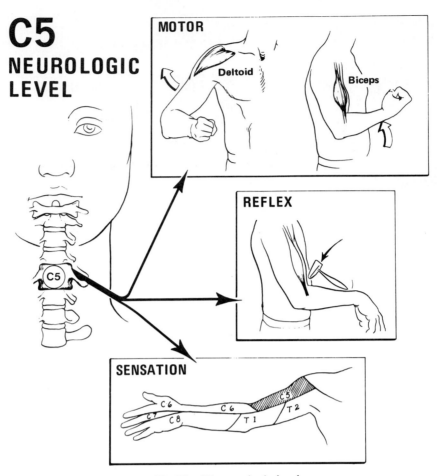

Fig. 33. The C5 neurologic level.

Biceps: C5–C6 Musculocutaneous Nerve

The biceps acts as a flexor for the shoulder and elbow and as a supinator for the forearm. Test the biceps strength relative to elbow flexion to determine its neurologic integrity. Since the brachialis muscle (the other main flexor of the elbow) is also innervated by the musculocutaneous nerve, a flexion test of the elbow should provide an adequate indication of C5 integrity.

To test elbow flexion, instruct your patient to flex his elbow slowly with his forearm supinated as you resist his motion. For further details, see page 52 (Fig. 38, Elbow Chapter).

Reflex Testing

Biceps Reflex

The biceps reflex primarily indicates the neurologic integrity of C5. However, the reflex also has a C6 component.

Since the muscle has two major levels of innervation, even a slightly diminished reflex (in comparison to the opposite side) indicates pathology.

Methodology for testing the biceps reflex is given on page 55.

Sensation Testing

Lateral Arm: Axillary Nerve

The C5 neurologic level supplies sensation to the lateral arm. The purest patch of axillary nerve sensation is located on the lateral arm, in the skin covering the lateral portion of the deltoid muscle. This localized area is useful in diagnosis of injuries to the axillary nerve or of general C5 nerve root injury (Fig. 33).

NEUROLOGIC LEVEL C6 (Fig. 34)

Muscle Testing

Neither of the C6 muscle tests is pure; the wrist extensor group is innervated partially by C6 and partially by C7, while the biceps has both C5 and C6 innervation.

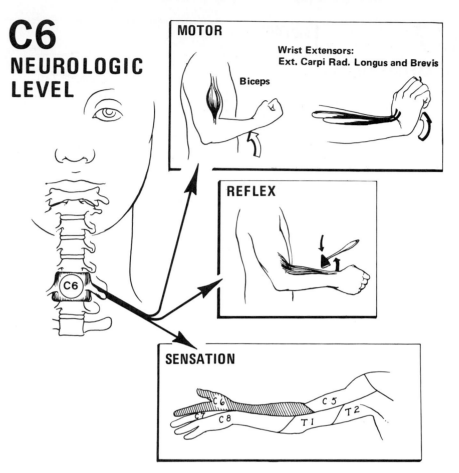

Fig. 34. The C6 neurologic level.

Wrist Extensor Group: C6, Radial Nerve

The wrist extensor group is composed of three muscles: (1) the extensor carpi radialis longus (C6), (2) the extensor carpi radialis brevis (C6), and (3) the extensor carpi ulnaris (C7). To accurately evaluate the strength of the wrist extensors, test bilaterally, noting the relative strength of the affected side in accordance with the muscle grading chart (Shoulder Chapter, page 26). For details, see pages 93 and 94.

Biceps: C6, Musculocutaneous Nerve

The biceps muscle test is given on page 52.

Reflex Testing

Brachioradialis Reflex

The brachioradialis reflex is tested proximal to the wrist, where the muscle becomes tendinous just before it inserts into the radius. For details, see page 55.

Biceps Reflex

Since the biceps is innervated by both C5 and C6, the strength of the reflex need only be slightly weaker than that of the opposite side to indicate neurologic problems. For details of testing, see page 55.

Sensation Testing

Lateral Forearm: Musculocutaneous Nerve

C6 supplies sensation to the lateral forearm, the thumb, the index, and one-half of the middle finger. To easily remember the C6 sensory distribution, form the number six with your thumb, index, and middle finger by pinching your thumb and index finger together and extending your middle finger.

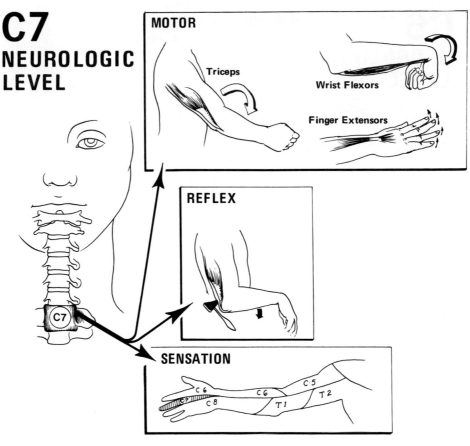

Fig. 35. The C7 neurologic level.

NEUROLOGIC LEVEL C7 (Fig. 35)

Muscle Testing

Triceps: C7, Radial Nerve

The triceps extends the elbow. To test it, instruct the patient to begin extension from a position of flexion as you resist his motion. For details, see page 52 (Fig. 39, Elbow Chapter).

Wrist Flexor Group: C7, Median and Ulnar Nerves

The wrist flexor group is composed of two muscles: (1) the flexor carpi radialis (median nerve), and (2) the flexor carpi ulnaris (ulnar nerve). The flexor carpi radialis (C7) is the more important of these two muscles, since it actually powers most of wrist flexion. The flexor carpi ulnaris, which is primarily innervated by C8, is less powerful.

To test wrist flexion, ask the patient to make a fist and to flex his wrist as you resist against the palmar aspect of his closed fist. Details of this test are given on page 94 (Fig. 99, Wrist and Hand Chapter).

Finger Extensors: C7, Radial Nerve

Finger extension is performed by three muscles: (1) the extensor digitorum communis, (2) the extensor digiti indicis, and (3) the extensor digiti minimi. To test finger extension, press on the dorsum of the patient's extended fingers. See page 94 for details (Fig. 100, Wrist and Hand Chapter).

All of the above muscle groups, although predominantly C7, have some C8 innervation.

Reflex Testing

Triceps Reflex

To test the triceps reflex, tap its tendon where it crosses the olecranon fossa at the elbow. See page 55 for details (Elbow Chapter).

Sensation Testing

Middle Finger

Sensation is supplied to the middle finger by C7. Occasionally, middle finger sensation is also supplied by C6 and C8.

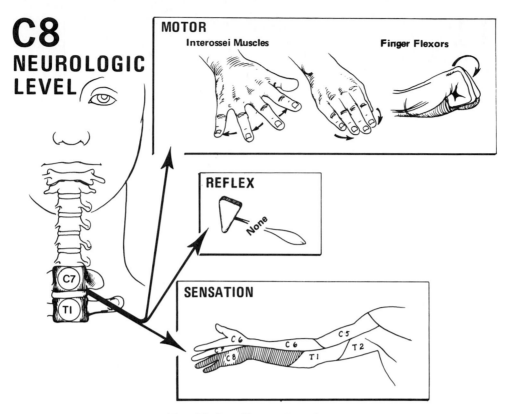

Fig. 36. The C8 neurologic level.

NEUROLOGIC LEVEL C8 (Fig. 36)

Since C8 has no reflex, muscle strength and sensation tests are utilized to determine its integrity.

Muscle Testing

Finger Flexors

The two muscles which flex the fingers are: (1) the flexor digitorum superficialis (which flexes the proximal interphalangeal joint), and (2) the flexor digitorum profundis (which flexes the distal interphalangeal joint). The flexor digitorum superficialis receives innervation from the median nerve, while the flexor digitorum profundis receives half its innervation from the ulnar nerve (on the ulnar side) and half from the median nerve (on the radial side).

To test finger flexion, curl or lock your fingers into the patient's flexed fingers and try to pull them out of flexion. Test the opposite side in the same manner and grade and record your findings (Fig. 101, Wrist and Hand Chapter).

Sensation Testing

C8 supplies sensation to the ring and little fingers of the hand and to the distal half of the forearm's ulnar side. The ulnar side of the little finger is the purest area for ulnar nerve sensation (predominantly C8) (Fig. 108, Wrist and Hand Chapter).

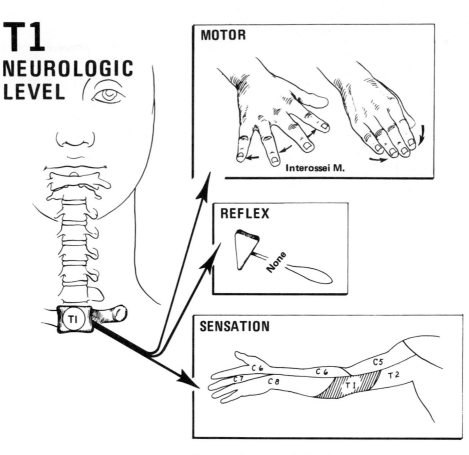

T1
NEUROLOGIC
LEVEL

MOTOR

Interossei M.

REFLEX

None

SENSATION

Fig. 37. The T1 neurologic level.

NEUROLOGIC LEVEL T1

Since T1, like C8, has no identifiable reflex, it is evaluated for its motor and sensory components (Fig. 37).

Muscle Testing

Finger Abductors

The finger abductors, innervated by the ulnar nerve, are: (1) the dorsal interossei, and (2) the abductor digiti quinti. Evaluate finger abduction by squeezing the abducted fingers together, as described on page 95 (Fig. 103, Wrist and Hand Chapter).

Sensation Testing

Medial Arm: Medial Brachial Cutaneous Nerve

Sensation is supplied to the medial side of the upper half of the forearm and the arm by T1.

The following chart summarizes the procedures and anatomy pertinent to the testing of neurologic levels (Table 1). The diagram in Table 1 further shows the clinical application of neurologic level testing to the pathology of herniated cervical discs.

It may be more feasible to evaluate all motor levels first, then all reflexes, and, finally, all sensory dermatomes of the upper extremity in the following manner:

Motor Levels		Reflexes		Sensory Levels	
Shoulder Abduction	C5	Biceps	C5	Lateral Arm	C5
Wrist Extension	C6	Brachioradialis	C6	Lateral Forearm	C6
Wrist Flexion	C7	Triceps	C7	Middle Finger	C7
Finger Extension	C7			Medial Forearm	C8
Finger Flexion	C8			Medial Arm	T1
Finger Abduction	T1				

Table 1. Neurology of the Upper Extremity

Disc	Root	Reflex	Muscles	Sensation
C4–C5	C5	Biceps Reflex	Deltoid Biceps	*Lateral Arm* Axillary nerve
C5–C6	C6	Brachioradialis Reflex (Biceps Reflex)	Wrist Extension Biceps	*Lateral Forearm* Musculocutaneous nerve
C6–C7	C7	Triceps Reflex	Wrist Flexors Finger Extension Triceps	*Middle Finger*
C7–T1	C8	—	Finger Flexion Hand Intrinsics	*Medial Forearm* Med. Ant. Brach. Cutaneous nerve
T1–T2	T1	—	Hand Intrinsics	*Medial Arm* Med. Brach. Cutaneous nerve

TESTING OF MAJOR PERIPHERAL NERVES

After upper extremity innervation has been evaluated by neurologic levels, the individual peripheral nerves may be assessed, using the following chart as a guide (Table 2).

Table 2. The Major Peripheral Nerves

Nerve	Motor Test	Sensation Test
Radial Nerve	Wrist Extension Thumb Extension	Dorsal web space between thumb and index finger
Ulnar Nerve	Abduction—little finger	Distal ulnar aspect—little finger
Median Nerve	Thumb pinch Opposition of thumb Abduction of thumb	Distal radial aspect—index finger
Axillary Nerve	Deltoid	Lateral Arm—Deltoid patch on upper arm
Musculocutaneous Nerve	Biceps	Lateral Forearm

SPECIAL TESTS

Five special tests are directly related to the cervical spine: (1) the distraction test, (2) the compression test, (3) the Valsalva test, (4) the swallowing test, and (5) the Adson test.

DISTRACTION TEST. This test demonstrates the effect that neck traction might have in relieving pain. Distraction relieves pain due to a narrowing of the neural foramen (and the resultant nerve root compression) by widening the foramen. Distraction also relieves pain in the cervical spine by decreasing pressure on the joint capsules around

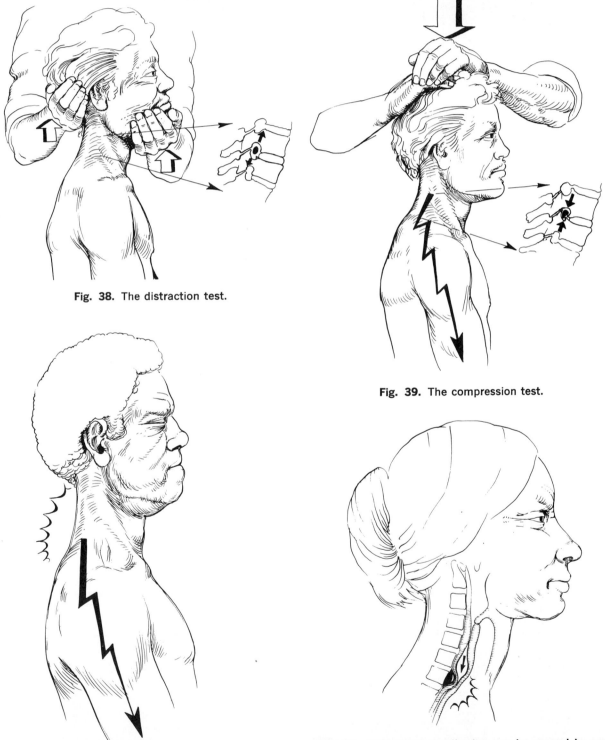

Fig. 38. The distraction test.

Fig. 39. The compression test.

Fig. 40. The Valsalva test.

Fig. 41. Difficulty in swallowing can be caused by cervical spine pathology.

the facet joints. In addition, it may help to alleviate muscle spasm by relaxing the contracted muscles.

To perform the cervical spine distraction test, place the open palm of one hand under the patient's chin, and the other hand upon his occiput. Then, gradually lift (distract) the head to remove its weight from the neck (Fig. 38).

COMPRESSION TEST.
A narrowing of the neural foramen, pressure on the facet joints, or muscle spasm can cause increased pain upon compression. In addition, the compression test may faithfully reproduce pain referred to the upper extremity from the cervical spine, and, in doing so, may help locate the neurologic level of any existing pathology.

To perform the compression test, press down upon the top of the patient's head while he is either sitting or lying down. If there is an increase in pain in either the cervical spine or the extremity, note its exact distribution and whether it follows any previously described dermatome (Fig. 39).

VALSALVA TEST.
This test increases intrathecal pressure. If a space-occupying lesion, such as a herniated disc or a tumor, is present in the cervical canal, the patient may develop pain in the cervical spine secondary to increased pressure. The pain may also radiate to the dermatome distribution that corresponds to the neurologic level of the cervical spine pathology.

To perform the Valsalva test, have the patient hold his breath and bear down as if he were moving his bowels. Then ask whether he feels any increase in pain, and, if so, whether he can describe the location (Fig. 40). Note that the Valsalva test is a subjective test which requires accurate response from the patient.

SWALLOWING TEST.
Difficulty or pain upon swallowing can sometimes be caused by cervical spine pathology such as bony protuberances, bony osteophytes, or by soft tissue swelling due to hematomas, infection, or tumor in the anterior portion of the cervical spine (Fig. 41).

ADSON TEST.
This test is used to determine the state of the subclavian artery, which may be compressed by an extra cervical rib or by tightened scalenus anticus and scalenus medius muscles, which can compress the artery where it passes between them on its way to the upper extremity.

To perform the Adson test, take the patient's radial pulse at the wrist. As you continue to feel the pulse, abduct, extend, and externally rotate his arm. Then instruct him to take a deep breath and to turn his head toward the arm being tested (Figs. 42, 43). If there is compression of the subclavian artery, you will feel a marked diminution or absence of the radial pulse.

EXAMINATION OF RELATED AREAS

In most cases, it is the cervical spine which refers pain to other areas of the upper extremity. However it is possible for pathology of the temporomandibular joint, infections of the lower jaw, teeth, or scalp infections to refer pain to the neck.

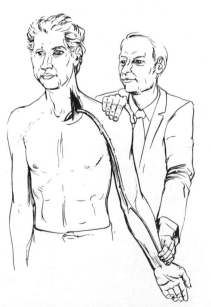

Fig. 42. The Adson test.

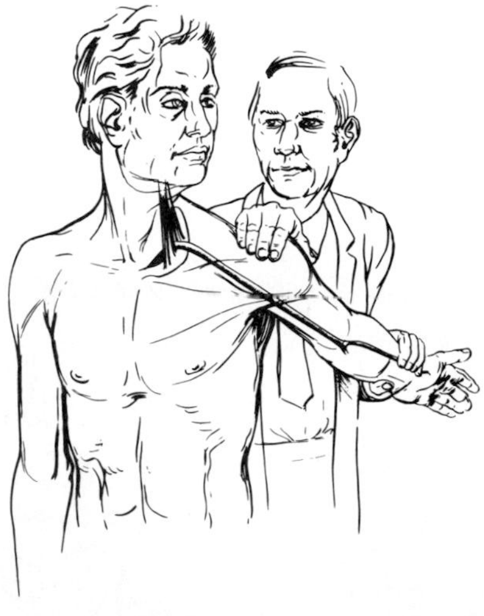

Fig. 43. The Adson Test: When the patient turns his head, an absent or diminished pulse indicates compression of the subclavian artery.

The Temporomandibular Joint

The temporomandibular joint is the joint most used in the body; it opens and closes approximately 1,500 to 2,000 times a day during its various motions of chewing, talking, swallowing, yawning, and snoring.

INSPECTION

Located just anterior to the external auditory canal, the temporomandibular joint etches no distinct surface contours on the skin since its external surface is well clothed with muscles. During inspection, observe the mandible in motion; note that it has two joints, one at either end.

Like the lower extremity, the temporomandibular joint has two phases to its gait pattern: (1) a swing phase, when the joint is in motion, and (2) a stance phase, when the mouth is closed.

In swing phase, notice the rhythm of the opening and closing of the jaw. Normally, the arc of motion is continuous and unbroken, with no evidence of asymmetrical or sideways mandibular motion. The mandible should open and close in a straight line, with the teeth coming together and separating easily (Fig. 44). In abnormal circumstances, the mouth will open and close awkwardly, with a break in the arc of motion or with obvious movement to one side or the other (Fig. 45). Such abnormality may result from pathology in one or both of the joints, or from improper dentition. An affected joint may be incapable of moving through a natural range of motion, in which case the patient must substitute an inefficient, asymmetrical motion for one that was efficient, but has since become restricted or painful.

In the stance phase, the jaw is normally centered and the teeth close symmetrically in the midline (Fig. 44). Since weight is transferred through the teeth to the maxilla, the temporomandibular joint, in its stance phase, is not a true weight-bearing joint. However, poor dentition or occlusion may compel the joint to bear weight. When a patient having poor dentition is placed into cervical traction, his temporomandibular joint is often converted into a weight-bearing joint, causing problems such as pain and headache.

As you inspect the temporomandibular joint, notice the way in which the joint motions of hinge and glide function. The joint hinges within the glenoid fossa and glides forward to the eminentia (Fig. 46). As in other joints having more than one type of motion, the meniscus intercedes, dividing the joint cavity into two portions, an upper portion used for hinge motion, and a lower portion used for glide. To accomplish this, the dual heads of each of the external pterygoid muscles act asynchronously, with one head pulling the meniscus forward as the second opens the joint (Fig. 47).

BONY PALPATION

To palpate the temporomandibular joint, place your index finger into the patient's external auditory canal and press anteriorly (Fig. 48). Instruct him to open and close his mouth slowly. As he does so, the motion of the mandibular condyle becomes palpable at the tip of your finger (Fig. 49). Both sides should be palpated simultaneously. The motion should feel smooth and bilaterally symmetrical; any deviations from the normal pattern of motion should be noted (Fig. 50). A palpable crepitation or clicking may be due to a damaged meniscus in the temporomandibular joint or to synovial swelling secondary to

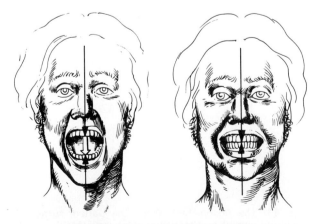

Fig. 44. Normal mandibular motion.

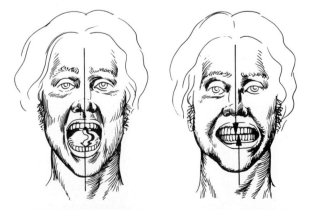

Fig. 45. Asymmetrical mandibular motion. **Left.** Swing phase. **Right.** Stance phase.

trauma. Ask the patient to open his mouth as wide as possible, to see whether or not his temporomandibular joints dislocate (Fig. 51). Alternately, you may palpate the condyles by placing your index finger just anterior to the ear and asking the patient to open his mouth.

SOFT TISSUE PALPATION

The temporomandibular joint is vulnerable to various types of traumatic injury, usually when the joint dislocates or is forced to bear weight. This may occur when acceleration–deceleration or bobbing injuries force the head into extreme hyperextension, whipping the mouth open in an uncontrolled movement and forcing the temporomandibular joint to dislocate (Fig. 52). Such dislocation causes soft tissue damage to the joint capsule and to the ligaments. It may also tear the joint's meniscus. In addition, the external pterygoid muscle may be stretched, with resultant muscle spasms. Many patients are then placed into cervical halter traction because of the associated neck injury. Traction may overload the already traumatized joint and force it to bear further weight, resulting in more pain and discomfort for the patient (Fig. 53). This is especially true in patients with poor dentition.

Asymmetrical dentition or poor occlusion alone also can overload the joint and cause a palpable clicking in the external auditory canal (Fig. 54). A constant grinding or clenching of the teeth (bruxism) also may overload the joint and eventually cause clinical problems.

External Pterygoid Muscle.   This muscle is palpated for spasm or tenderness. Place your index finger in the patient's mouth between the buccal mucosa and the superior gum and point the tip of your index finger posteriorly, past the last upper molar to the neck of the mandible. Then ask the patient to open and close his mouth slowly. As the neck of the mandible swings forward and the mouth opens, you will feel for the external pterygoid muscle tighten against your fingertip (Fig. 55). If the external pterygoid has been traumatized or is in spasm, the patient may feel some pain or tenderness. The external pterygoid has clinical importance, for if it is traumatized secondary to stretch injury, it may go into spasm and cause temporomandibular joint pain, as well as an asymmetrical, sideways motion of the jaw.

RANGE OF MOTION

Active Range of Motion

Instruct the patient to open and close his mouth. Normally, he can open his mouth wide enough so that three fingers can be inserted between the incisor teeth (approximately 35 to 40 millimeters) (Fig. 56).

The temporomandibular joint also allows the jaw to glide forward or to protrude. Ask the patient to jut his jaw forward. Normally, it should protrude far enough so that he can place his bottom teeth in front of his top teeth.

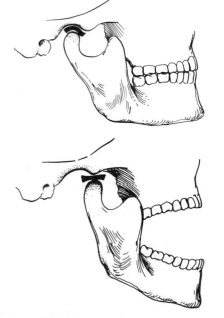

Fig. 46. The hinge and glide motions of the temporomandibular joint. The meniscus divides the joint into an upper and lower portion.

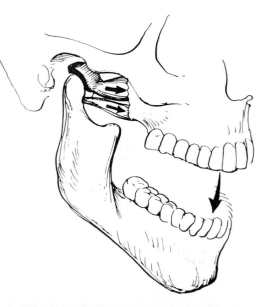

Fig. 47. The external pterygoid muscle's two heads act asynchronously to open the temporomandibular joint.

Passive Range of Motion

If a patient is unable to complete an active range of motion or if test results seem inconclusive, then test him passively in the following way: carefully place one finger upon the patient's lower incisor teeth, and push the mouth open as far as possible. Limitations in mandibular range of motion are generally secondary to rheumatoid arthritis, congenital bone anomalies, soft tissue or bony ankylosis, osteoarthritis involving the temporomandibular joint, or muscle spasm.

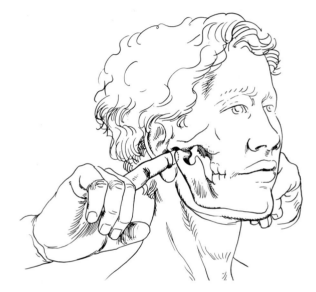

Fig. 48. To palpate the temporomandibular joint, place your index finger in the auditory canal.

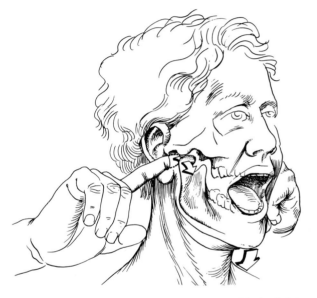

Fig. 49. The movement of the temporomandibular joint can be felt when the patient opens his mouth.

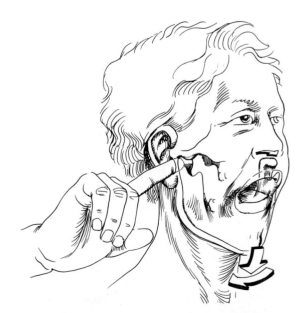

Fig. 50. A deviated pattern of motion in the temporomandibular joint.

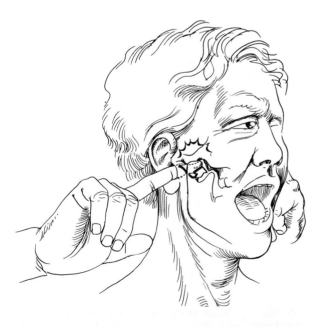

Fig. 51. Dislocation of the temporomandibular joint.

NEUROLOGIC EXAMINATION

Muscle Testing

OPENING THE MOUTH

Primary Opener:
1) External pterygoid muscle
   trigeminal nerve—mandibular division,
   pterygoid branch

Secondary Opener:
1) Hyoid muscles
2) Gravity

To test the muscles which open the mouth, place the open palm of your resisting hand under the patient's jaw, and ask him to open his mouth. As he does so, gradually increase the pressure of resistance until you have determined the amount of resistance he can overcome. Normally, he should be able to open his mouth against maximum resistance.

CLOSING THE MOUTH

Primary Closers:
1) Masseter muscle
   trigeminal nerve
2) Temporalis muscle
   trigeminal nerve

Secondary Closer:
1) Internal pterygoid muscle

The inability to close the mouth is more often a social problem than a clinical one. You may test closing by forcing the closed mouth into an open position with the palm of your hand.

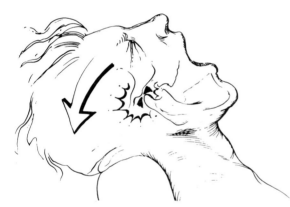

Fig. 52. Hyperextension injury can cause dislocation of the temporomandibular joint.

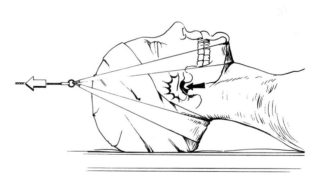

Fig. 53. In neck injury with associated mandibular dislocation, traction forces the joint to bear weight, and results in increased pain.

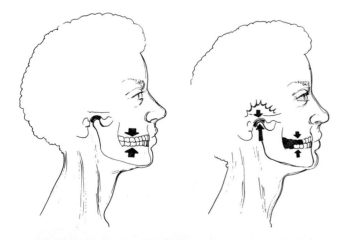

Fig. 54. Asymmetrical dentition (right) or poor occlusion can cause clicking in the temporomandibular joint.

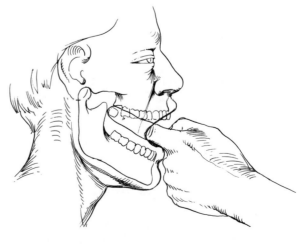

Fig. 55. Palpation of the external pterygoid muscles.

Reflex Testing

JAW REFLEX. The jaw reflex is a stretch reflex, involving the masseter and temporalis muscles. The fifth cranial (trigeminal) nerve innervates these muscles and mediates the reflex arc. To test the reflex, place one finger over the mental area of the chin while the mouth is in the physiologic rest position (slightly open). Then tap your finger with a neurologic hammer; the reflex elicited will close the mouth. If the reflex is absent or diminished, there may be pathology along the course of the fifth cranial nerve. A brisk reflex may be due to an upper motor neuron lesion (Fig. 57).

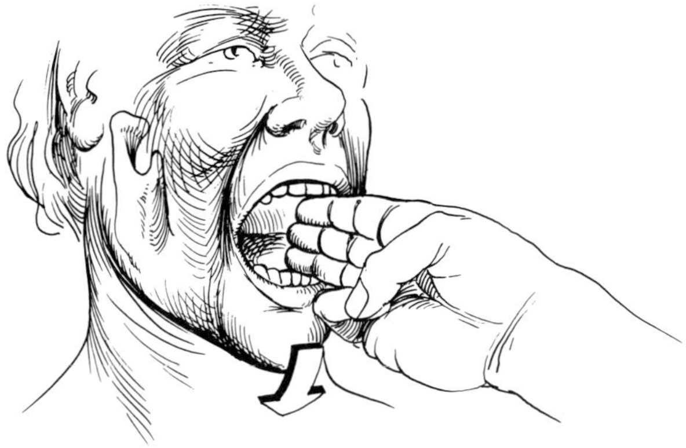

SPECIAL TESTS

CHVOSTEK TEST. This is a test of the seventh cranial nerve (facial nerve). Tap the area of the parotid gland overlying the masseter muscle. The facial muscles will contract in a twitch if blood calcium is low (Fig. 58).

RELATED AREAS

Pain is not usually referred to the temporomandibular joint; rather, the joint often refers pain to other areas. A tooth abscess of the lower jaw may refer pain to the joint and the neck, but more commonly, pathology and dysfunction of the temporomandibular joint refers pain to the head and neck and causes headache or mandibular pain.

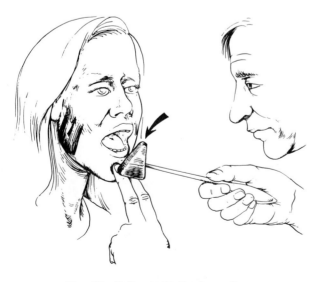

Fig. 56. The normal mouth span is wide enough to accommodate three fingers inserted between the incisor teeth.

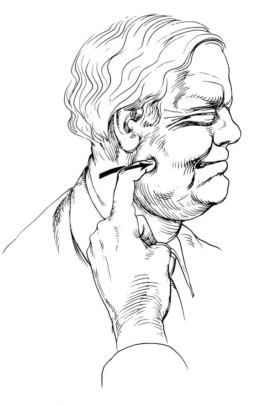

Fig. 57. Reflex test—the jaw reflex.

Fig. 58. The Chvostek test.

5
Examination of Gait

The lower extremity is dedicated to the vital tasks of weight bearing and ambulation; its health is essential to normal and efficient daily functioning. Since pathology that affects the lower extremity often manifests itself most clearly in gait, we must consider the gait's normal and abnormal parameters so that we can recognize and treat characteristic pathologies when they occur.

There are two phases to the normal walking cycle: stance phase, when the foot is on the ground; and swing phase, when it is moving forward. Sixty percent of the normal cycle is spent in stance phase (25 percent in double stance, with both feet on the ground) and 40 percent in swing phase. Each phase, in turn, is divided into its smaller components (Figs. 1, 2):

Stance Phase	Swing Phase
1. Heel Strike	1. Acceleration
2. Foot Flat	2. Midswing
3. Midstance	3. Deceleration
4. Push-off (Toe-off)	

Most problems become apparent in stance phase since, because it bears weight and constitutes the major portion of gait, it undergoes the greater stress.

Examination of gait begins as soon as the patient enters the examining room. Note any obvious limp or deformity of the extremity that may be affecting normal gait and try to determine in which phase and component the problem occurs. Since each component has its characteristic

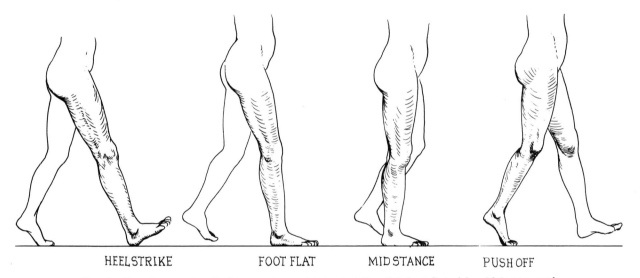

HEELSTRIKE   FOOT FLAT   MIDSTANCE   PUSH OFF

Fig. 1. The phases of gait. Stance phase: (a) heel strike, (b) foot flat, (c) midstance, and (d) push-off.

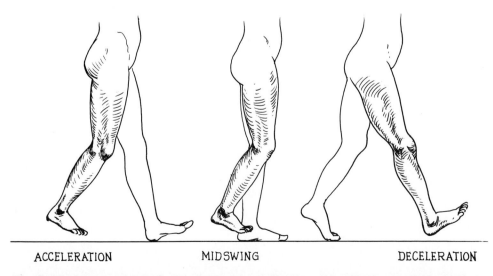

ACCELERATION   MIDSWING   DECELERATION

Fig. 2. The phases of gait. Swing phase: (a) acceleration, (b) midswing, and (c) deceleration.

physical pattern, pinpointing the involved component is an excellent first step in determining the etiology of the problem. As you examine the gait, take into account these additional measureable determinants (according to Inman):

1. *The width of the base* should not be more than two to four inches from heel to heel. If you note that the patient is walking with a wider base, you should suspect pathology. Patients usually widen their base if they feel dizzy or unsteady as a result, perhaps, of cerebellar problems or decreased sensation in the sole of the foot (Fig. 3).

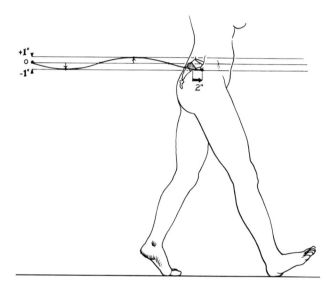

Fig. 4. The center of gravity oscillates vertically approximately 2 inches during gait.

Fig. 3. The width of a normal base measures from 2 to 4 inches. Normal step length is approximately 15 inches.

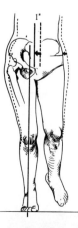

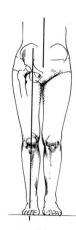

Fig. 5. The pelvis and trunk shift laterally approximately 1 inch during gait.

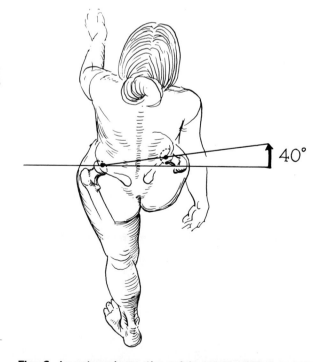

Fig. 6. In swing phase, the pelvis rotates 40° forward. The opposite hip joint acts as a fulcrum for this rotation.

2. *The body's center of gravity* lies two inches in front of the second sacral vertebra. In normal gait it oscillates no more than two inches in a vertical direction. Controlled vertical oscillation main-tains the smooth pattern of gait as the body advances. Increased vertical motion may indicate pathology (Fig. 4).

3. *The knee should remain flexed during all components of stance phase* (except heel strike) to prevent the excessive vertical displacement of the center of gravity. For example, in toe-off, when the ankle, with 20° of plantar flexion, tends to cause the center of gravity to rise, the knee flexes to approximately 40° to counterbalance it. Patients with their knees fused in extension may be unable to counteract excesses of ankle motion, losing the normal smooth pattern of gait.

4. *The pelvis and trunk shift laterally* approximately one inch to the weight-bearing side during gait to center the weight over the hip. If the pa-

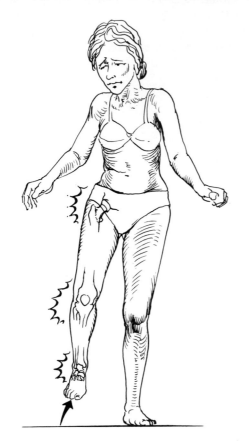

Fig. 7. By trying to avoid a painful component of gait, a patient walks with an antalgic gait.

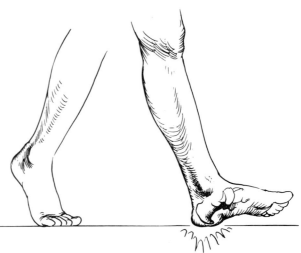

Fig. 8. A spike of bone protruding from the medial tubercle on the plantar surface of the os calcis is commonly referred to as a heel spur.

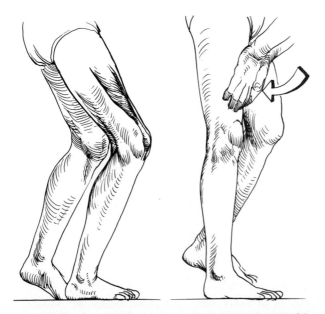

Fig. 9. Weak quadriceps cause the knee to be unstable at heel strike, and the patient may have to push his knee manually into extension.

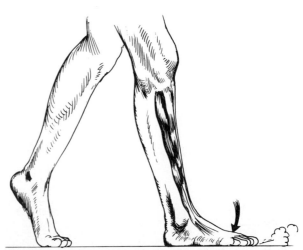

Fig. 10. Weak dorsiflexors cause the foot to slap down after heel strike.

tient has gluteus medius weakness, this lateral shift of trunk and pelvis is markedly accentuated (Fig. 5).

5. *The average length of a step is approximately 15 inches.* With pain, advancing age, fatigue, or pathology within the lower extremity, the length of the steps may decrease (Fig. 3).

6. *The average adult walks at a cadence of approximately 90 to 120 steps per minute,* with an average energy cost of only 100 calories per mile. Changes in this smooth, coordinated pattern markedly reduce efficiency and greatly increase the energy cost. With advancing age, fatigue, or pain, the number of steps per minute decreases. If the surface on which the patient is walking is slick, and if his footing is unsure, the number of steps per minute also decreases.

7. *During swing phase, the pelvis rotates 40° forward,* while the hip joint on the opposite extremity (which is in stance phase) acts as the fulcrum for rotation. Patients do not rotate normally around a hip joint that is stiff or painful (Fig. 6).

Let us now determine how a particular component of gait can be affected by pathology in each of the joints of the lower extremity during ambulation.

STANCE PHASE

Most of the problems in stance phase result in pain and cause the patient to walk with an *antalgic gait:* He remains on the involved extremity for as short a time as is possible, and he may try to avoid the painful component completely (Fig. 7).

Stance phase is also commonly affected by shoe problems, which may cause pain throughout stance. Pain may develop from nails sticking through the shoe's heel, from bent or roughened lining, from a loose object trapped in the shoe, or from the size of the shoe (it may be too small or too large, or the shoe's toe may be too narrow and constricted).

Proceed to examine stance phase by components, noting the characteristic problems of each joint.

Heel Strike

FOOT. Foot pains may be a result of a heel spur, a spike of bone that protrudes from the medial tubercle on the plantar surface of the os calcis. It usually causes a very sharp pain as the patient brings his heel down hard on the floor. In time, a protective bursa may develop over the spur; bursitis may follow, causing increased pain. To relieve the pain, the patient may try to hop onto the involved foot in an attempt to avoid heel strike completely (Fig. 8).

KNEE. The knee is normally extended at heel strike; if it is unable to extend as a result of weak quadriceps (unstable knee gait) or if the knee is fused in flexion, the patient may try to push it into extension with his hand. If he is unable to do so, the knee remains unstable during heel strike (Fig. 9).

Foot Flat

FOOT. The dorsiflexors of the foot (the tibialis anterior, extensor digitorum longus, and extensor hallucis longus) permit the foot to move into plantar flexion through eccentric elongation so that the foot flattens smoothly on the ground. Patients with weak or nonfunctioning dorsiflexors may slap their foot down after heel strike instead of letting it land smoothly. Patients with fused ankles may be unable to reach foot flat until midstance (Fig. 10).

Midstance

FOOT. Normally, weight is borne evenly on all aspects of the foot. Patients with rigid pes planus and subtalar arthritis may develop pain when walking on uneven ground; those with fallen transverse arches of the forefoot may develop painful calluses over the metatarsal heads (Figs. 11, 12). Corns formed on the dorsum of the toes may also become painful in midstance, since they may rub against the shoe as the toes begin to grip the ground (Fig. 13).

KNEE. The quadriceps muscles contract to hold the knee stable, since it is not normally straight. Weakened quadriceps may result in excessive flexion and a relatively unstable knee.

HIP. During midstance there is approximately one inch of lateral displacement of the hip to the weight-bearing side. A weakened gluteus medius muscle forces the patient to lurch toward the involved side to place the center of gravity over the hip; such movement is called an abduction, or gluteus medius, lurch (Fig. 14).

If the gluteus maximus muscle is weakened, the patient must thrust his thorax posteriorly to maintain hip extension (an extensor, or gluteus maximus, lurch) (Fig. 15).

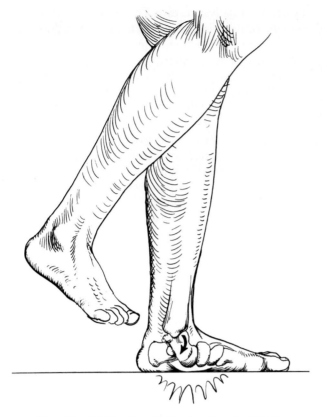

Fig. 11. A fallen longitudinal arch, pes planus.

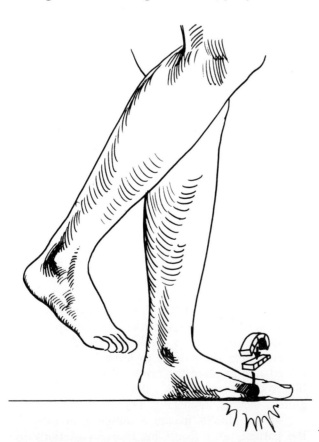

Fig. 12. Calluses formed over the metatarsal heads secondary to a fallen transverse arch can be very painful.

Push-off

FOOT. If the patient has osteoarthritis or a partially or fully fused metatarsophalangeal joint (hallux rigidus), he may be unwilling or unable to hyperextend the metatarsophalangeal joint of his great toe, and may be forced to push off from the lateral side of his forefoot, a maneuver which eventually causes pain. Pain may be increased as a result of the increased pressure on the metatarsal heads if callosities have developed secondary to a dropped head (metatarsalgia). Soft corns between the fourth and fifth toes may also become excessively painful as a result of the added pressure. You can often diagnose this condition by examining the shoe; instead of the normal transverse crease over the toes, an oblique crease, cutting across the toes and forefoot, may develop (see Foot and Ankle Chapter, Fig. 78).

KNEE. The gastrocnemius, soleus, and flexor hallucis longus are vital to push-off; weakness of these muscles can result in a flat-footed or calcaneal gait.

SWING PHASE

Fewer problems become evident in swing phase than in stance phase, since the extremity is no longer subjected to the stresses of weight bearing and support.

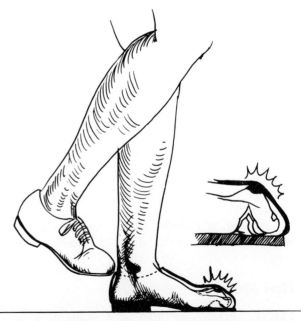

Fig. 13. A corn on the dorsum of a claw toe causes pain in stance phase.

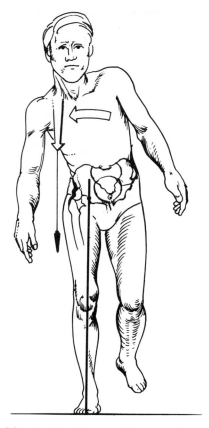

Fig. 14. An abduction, or gluteus medius, lurch.

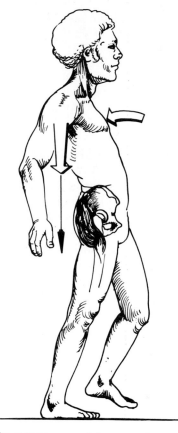

Fig. 15. An extensor, or gluteus maximus, lurch.

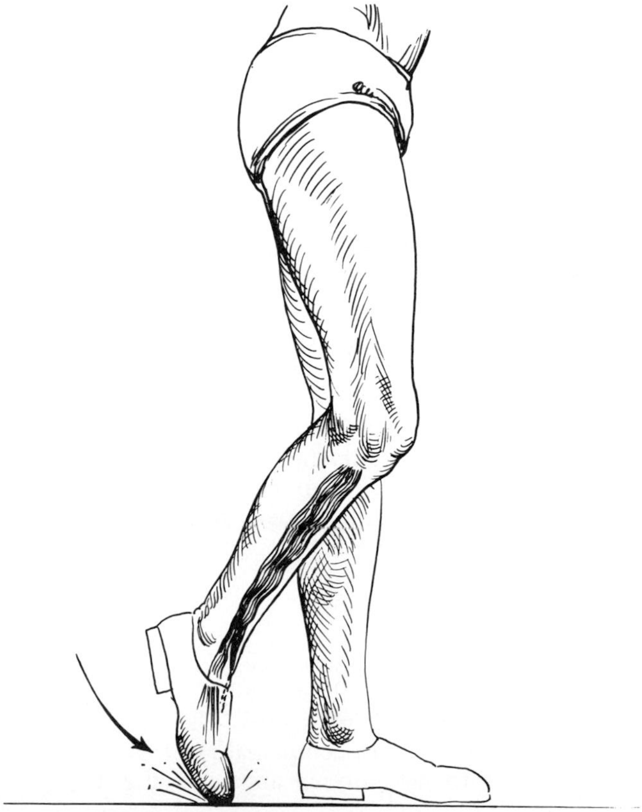

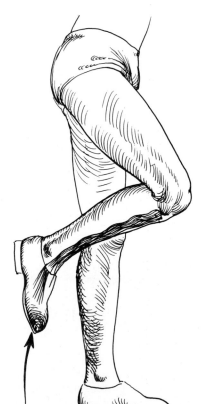

Fig. 16. Loss of ankle dorsiflexion can cause the patient to scrape the toe of his shoe on the floor.

Fig. 17. Steppage gait: the knee is lifted higher than normal to enable the foot to clear the floor.

Acceleration

FOOT. The dorsiflexors of the ankle are active during the entire swing phase. They help shorten the extremity so that it can clear the ground by holding the ankle neutral.

KNEE. The knee reaches its maximum degree of flexion between toe-off and midswing, approximately 65°. It further serves to shorten the extremity so that it can clear the ground.

HIP. The quadriceps muscle begins to contract just before toe-off to help initiate the forward swing of the leg. If the patient has poor quadriceps strength, he may rotate the pelvis anteriorly in an exaggerated motion to provide forward thrust for the leg.

Midswing

FOOT. When the ankle dorsiflexors are not working, the toe of the shoe scrapes the ground to produce a characteristic shoe scrape (Fig. 16). To compensate, the patient may flex his hip excessively to bend the knee, permitting the foot to clear the ground (steppage gait) (Fig. 17).

Deceleration

KNEE. The hamstring muscles contract to slow down the swing just prior to heel strike so that the heel can strike the ground quietly in a controlled motion. If the hamstrings are weak, heel strike may be excessively harsh, causing thickening of the heel pad, and the knee may hyperextend (back knee gait).

SUMMARY

Stance Phase

MUSCLE WEAKNESS

1) Patients with muscle weakness of the tibialis anterior (L4) may have a drop foot gait (Fig. 16, 17).
2) Patients with muscle weakness of the gluteus medius (L5) may have an abductor, or gluteus medius, lurch (Fig. 14).

3) Patients with gluteus maximus weakness (S1) may have an extensor, or gluteus maximus, lurch (Fig. 15).
4) Patients with muscle weakness of the gastroc-soleus group (S1, S2) may have a flat foot gait with no forceful toe-off (Fig. 18).
5) Patient with quadriceps weakness (L2, 3, 4) may walk with a back knee gait to lock their knees in extension (Fig. 9).

INSTABILITY

1) Patients with instability widen the base of their gait more than four inches.
2) Patients with decreased sensation on the soles of their feet (caused by diabetes, syphilis, or any peripheral neuropathy) broaden their gait to gain stability. In addition, they may look at their feet to orient themselves in relation to space and the ground.
3) Patients with cerebellar problems may have difficulty in maintaining their balance, and, as a result, may widen their base.
4) Patients with dislocating knee caps have unstable knees which may suddenly fall into marked flexion.
5) Patients with torn menisci have unstable knees which may buckle.
6) Patients with torn collateral ligaments have unstable knees which may buckle.

PAIN

1) Patients with shoe problems may have pain in all portions of stance phase, resulting in an antalgic gait.
2) Patients with heel spurs may have pain in the heel strike position of stance phase (Fig. 8).
3) Patients with osteoarthritis of the knee or hip may have pain in all phases of stance. In general, they spend as little time in stance phase as possible because of the pain (antalgic gait).
4) Patients with hallux rigidus may not be able to push off properly because of the pain, causing a flat-foot gait.

FUSED JOINTS

1) Patients with fused ankles, knees, or hips may have difficulties in all phases of gait. If only one joint is fused, the patient is usually able to compensate so that gross disturbances are not apparent (Fig. 19).

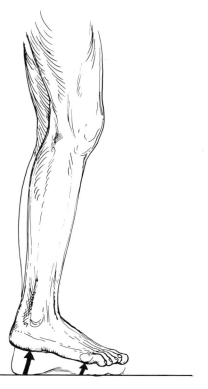

Fig. 18. Flat-footed gait with no push-off.

Swing Phase

MUSCLE WEAKNESS

1) Patients with weak dorsiflexors of the foot and ankle may develop a steppage gait, in which they lift the knee higher than normal so that the foot can clear the ground (Figs. 16, 17).
2) Patients with quadriceps weakness may not be able to accelerate without abnormal hip rotation (Fig. 19).
3) Patients with hamstring weakness may not be able to decelerate properly just before heel strike.

FUSED JOINTS

1) A fused knee may force the patient to hike his hip up on the involved side so that the foot can clear the ground (Fig. 20).

The examination of the patient's gait should be integrated with the examination of the entire lower extremity.

The upper extremity is involved in gait in that the arm swings in tandem with the opposite leg in the lower extremity to produce a smooth-flowing, balanced gait.

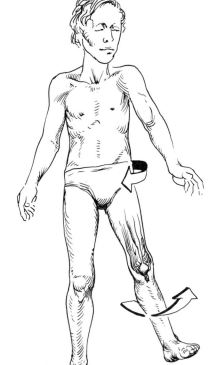

Fig. 19. Compensation in gait for a fused joint.

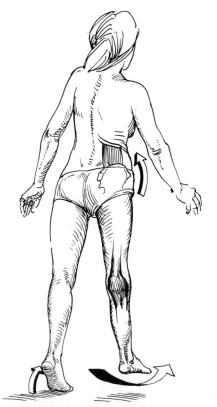
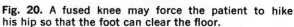

Fig. 20. A fused knee may force the patient to hike his hip so that the foot can clear the floor.

6

Physical Examination of the Hip and Pelvis

INSPECTION
BONY PALPATION
   Anterior Aspect
      Anterior Superior Iliac Spines
      Iliac Crest
      Iliac Tubercle
      Greater Trochanter
      Pubic Tubercles
   Posterior Aspect
      Posterior Superior Iliac Spines
      Greater Trochanter
      Ischial Tuberosity
      Sacroiliac Joint (S2)
SOFT TISSUE PALPATION
   Zone I   — Femoral Triangle
   Zone II — Greater Trochanter
   Zone III — Sciatic Nerve
   Zone IV — Iliac Crest
   Zone V — Hip and Pelvic Muscles
RANGE OF MOTION
   Active Range of Motion Tests
   Passive Range of Motion Tests
   Flexion (Thomas Test) — 120°
      Extension _____ 30°
      Abduction _____ 45°–50°
      Adduction _____ 20°–30°
      Internal Rotation ____ 35°
      External Rotation ____ 45°
NEUROLOGIC EXAMINATION
   Muscle Testing
   Sensation Tests
SPECIAL TESTS
   Trendelenburg Test
   Tests for Leg Length Discrepancy
      True Leg Length Discrepancy
      Apparent Leg Length Discrepancy
   Ober Test for Contraction of the Iliotibial Band
   Thomas Test for Flexion Contracture
   Tests for Congenital Dislocation of the Hip
      Ortolani Click
      Telescoping
      Adduction Contracture
EXAMINATION OF RELATED AREAS
   Rectal Examination

The pelvic girdle is composed of three joints: (1) the hip joint (acetabularfemoral joint), (2) the sacroiliac joint, and (3) the pubic symphysis, all of which work in unison to provide mobility and stability for the body. The ball-and-socket configuration of the hip is designed particularly to fulfill that dual function.

For all intents and purposes, the sacroiliac and the pubic symphysis are practically immovable joints, and, while they may become involved pathologically, they seldom restrict function or cause pain. On the other hand, the hip joint is mobile, and pathology affecting it becomes immediately perceptible during walking as pain or limited motion.

INSPECTION

When the patient enters the examination room, particular attention should be paid to his gait, for, as was discussed in the previous chapter, many hip problems manifest themselves most clearly during ambulation.

To ensure a thorough examination of the hip joint and related areas, it is preferable that the patient disrobe completely. However, if doing so causes him discomfort or embarrassment, he may keep his underwear on. While the patient undresses, note whether he performs any particular maneuver that seems painful or inefficient. Quite often, an efficient movement is sacrificed for one that is less efficient but less painful.

Also check the hip and pelvic area for abrasions, discolorations, birth marks, blebs, open sinus drainage, and particularly for abnormal swellings, bulges, or skin folds.

Next, observe the patient's stance, checking to see if the anterior superior iliac spines are in the same horizontal plane. If they are not, there may be some pelvic obliquity (tilted pelvis) secondary to leg length discrepancy.

When observed from the side, the lumbar portion of the spine normally exhibits a slight lordosis (anterior curvature of the spine), neither unduly lordotic nor flat. An absence of the normal lordosis may suggest paravertebral muscle spasms. If the spine exhibits an exaggerated curve, the anterior abdominal muscles may be weak, since they help to prevent the lumbar spine from becoming increasingly lordotic. Increased lumbar lordosis may also be caused by a fixed flexion deformity of the hip. Excessive lordosis in this case occasionally substitutes for true hip extension.

While observing the posterior aspect of the hip, notice that the lower borders of the buttocks are marked by the gluteal folds (lateral and slightly inferior to the approximate midline of the thigh). The size and depth of the folds increase upon hip extension and decrease upon hip flexion.

In infants, skin folds are situated symmetrically around the groin and along the thigh. Asymmetrical folds may be due to a congenital dislocation of the hip, muscular atrophy, pelvic obliquity, or a leg length discrepancy.

Observe the two discernible dimples which overlie the posterior superior iliac spine directly above the buttocks. They should lie along the same horizontal plane. If they do not, there is evidence of pelvic obliquity.

BONY PALPATION

The patient may either stand or lie down, whichever is more comfortable. If it is possible, some portion of this examination should be conducted while he is standing, since pathology overlooked in a non-weight-bearing position may become patently obvious under the stress of weight bearing.

Anterior Aspect

Your first contact should be gentle, yet firm. As you palpate, gauge the skin temperature and take note of any tenderness elicited. It is best to palpate both sides at the same time to facilitate bilateral comparison.

Anterior Superior Iliac Spines. Stand in front of the patient and place your hands upon the sides of his waist with your thumbs on the anterior superior iliac spines and your fingers on the anterior portion of his iliac crests (Fig. 1). In thin patients, these bony prominences are subcutaneous, but in obese patients, they are covered by adipose tissue and may be somewhat more difficult to find.

Iliac Crest. The iliac crest is subcutaneous, and serves either as a point of origin or of insertion for a variety of muscles. None of these muscles cross the bony linear crest and it remains available for palpation. Normally, the iliac crests are level in relation to each other. When they are not, it is usually because of pelvic obliquity (Fig. 5).

Iliac Tubercle. Keep your thumb upon the anterior superior iliac spine and move your fingers posteriorly along the lateral lip of the iliac crest. About three inches from the top of the crest, you can palpate the iliac tubercle, which marks the widest point on the crest (Fig. 2).

Greater Trochanter. With your thumbs still in place on the anterior superior spines, move your fingers down from the iliac tubercles to the greater trochanters of the femurs (Fig. 3). The posterior edge of the greater trochanter is relatively uncovered, and, as such, is easily palpable. The anterior and lateral portions are covered by the tensor fascia lata and the gluteus medius muscle and are less accessible to palpation. Normally, the trochanters are level. A congenital dislocation of the hip or a hip fracture that has healed in a poor position are two pathologies that could make the levels of the trochanters unequal.

Pubic Tubercles. With your fingers anchored on the trochanters, move your thumbs along the inguinal creases medially and obliquely downward until you can feel the pubic tubercles (Fig. 4). Although they are hidden under pubic hair and the pubic fat pad (mons pubis), the pubic tubercles are palpable bony protuberances. Note that they are on the same level as the top of the greater trochanters.

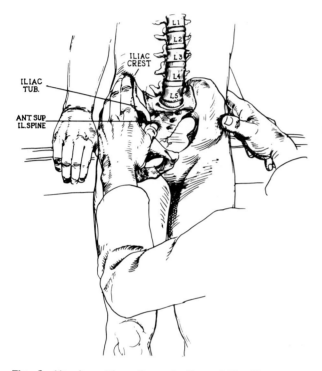

Fig. 1. Hand positions for palpation of the iliac crest.

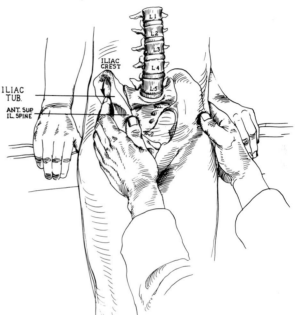

Fig. 2. The iliac tubercle is the widest point on the crest.

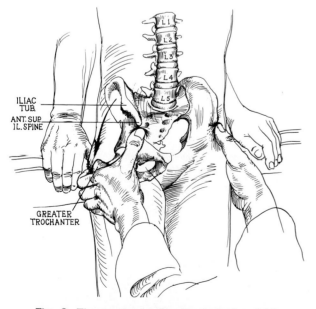

Fig. 3. The greater trochanter (anterior view).

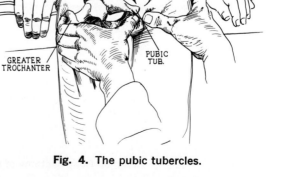

Fig. 4. The pubic tubercles.

Posterior Aspect

For this portion of the hip examination, the patient should lie on his side with his hip flexed (Fig. 6).

Posterior Superior Iliac Spines. These are easily located, for they lie directly underneath the visible dimples just above the buttocks. The spines are subcutaneous and easily palpable. With the patient lying on his side, anchor your thumb upon the upper spine and palpate along the posterior iliac crest to the iliac tubercle (Fig. 7). The entire edge of the iliac crest is subcutaneous, from the posterior to the anterior superior iliac spines.

Greater Trochanter. Keeping your thumb upon the posterior superior iliac spine, move your fingers downward and you can again palpate the posterior aspect of the greater trochanter (Fig. 8).

Ischial Tuberosity. The ischial tuberosity is located in the middle of the buttock at the approximate level of the gluteal fold (Fig. 9). With your fingers in place upon the greater trochanter, move your thumb from the posterior superior iliac spine to the ischial tuberosity. The tuberosity is difficult to palpate if the hip joint is extended, since the gluteus maximus muscle and fat pads cover it. However, if the hip is flexed, the gluteus maximus moves upward and the ischial tuberosity becomes easily palpable. The tuberosities lie in the same horizontal plane as the lesser trochanters of the femurs.

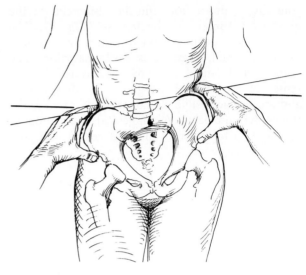

Fig. 5. Pelvic obliquity.

Sacroiliac Joint. The sacroiliac joint is not palpable, due to the overhang of the ilium and the obstruction of the supporting ligaments. It is rarely involved pathologically. The center of the joint, at S2, is crossed by an imaginary line drawn between the posterior superior iliac spines; a line drawn across the top of the iliac crests crosses the spine between the spinous processes of L4 and L5 (Fig. 10). These anatomic guidelines are also helpful in making a precise identification of the lumbar spinous processes (Fig. 11).

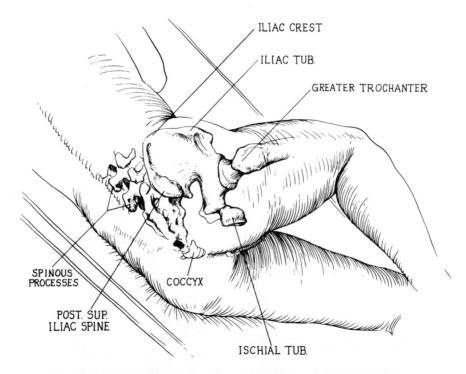

ILIAC CREST

ILIAC TUB.

GREATER TROCHANTER

SPINOUS PROCESSES

COCCYX

POST. SUP. ILIAC SPINE

ISCHIAL TUB.

Fig. 6. Bony anatomy of the hip and pelvis (posterior aspect).

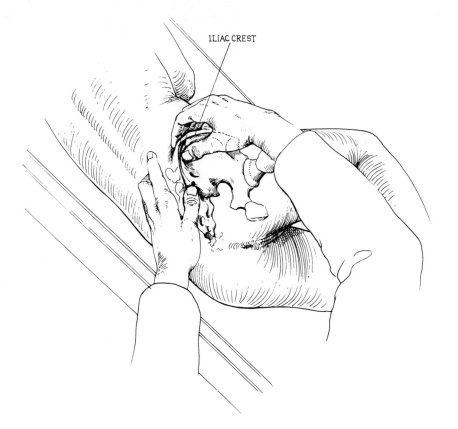

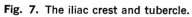

Fig. 7. The iliac crest and tubercle.

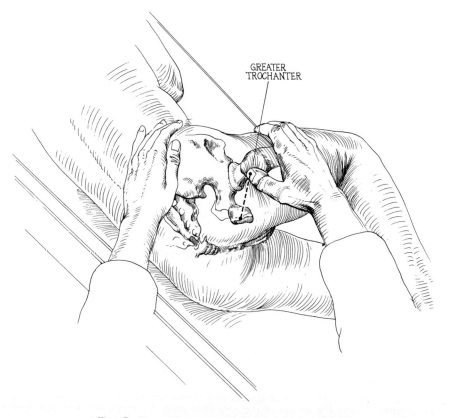

Fig. 8. The greater trochanter (posterior aspect).

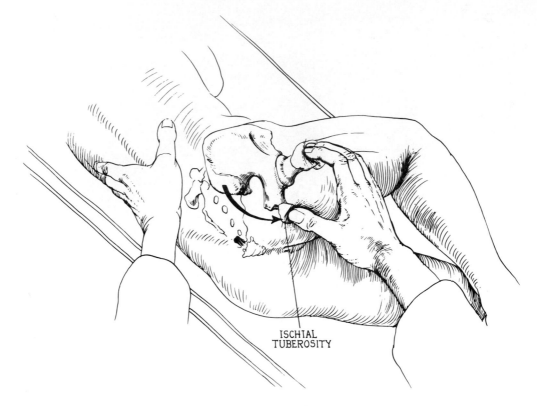

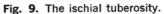

ISCHIAL
TUBEROSITY

Fig. 9. The ischial tuberosity.

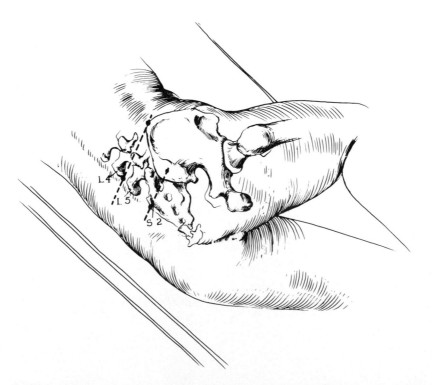

Fig. 10. The sacroiliac joint. An imaginary line drawn between the posterior superior iliac spines crosses S2 and the center of the sacroiliac joint. An imaginary line connecting the tops of the posterior iliac crests crosses the spine between the L4 and L5 vertebrae.

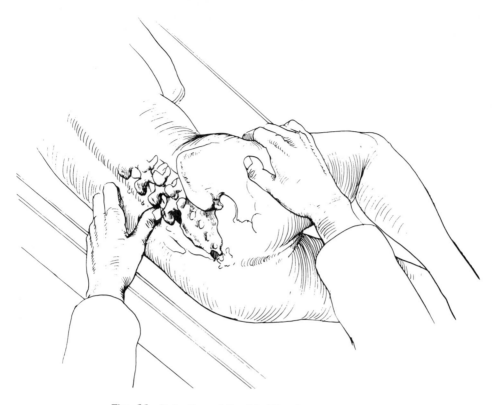

Fig. 11. Palpation of the L4–L5 spinous processes.

Because the hip joint lies deep and is heavily clothed by muscles, neither its components nor any possible abnormalities, such as a fracture of the proximal end of the femur or acetabulum, are palpable. However, the combination of a visibly shortened extremity, external hip rotation, and pain upon motion strongly suggest a fractured hip.

SOFT TISSUE PALPATION

The examination of the hip and pelvic region is divided into five clinical zones: (1) the femoral triangle, (2) the greater trochanter, (3) the sciatic nerve, (4) the iliac crest, and (5) the hip and pelvic muscles.

Zone I—Femoral Triangle

The femoral triangle is defined superiorly by the inguinal crease, medially by the adductor longus muscle, and laterally by the sartorius muscle ridge (Fig. 12). The floor of the triangle is formed by portions of the adductor longus, the pectineus, and the iliopsoas muscles. The femoral artery and lymph glands are superficial to the iliopsoas muscle, and the psoas bursa and hip joint lie deep to it.

The soft tissues of the femoral triangle are most efficiently examined when the patient is supine, with the heel of the leg being examined resting upon the opposite knee. This position puts the hip in flexion, abduction, and external rotation.

Inguinal Ligament. The inguinal ligament is located between the anterior superior iliac spines and the pubic tubercles. Any unusual bulges along the course of this ligament may indicate an inguinal hernia (Fig. 13).

Femoral Artery. The femoral artery passes under the inguinal ligament at about its midpoint. Its pulse is palpable just inferior to the inguinal ligament, at a point halfway between the anterior superior iliac spine and the pubic tubercle (Fig. 14). Normally the pulse is quite strong, but if the common iliac or external iliac artery is partially occluded, the pulse may be diminished. The femoral head lies deep to the femoral artery, but because it is covered by the thick anterior joint capsule (iliofemoral ligament) and the tendon and fibers of the psoas muscle, it is not palpable.

Femoral Nerve. The femoral nerve lies lateral to the femoral artery; it is not palpable.

Femoral Vein. The femoral vein, medial to the artery, is a clinical site for venous puncture. Under normal circumstances, it is not palpable (Fig. 15).

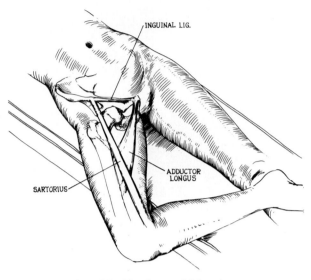

Fig. 12. The femoral triangle.

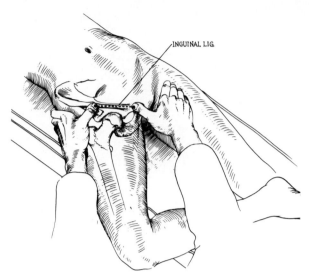

Fig. 13. The inguinal ligament.

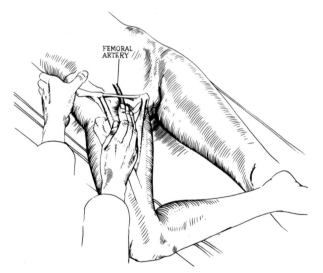

Fig. 14. Palpation of the pulse of the femoral artery.

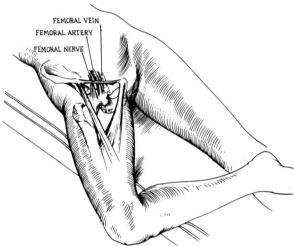

Fig. 15. Normally, the femoral vein and nerve are not palpable.

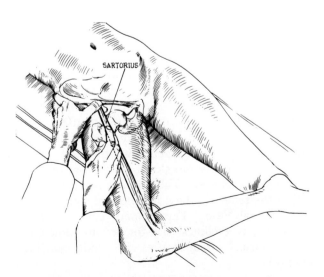

Fig. 16. Palpation of the sartorius muscle.

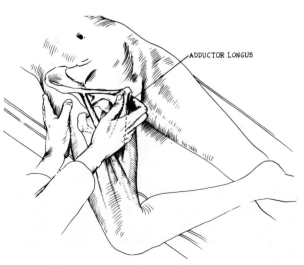

Fig. 17. Palpation of the adductor longus muscle.

Sartorius Muscle. The sartorius muscle, which forms the lateral border of the femoral triangle, is the longest muscle of the body. It is palpable at its origin (slightly inferior to the anterior superior iliac spine), and is rarely pathologically involved (Fig. 16).

Adductor Longus Muscle. This muscle is palpable when the legs are abducted away from the midline. It then forms a distinct ridge, extending from the area of the pubic symphysis toward the middle of the thigh. The proximal cordlike terminus of the muscle is particularly prominent. The adductor longus is frequently pulled during strenuous activity or athletic endeavor, and may be tender to palpation. Occasionally, in spastic children, this muscle must be tenotomized to release the extremity from severe adduction and to prevent possible hip dislocation (Fig. 17).

The general area within the triangle should also be probed for enlarged lymph nodes, which may be a sign of an infection ascending from the lower extremity, or of local pelvic problems (Fig. 18). The lymph nodes are the most medial structure in the triangle.

Zone II—Greater Trochanter

To palpate the area of the greater trochanter, have the patient turn over on his side.

Trochanteric Bursa. The soft tissues that cross the bony posterior portion of the greater trochanter are protected from it by the trochanteric bursa (Fig. 19). Palpate the trochanter for any tenderness that might indicate trochanteric bursitis. The bursa itself is not palpable unless it is distended or inflamed. If it is inflamed, the area around it feels boggy and may be tender to palpation.

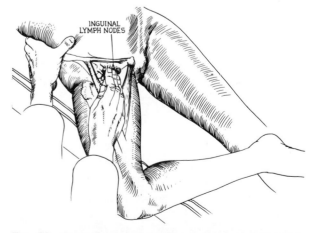

Fig. 18. Tenderness and swelling in the femoral triangle may indicate enlarged lymph nodes as a result of an ascending infection or local pelvic problems.

Gluteus Medius Muscle. This muscle inserts into the upper lateral portion of the trochanter. Occasionally, when the hip is flexed, adducted, and bearing weight, the tensor fascia lata can ride anteriorly over the greater trochanter; an audible and palpable snap becomes perceptible when it returns to a neutral position. This snap usually occurs in activities such as climbing or walking up stairs. While the condition can generate a mild aching sensation or trochanteric bursitis, snapping hip is rarely a problem of any magnitude.

Zone III—Sciatic Nerve

To palpate the soft tissues in this zone, have the patient remain on his side, with his back to you.

Sciatic Nerve. The sciatic nerve is located midway between the greater trochanter and the ischial tuberosity. When the hip is extended, the sciatic nerve is covered by the gluteus maximus muscle, but when it is flexed, the gluteus maximus moves out of the way. Palpate the greater trochanter and the ischial tuberosity again to determine the midpoint between them. If you press firmly into the soft tissue depression at that midpoint, you may be able to feel the sciatic nerve underneath the fatty tissue (Figs. 20 to 22). Tenderness of the nerve may be due to a herniated disc in the lumbar spine, a pyriformis muscle spasm, or direct trauma to the nerve itself, such as a misplaced injection. Note that there is a bursa overlying the ischial tuberosity. Tenderness elicited during palpation of the tuberosity may possibly result from ischial bursitis, a rare finding. Sciatic pain can be easily confused with ischial bursitis and the two structures must be isolated and the precise area of tenderness identified to avoid such an error (Fig. 23).

Zone IV—Iliac Crest

The iliac crest area is clinically significant, first because the cluneal nerves cross it, and second because the gluteus and sartorius muscles originate just below it.

Cluneal Nerves. The cluneal nerves supply sensation to the skin over the iliac crest, between the posterior superior iliac spines and the iliac tubercles. When an iliac bone graft is taken, these nerves are often cut, and the crest should be palpated for possible neuromas in the cluneal nerves (Fig. 24). On occasion, fibro-fatty nodules may be found along the iliac crest. Such palpable enlargements are painful and very tender to the touch (Lumbar Spine Chapter, Fig. 22, page 245).

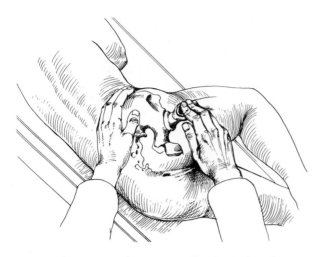

Fig. 19. The trochanteric bursa: Trochanteric pain may be confused with sciatic pain.

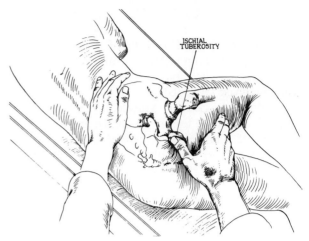

Figs. 20, 21, 22. Palpation of the sciatic nerve: The sciatic nerve is located halfway between the ischial tuberosity and the greater trochanter.

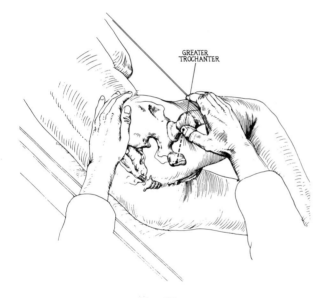

Fig. 21.

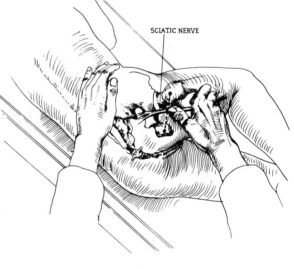

Fig. 22.

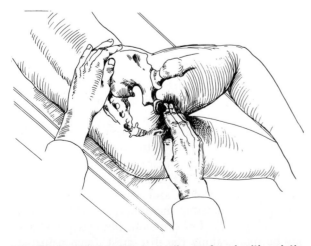

Fig. 23. Ischial bursitis is easily confused with sciatic pain, unless the structures are isolated, and the precise area of pain identified.

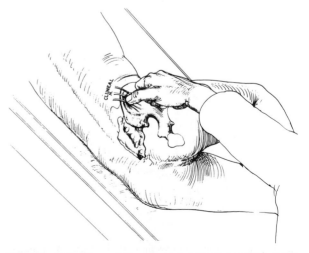

Fig. 24. Palpation of the cluneal nerves as they cross the iliac crest.

Zone V—Hip and Pelvic Muscles

The superficial muscles of the hip and pelvic region lie in quadrants, according to their position and function (Fig. 25):

1) Flexor grouping—anterior quadrant
2) Adductor grouping—medial quadrant
3) Abductor grouping—lateral quadrant
4) Extensor grouping—posterior quadrant

Flexor Grouping

Iliopsoas Muscle. The iliopsoas muscle is the primary hip flexor. It is not palpable, since it lies deep to other muscles and fascia. The psoas bursa lies underneath the iliopsoas, and occasionally the iliopsoas contracting over an inflamed bursa causes pain in the inguinal area (Fig. 26). (Osteoarthritis of the hip commonly causes inflammation of the psoas bursa.) An abnormal contracture of the iliopsoas may lead to a flexion deformity of the hip.

Sartorius Muscle. The sartorius muscle is a long, straplike muscle that runs obliquely down the anterior aspect of the thigh (Fig. 16). For its palpation, see page 151.

Rectus Femoris. The rectus femoris crosses both the hip joint and the knee joint, acting as a flexor for the hip and an extensor for the knee (Fig. 27). It is the only two-joint muscle in the quadriceps group. The rectus femoris has a dual origin, a direct head and an indirect head. Neither head is distinctly palpable, since the muscle disappears proximally in the depression between the sartorius and the tensor fascia lata. Either head (or both) can be torn from its attachments, and the area should be palpated for tenderness. The direct head, which takes origin from the anterior inferior iliac spine, is the more commonly avulsed, usually from sport injuries.

Although it is difficult to distinguish the rectus femoris from the other quadriceps, it is possible to detect an obvious deficit or rupture in the belly of the muscle. The other three muscles of the quadriceps group, the vastus lateralis, the vastus medialis, and the vastus intermedius, are discussed in the Knee Chapter, page 178 (Fig. 28).

Adductor Grouping

The adductor group consists of five muscles: (1) the gracilis, (2) the pectineus, (3) the adductor longus, (4) the adductor brevis, and (5) the adductor magnus. Of these, the adductor longus is the most superficial and the only muscle accessible to palpation. Details for its examination are given on page 151 (Fig. 17).

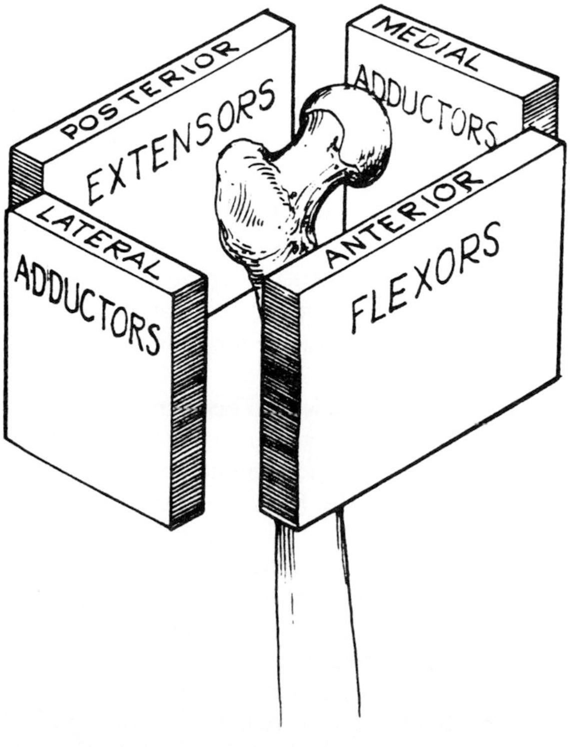

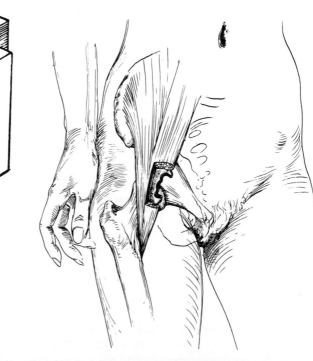

Fig. 25. The superficial hip and pelvic muscles visualized in quadrants, relative to position and function.

Fig. 26. The iliopsoas muscle, contracting over an inflamed bursa, causes inguinal pain.

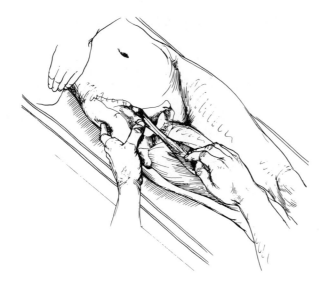

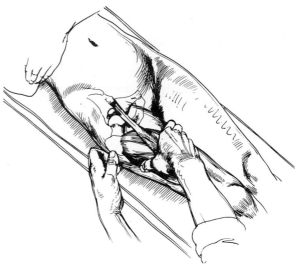

Fig. 27. Palpation of the rectus femoris muscle; there are two heads of origin.

Fig. 28. Palpation of the quadriceps muscle.

Abductor Grouping

The abductor group consists primarily of the gluteus medius and minimus muscles. The minimus lies deep to the medius and is not palpable.

Gluteus Medius Muscle. The gluteus medius muscle is the main hip abductor. It is most easily palpable when the patient lies on his side with his free leg raised in a few degrees of abduction. This position makes the muscle stand out clearly (Fig. 51). Palpate the origin of the gluteus medius, just below the iliac crest, and note any tenderness due to tears or gapping.

The muscle belly is palpable to its insertion into the anterior and lateral aspects of the greater trochanter. Weakness of this muscle results in a "gluteus medius lurch." (See the Gait Chapter, page 137).

Extensor Grouping

The extensor grouping consists of the gluteus maximus and the hamstring muscles.

Gluteus Maximus. The gluteus maximus, a massive, coarse-grained muscle, is the primary hip extensor. Its origin and insertion are difficult to palpate. The outline of the gluteus maximus can be roughly estimated by using some of the bony landmarks located during bony palpation: An imaginary line drawn from the coccyx to the ischial tuberosity represents the maximus' lower border; another line drawn from the posterior superior iliac spine to slightly above the greater trochanter represents the muscle's upper border; and a third line between the posterior superior iliac spine and the coccyx completes the outline (Fig. 29).

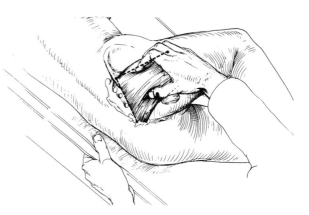

Fig. 29. The origin of the gluteus maximus muscle.

The gluteus maximus is most palpable when the patient is in the prone position, with his buttocks squeezed together. The muscle also becomes prominent when the patient, while prone, extends his hip and flexes his knee (Fig. 50). Both gluteus maximus muscles should be palpated simultaneously to provide instant comparison of tone, size, shape, and quality.

Hamstring Muscles. The hamstring muscles consist of the biceps femoris on the lateral side and the semitendinosus and semimembranosus on the medial side. (See the Knee Chapter, Figs. 35, 39, and 54.) They are palpable from origin to insertion. To palpate their common origins on the ischium, ask the patient to turn on his side, and to bring his knees to his chest. The muscles should be palpated bilaterally and compared for consistency and symmetry of size and shape.

Any tenderness elicited while examining the hamstrings may result from ischial bursitis, or, in the case of a severe injury, from direct damage to the hamstrings. General tenderness or spasm of the muscles may be a result of excessive athletic activity (pulled hamstring). In addition, the hamstrings may go into spasm secondary to a herniated disc in the lower lumbar spine, or to slippage of one lumbar vertebra on another (spondylolisthesis).

RANGE OF MOTION

Active Range of Motion Tests

There are several quick tests designed to determine whether or not there is a gross restriction in the range of hip motion.

ABDUCTION. Ask the patient to stand and to spread his legs apart as far as he can. He should be able to abduct each leg at least 45° from the midline.

ADDUCTION. Instruct the patient to bring his legs together from the abducted position, and alternately cross them, first with the right leg in front, then with the left. He should be able to achieve at least 20° of adduction.

FLEXION. Instruct the patient to draw each knee toward his chest as far as he can without bending his back. He should be able to bring his knees almost to his chest (approximately 135° of flexion).

FLEXION AND ADDUCTION. Have the patient sit in a chair and ask him to cross one thigh over the other.

FLEXION, ABDUCTION, AND EXTERNAL ROTATION. Then, instruct the patient to uncross his thighs and place the lateral side of his foot upon the opposite knee.

EXTENSION. Ask the patient to fold his arms across his chest, and, keeping his back straight, to get up from the chair.

INTERNAL AND EXTERNAL ROTATION. There are no specific, quick active tests for range of internal and external rotation of the femur; however, these functions have been adequately tested in conjunction with the previous tests.

Passive Range of Motion Tests

On occasion, a patient may substitute motion of the pelvis and lumbar spine to compensate for decreased range of hip motion. To accurately evaluate range of hip motion, such compensatory motion must be prevented; the pelvis must be stabilized throughout the following tests.

FLEXION (THOMAS TEST)—120°. Although the Thomas test is a specific test designed to detect flexion contractures of the hip, it may also be used to evaluate range of hip flexion.

The patient should be supine on the examining table, with his pelvis level and square to his trunk so that an imaginary line drawn between the anterior superior iliac spines is perpendicular to the axis of his body. Stabilize the pelvis by placing your hand under the patient's lumbar spine and flexing his hip, bringing his thigh up onto his trunk. As you flex the hip, notice at what point his back touches your hand. The previous lordosis of the lumbar spine is then flattened, the pelvis is stabilized, and further flexion can originate only in the hip joint (Figs. 30, 31). Flex the hip as far as possible. Normal flexion limits allow the anterior portion of the thigh to rest against the abdomen, almost touching the chest wall (Fig. 32). Flex the other hip in a similar manner. Then have the patient hold one leg on his chest and let his other leg down until it is flat on the table. If the hip does not extend fully, the patient may have a fixed flexion contracture of that hip (Fig. 33). If he rocks forward, lifting his thoracic spine from the table, or arches his back to reform the lumbar lordosis when he lowers his leg, a fixed flexion deformity is again indicated, since rocking and arching of the back are compensatory mechanisms to facilitate lowering of a contracted hip. The extent of a flexion contracture can be approximated if you observe the patient from the side and estimate the angle between his leg and the table at the point of greatest extension (Fig. 34).

EXTENSION—30°. Ask the patient to lie prone upon the examining table, and stabilize the pelvis by placing your arm over the iliac crest and lower lumbar spine. Have the patient then bend his knees slightly to relax the hamstring muscles so that they will not be active in hip extension. Now, place your other hand under the thigh and lift his leg upward (Fig. 35). If the hip cannot extend, a flexion contracture is a probable cause. Repeat the test on the opposite side, and compare the ranges of motion.

ABDUCTION—45°-50°. With the patient supine and his legs in the neutral position, stabilize the pelvis by placing your forearm across the abdomen and your hand upon the opposite anterior superior iliac spine. Then, hold one ankle and gently abduct the leg as far as it will go (Fig. 36).

You can feel the pelvis begin to move at the end point of hip abduction. Abduction of both hips can be easily compared if the leg remains in this position while you repeat the same maneuver on the other leg.

Hip abduction can be measured accurately by recording the degrees of abduction for each leg, and measuring the intermalleolar separation during full abduction (Fig. 38). Abduction is more often limited by pathology than adduction.

ADDUCTION—20°–30°. With the patient still supine, continue to stabilize the pelvis and, by holding one ankle, guide the leg across the midline of the body and over the opposite extremity. You can feel the pelvis begin to move at the end point of hip adduction. Measure the range of adduction and repeat the procedure for the opposite hip (Fig. 37). Note that heavy thighs can offer some soft tissue resistance to a full range of adduction.

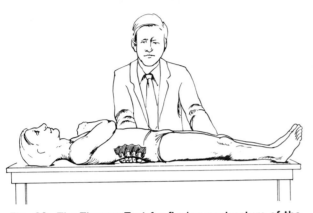

Fig. 30. The Thomas Test for flexion contracture of the hip.

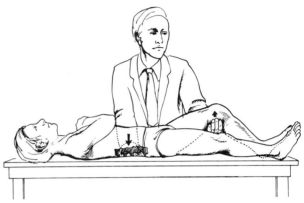

Fig. 31. With the hip flexed, the lumbar spine flattens and the pelvis is stabilized. Further flexion can then only originate in the hip joint.

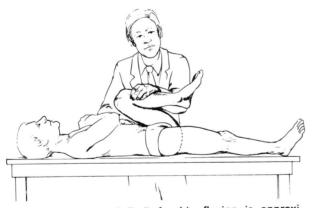

Fig. 32. The normal limit for hip flexion is approximately 135°.

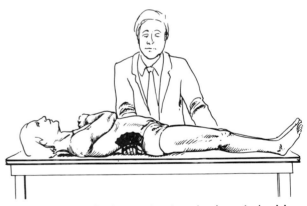

Fig. 33. A fixed flexion contracture is characterized by the inability to extend the leg straight without arching the thoracic spine.

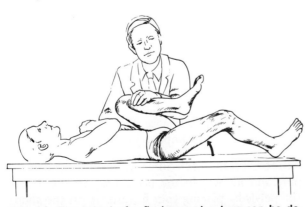

Fig. 34. The extent of a flexion contracture can be determined by estimating the angle between the table and the patient's leg.

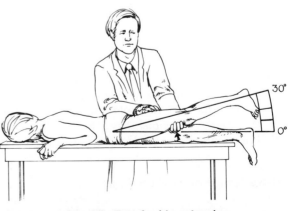

Fig. 35. Test for hip extension.

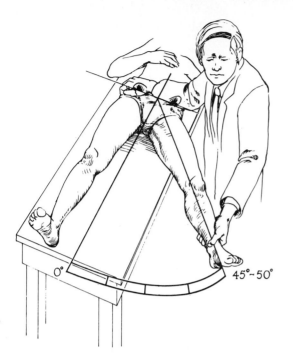

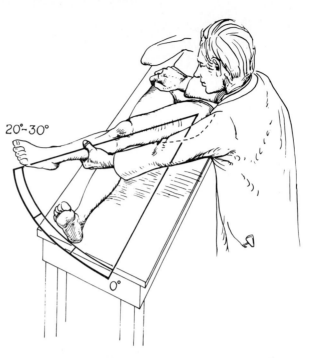

Fig. 36. Normal limits for hip abduction are 45°–50°.   **Fig. 37.** Normal limits for hip adduction are 20°–30°.

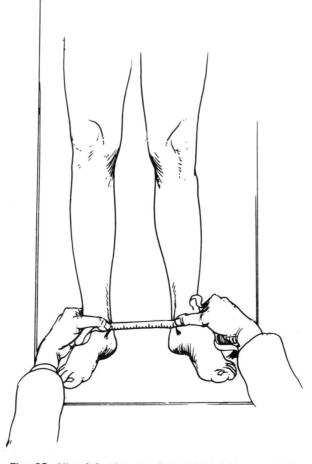

Fig. 38. Hip abduction can be evaluated by measuring the intermalleolar separation.

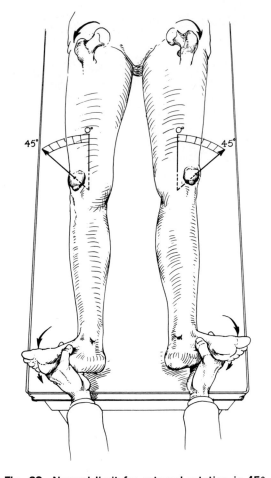

Fig. 39. Normal limit for external rotation is 45°.

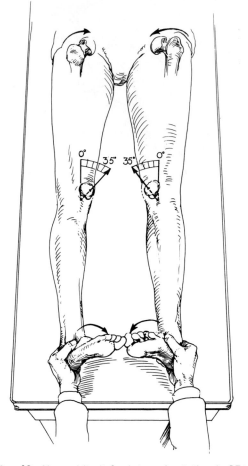

Fig. 40. Normal limit for internal rotation is 35°.

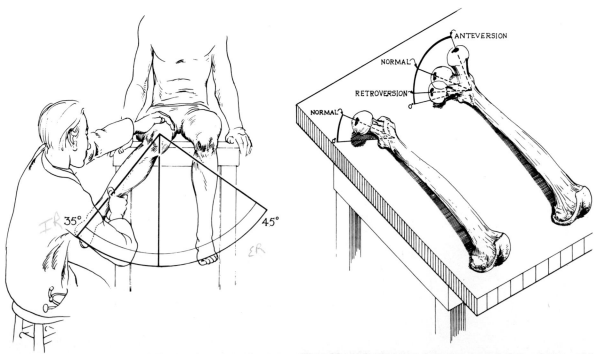

Fig. 41. Test for internal and external femoral rotation in the flexed position.

Fig. 42. Left. Normal anterior angulation of the neck of the femur. **Right.** Anteversion and retroversion of the neck of the femur.

INTERNAL ROTATION—35°
EXTERNAL ROTATION—45°

It is important that the range of femoral rotation be tested with the patient's hip both extended and flexed, since rotation can exist in one position, but be limited in the other. It is perhaps more important that rotation be tested when the hip is extended since hip extension is vital to ambulation.

Have the patient assume a supine position, with his legs extended. Stand at the foot of the table, hold his feet just above the malleoli, and rotate the legs externally and internally, using the proximal end of the patella as a guideline to evaluate range of rotation (Figs. 39, 40).

Alternate Test Method. Keep the patient supine and have him hang his legs over the end of the table with his knees flexed. Stabilize his thigh so that the femur is not pulled from side to side during the test. Then grip the lower end of the tibia and rotate the whole limb externally and internally, using the tibia and fibula as levers. In this position, the tibia will act as a useful pointer and will exaggerate any slight differences of rotation. The procedure should be repeated on the opposite extremity and the findings compared.

Occasionally, the rotation range of an extended hip may differ from that of a flexed hip. To test rotation of the hip in flexion, ask the patient to sit up on the end of the table so that both hips and knees are in 90° of flexion. Stabilize the femur so that it cannot move from side to side during the test. Then grasp the lower end of the tibia and rotate the leg, externally and internally using the tibia and fibula as levers, as in the previous test (Fig. 41).

One possible cause of excessive internal or external hip rotation is femoral neck anteversion or retroversion. Normally the neck of the femur is angled 15° anterior to the long axis of the shaft of the femur and the femoral condyles (Figs. 42, 43). Any increase in this anterior angulation (excessive anteversion) results in a greater internal rotation. Patients who toe-in may have excessive anteversion. Conversely, a decreased anterior angulation (retroversion) results in a greater degree of external rotation. Patients who toe-out may have an excessive retroversion. Ordinarily, infants have a greater degree of anteversion than adults (Figs. 44–48). Also, during the rapid growth period of puberty, the young patient may develop a slipped capital femoral epiphysis (inferior and posterior slipping of the upper femoral epiphysis), which usually results in a relative retroversion, limiting internal rotation and increasing external rotation.

Osteoarthritis can limit motion in all planes, but it most often affects internal rotation and abduction.

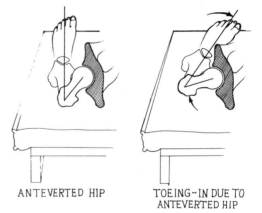

ANTEVERTED HIP   TOEING-IN DUE TO
                        ANTEVERTED HIP

Fig. 44. Excessive femoral neck anteversion can cause a toe-in gait.

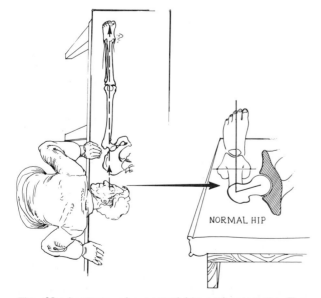

NORMAL HIP

Fig. 43. Anatomy of a normal hip and extremity. Tunnel view.

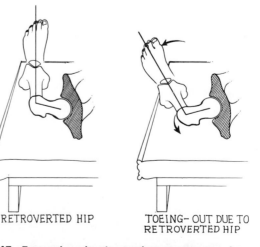

RETROVERTED HIP   TOEING-OUT DUE TO
                        RETROVERTED HIP

Fig. 45. Femoral neck retroversion can cause a toe-out gait.

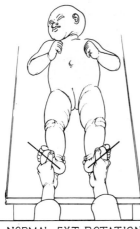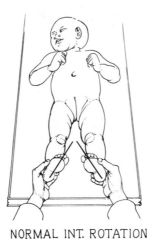

NORMAL EXT. ROTATION   NORMAL INT. ROTATION

Fig. 46. Normal femoral rotation in infants.

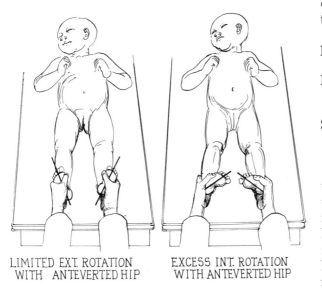

LIMITED EXT. ROTATION   EXCESS INT. ROTATION
WITH ANTEVERTED HIP   WITH ANTEVERTED HIP

Fig. 47. Excessive anteversion is more common in infants than in adults.

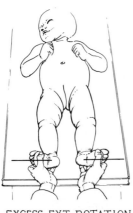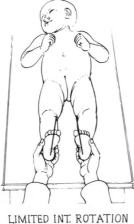

EXCESS EXT. ROTATION   LIMITED INT. ROTATION
WITH RETROVERTED HIP   WITH RETROVERTED HIP

Fig. 48. Excessive femoral retroversion.

NEUROLOGIC EXAMINATION

The neurologic examination of the hip is divided into two parts: (1) muscle testing and (2) sensation testing.

Muscle Testing

The muscles will be tested in functional groups: Flexors, extensors, adductors, and abductors. This type of testing is important for clinical reasons since each functional group receives innervation from a different peripheral nerve, and, in most instances, from a different neurologic level. The integrity of the nerve supply from the spinal cord to the muscle can be partially evaluated by testing the strength of that muscle.

FLEXORS

Primary Flexor
    Iliopsoas
        Femoral Nerve L1,2,3
Secondary Flexor
    Rectus Femoris

To test the iliopsoas muscle, instruct the patient to sit upon the edge of the examining table with his legs dangling. Stabilize the pelvis by placing your hand over the iliac crest, and then ask him to raise his thigh from the table. Place your free hand over the distal end of the thigh and ask him to raise his thigh further, while you offer resistance (Fig. 49). After determining the maximum resistance he can overcome, repeat the test for the opposite iliopsoas muscle, so that muscle strengths can be compared. The iliopsoas is often weakened by reflex action following knee surgery. An abscess formation (from tuberculosis or staphylococcus infection) within its substance also weakens the muscle. After you have determined the maximum resistance the patient may overcome record your findings in accordance with the muscle grading chart (Table 1).

| Table 1. Muscle Grading Chart ||
Muscle Gradations	Description
5—Normal	Complete range of motion against gravity with full resistance
4—Good	Complete range of motion against gravity with some resistance
3—Fair	Complete range of motion against gravity
2—Poor	Complete range of motion with gravity eliminated
1—Trace	Evidence of slight contractility. No joint motion
0—Zero	No evidence of contractility

EXTENSORS

Primary Extensors
    Gluteus Maximus
        Inferior Gluteal Nerve, S1
Secondary Extensor
    Hamstrings

To test the gluteus maximus muscle, ask the patient to lie prone and to flex his knee to relax the hamstring muscle so that it cannot assist the maximus in hip extension. Place your forearm over the iliac crests to stabilize the pelvis, and ask him to raise his thigh from the table. With your other hand, offer resistance to his motion by pushing down on the posterior aspect of the thigh just above the knee joint. The gluteus maximus muscle should be palpated for tone during the test (Fig. 50). Test the opposite side and compare your findings.

The hamstring muscle test is given in the Knee Chapter on page 189.

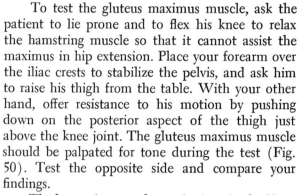

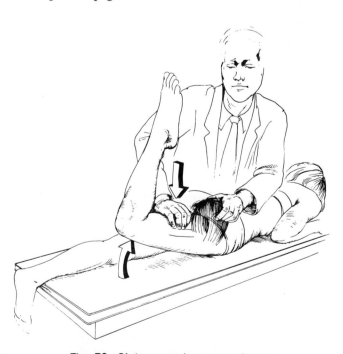

Fig. 49. Flexion muscle test for the iliopsoas muscle.

Fig. 50. Gluteus maximus muscle test.

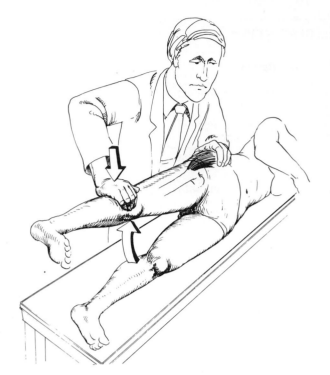

Fig. 51. Muscle test for abduction.

ABDUCTORS

Primary Abductor
    Gluteus Medius
        Superior Gluteal Nerve, L5
Secondary Abductor
    Gluteus Minimus

To test abduction, have the patient turn on his side. Stabilize his pelvis by placing your hand over the iliac crest and tubercle. Then instruct him to abduct his leg. When he has done so, try to return it to adduction by pushing against the lateral side of the thigh. Palpate the gluteus medius muscle as you perform this test (Fig. 51).

Alternate Test Method. With the patient supine and his legs abducted about 20°, place your hands on the lateral sides of his knees and offer resistance to further abduction. In this way, the abductors can be compared simultaneously (Fig. 52).

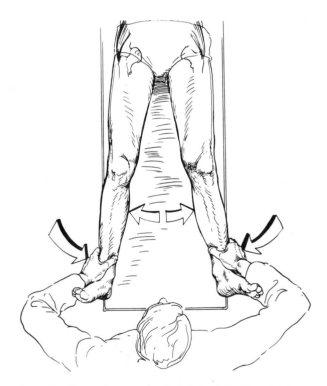

Fig. 52. Alternate muscle test for abduction (gluteus medius).

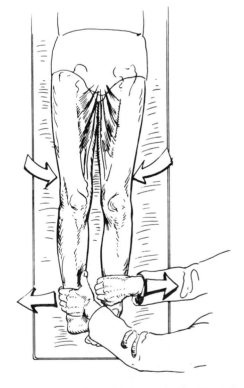

Fig. 53. Test for adductor muscle strength.

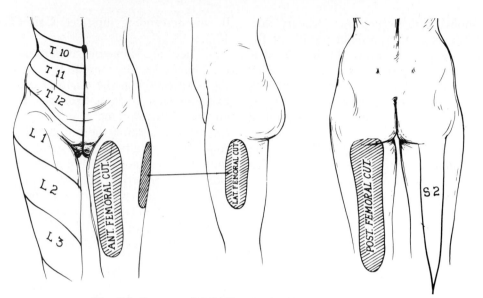

Fig. 54. Sensory distribution to the hip and pelvis.

ADDUCTORS

Primary Adductor
    Adductor Longus
        Obturator Nerve, L2,3,4
Secondary Adductors
    Adductor brevis
    Adductor magnus
    Pectineus
    Gracilis

Have the patient lie on his side and abduct his leg. Then place your hand on the medial side of his knee, and ask him to try to pull his leg back toward the midline of the body against your resistance. After you have determined the maximum resistance he can overcome, test the opposite side and compare your findings.

Alternate Test Method. The patient should either be seated or lying supine with legs abducted. Have him adduct his legs while you exert resisting pressure on the medial aspects of both knees. This test permits direct comparison of the strength of the adductors (Fig. 53).

Sensation Tests

Sensation is supplied to the hip, pelvic region, and thigh by nerves taking origin from roots in the lower thoracic, lumbar, and sacral spines. The

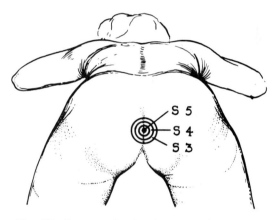

Fig. 55. Sensory distribution around the anus.

areas supplied by each particular neurologic level are broadly defined as bands, or dermatomes, which cover certain areas of skin. Roughly, the dermatomes of the anterior abdominal wall run in transverse, slightly oblique bands: The strip approximately level with the umbilicus is supplied by T10, the strip immediately above the inguinal ligament is supplied by T12, and the area in between is supplied by T11. The sensory area of L1 lies immediately below the inguinal ligament and parallel to it on the upper anterior portion of the thigh. An oblique band immediately above the kneecap represents L3, and the area between L1 and L3 on the midthigh is supplied by L2 (Fig. 54).

The cluneal nerves (posterior primary divisions of L1,2,3) cross the posterior portion of the iliac crest and supply sensation: (1) over the iliac crest, (2) between the posterior superior iliac spine and the iliac tubercle, and (3) over the buttocks (Fig. 24). The posterior cutaneous nerve of the thigh (S2) supplies sensation to a longitudinal band on the posterior aspect of the thigh, extending from the gluteal crease to beyond the popliteal fossa. The lateral cutaneous nerve of the thigh (S3) supplies sensation to a broad, oval area on the lateral aspect of the thigh (Fig. 54).

The dermatomes around the anus are arranged in three concentric rings, receiving innervation from S2 (the outermost ring), S3, and S4 (the innermost ring) (Fig. 55).

SPECIAL TESTS

TRENDELENBURG TEST. This procedure is designed to evaluate the strength of the gluteus medius muscle. Stand behind the patient and observe the dimples overlying the posterior superior iliac spines. Normally, when the patient bears weight evenly on both legs, these dimples appear level. Then ask the patient to stand on one leg. If he stands erect, the gluteus medius muscle on the supported side should contract as soon as the leg leaves the ground and should elevate the pelvis on the unsupported side. This elevation indicates that the gluteus medius muscle on the supported side is functioning properly (negative Trendelenburg sign) (Fig. 56). However, if the pelvis on the unsupported side remains in position or actually descends, the gluteus medius muscle on the supported side is either weak or nonfunctioning (positive Trendelenburg sign) (Fig. 56).

During gait, the gluteus medius acts much as a tie rod since it prevents the unsupported hip from dropping and causing instability. If the gluteus medius muscle is weak, the patient may exhibit the characteristic Trendelenburg, or gluteus medius, lurch to counteract the imbalance caused by his descending hip (see Gait Chapter, page 137).

There are numerous conditions that weaken the gluteus medius muscle. For instance, any pathology that brings the origin of the muscle closer to its insertion, such as coxa vara, fractures of the greater trochanter, or a slipped capital femoral epiphysis, can cause the muscle to become weak. Another possibility is a congenital dislocation of the hip, which not only brings the muscle's origin closer to its insertion, but also destroys the normal fulcrum around which it functions. In addition, neurologic problems, including poliomyelitis, meningomyelocele, or a root lesion within the spinal canal, may cause denervation of the gluteus medius muscle.

TESTS FOR LEG LENGTH DISCREPANCY. If, during the inspection portion of your examination, you suspect that one of your patient's legs might be shorter than the other, the following procedures will assist you in determining whether the discrepancy is true or only apparent.

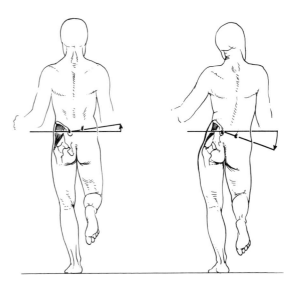

Fig. 56. The Trendelenburg Test. **Left.** Negative. **Right.** Positive.

True Leg Length Discrepancy. To determine true leg length, first place the patient's legs in precisely comparable positions and measure the distance from the anterior superior iliac spines to the medial malleoli of the ankles (from one fixed bony point to another) (Fig. 57). Begin measurement at the slight concavity just below the anterior superior iliac spine, for the tape measure may slide if pressed directly onto the spine. Unequal distances between these fixed points verify that one lower extremity is shorter than the other (Fig. 58).

To determine in short order where the discrepancy lies (whether in the tibia or in the femur), ask the patient to lie supine, with his knees flexed to 90° and his feet flat on the table. If one knee appears higher than the other, the tibia of that extremity is longer (Fig. 59A). If one knee projects further anteriorly than the other, the femur of that extremity is longer (Fig. 59B). A

true shortening may be the result of poliomyelitis, or of a fracture that crossed the epiphyseal plate during childhood.

Apparent Leg Length Discrepancy. Establish that there is no true leg length discrepancy before testing for an apparent discrepancy, in which there is no true bony inequality. Apparent shortening may stem from pelvic obliquity or from adduction or flexion deformity in the hip joint. During inspection, pelvic obliquity manifests itself as uneven anterior or posterior superior iliac spines while the patient is standing.

Have the patient lie supine with his legs in as neutral position as is possible, and take a measurement from the umbilicus (or xiphisternal juncture) to the medial malleoli of the ankle (from a nonfixed point to a fixed bony point) (Fig. 60). Unequal distances signify an apparent leg length discrepancy (Fig. 61), particularly if the true leg length measurements are equal (Fig. 62).

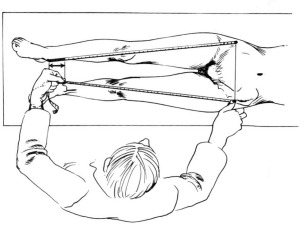

Fig. 57. Measure from one fixed bony point to another to find true leg length.

Fig. 58. True leg length discrepancy.

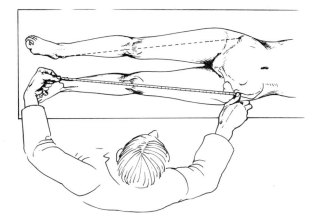
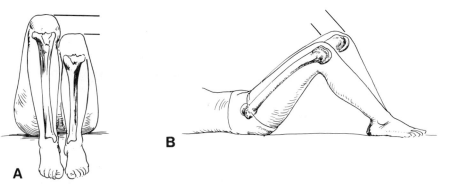

Fig. 59. A. Tibial length discrepancy. B. Femoral length discrepancy.

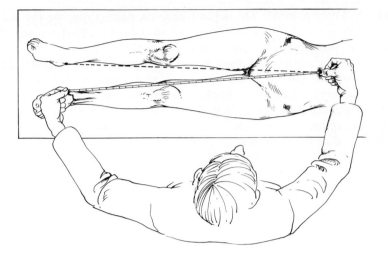

Fig. 60. Measure from a nonfixed point to a fixed point to determine an apparent leg length discrepancy.

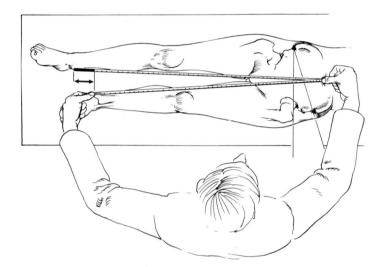

Fig. 61. An apparent leg length discrepancy associated with pelvic obliquity.

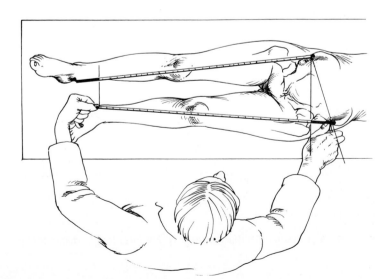

Fig. 62. True leg length measurements are equal despite the apparent leg length discrepancy.

OBER TEST FOR CONTRACTION OF THE ILIOTIBIAL BAND.

Have the patient lie on his side with his involved leg uppermost. Abduct the leg as far as possible and flex the knee to 90° while keeping the hip joint in the neutral position to relax the iliotibial tract (Fig. 63). Then release the abducted leg. If the iliotibial tract is normal, the thigh should drop to the adducted position (Fig. 64). However, if there is a contracture of the fascia lata or iliotibial band, the thigh remains abducted when the leg is released (Fig. 65). Such continued abduction (a positive Ober Test) may be caused by poliomyelitis or meningomyelocele.

THOMAS TEST FOR FLEXION CONTRAC-TURE.

The Thomas Test has been described previously in the passive test for range of hip flexion, page 155.

TESTS FOR CONGENITAL DISLOCATION OF THE HIP

Ortolani Click. If, in conjunction with a congenitally dislocated hip, the flexed thigh is abducted and externally rotated, the femoral head can slide over the acetabular rim, reducing the hip and producing a palpable click, or jerk. The click may also be audible as the femoral head enters and leaves the acetabular. A congenitally dislocated hip limits abduction on the involved side (Figs. 66, 67).

Telescoping. Congenital dislocation of the hip may be diagnosed by pushing and pulling the femur in relation to the pelvis. With one hand, apply traction to the femur at the level of the knee. With the other hand, stabilize the pelvis and place your thumb on the greater trochanter. You may be able to feel the greater trochanter move distally when you apply traction to the femur and return to its previous position upon the release of traction. This abnormal to-and-fro motion of the greater trochanter is called "telescoping." It indicates congenital dislocation of the hip (Fig. 68).

Adduction Contracture. Flex the patient's hips to 90° and abduct them. Normally, you should obtain 90° of bilateral abduction. Infants with congenitally dislocated hips have a limited abduction of 20° or less. If a baby has a unilateral hip dislocation, you should be able to see the difference in the abduction ranges of the two hips (Fig. 67).

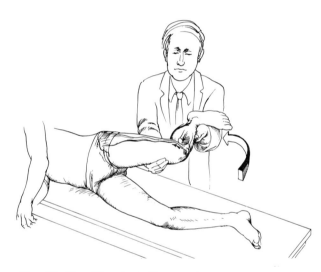

Fig. 63. The Ober test: To test for contraction of the fascia lata.

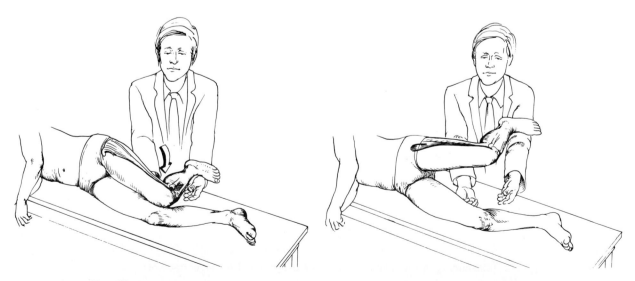

Fig. 64. A negative Ober.

Fig. 65. A positive Ober.

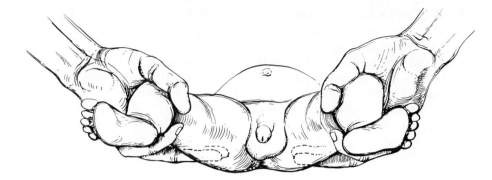

Fig. 66. In the newborn, both hips can be equally flexed, abducted, and externally rotated without producing a "click."

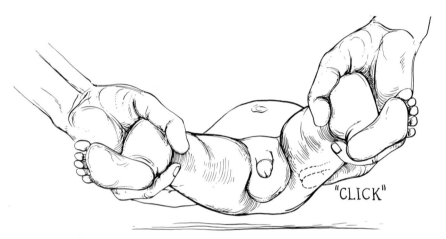

Fig. 67. A diagnosis of a congenital dislocation of the hip may be confirmed by the Ortolani "click" test. The involved hip is not able to be abducted as far as the opposite one, and there is a "click" as the hip reduces.

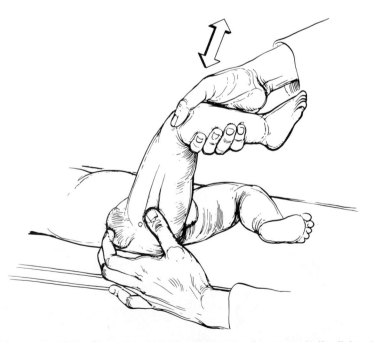

Fig. 68. Telescoping of the femur to aid in the diagnosis of a congenitally dislocated hip.

EXAMINATION OF RELATED AREAS

Most often, primary hip pain is perceived as inguinal pain. Symptoms of pain in the hip's posterior aspect are usually referred from the lumbar spine, and run along the course of the sciatic nerve. In some instances, pain may also be referred to the hip from the knee (Fig. 69).

Rectal Examination

This is an essential part of an examination of the pelvic area, since it is the best way to directly palpate the coccyx and the sacrococcygeal joint. To examine the rectum, ask the patient to lie on his side. Initially the anus should be checked for the normal corrugated appearance. If sphincter tone is absent, the anus appears flattened out and there is no corrugation of the skin and muscle around it (patulous anus).

Put on a surgical glove and lubricate the index finger. At first touch, notice whether or not the superficial anal reflex (S2, 3, 4) is present. Then, have the patient bear down as if he were moving his bowels to relax the anal sphincter muscles and allow your finger to enter the rectum without too much discomfort. The internal contours of the anus should be smooth. As you palpate, you should be able to feel the deep sphincter muscle grip your finger (deep anal reflex, S5). The absence of the deep anal reflex indicates an S5 defect.

Insert your finger into the rectum as far as possible, then rotate it so that its palmar surface rests against the coccyx. Palpate the coccyx with your thumb outside the rectum and your index finger inside, and move it as a unit, rocking it at the sacrococcygeal joint (Fig. 70). Any major points of tenderness (coccydynia) should be noted.

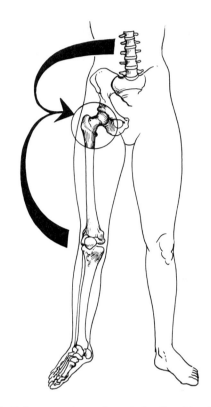

Fig. 69. Pain may be referred to the hip from the lumbar spine and from the knee.

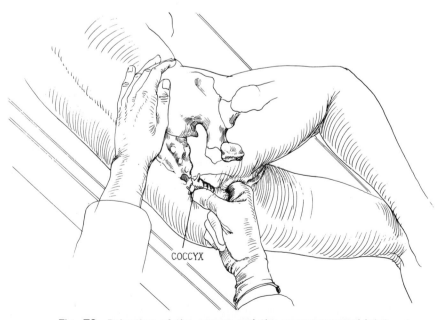

COCCYX

Fig. 70. Palpation of the coccyx and the sacrococcygeal joint.

7

Physical Examination of the Knee

The knee is the largest joint in the body. It is a ginglymus (modified hinge) joint, and as such provides a fairly wide range of motion. Like the elbow, the knee's greatest range of motion is in flexion.

The knee is usually susceptible to traumatic injury primarily because it is subject to maximum stress, located as it is at the end of two long lever arms, the tibia and the femur. In addition, since the knee is not protected by layers of fat or muscle, its exposure, both environmentally and anatomically, contributes to its high incidence of injury.

The bony contours of the knee are prominent and easily palpable, and the diagnostic process is far easier for it than for the other joints.

INSPECTION

When the patient first walks into the examination room, his gait should flow in a smooth, rhythmic motion. As stated in Chapter 5, the knee is bent during swing phase; the quadriceps then contract to begin lower limb acceleration. After the midpoint of swing phase, the hamstrings contract to decelerate the leg in preparation for heel strike. The knee should be fully extended at heel strike. It then remains flexed during all stages of stance phase.

After analyzing the patient's gait, ask him to remove his clothing from the waist down (the underwear need not be removed). While he is in the process of undressing, watch carefully when he bends to remove his shoes and stockings and note any abnormal movement used to compensate for pain or stiffness in the knee joint.

In the knee, swelling is classified as one of two types, either localized (bursal) or generalized (intra-articular). A bursal swelling is more frequently found over the patella (prepatellar bursitis), or over the tibial tubercle (infrapatellar bursitis). Occasionally, a bursal swelling may present in the popliteal fossa (due to a cyst) or over the medial aspect of the tibial tubercle (pes anserine bursitis).

Intra-articular hemorrhage, irritation of the synovium (synovitis) causing secretion of synovial fluid, or synovial thickening all can precipitate a generalized swelling which affects the entire knee. Generalized swelling either partially or fully obscures the knee's normal contour; the knee is usually slightly flexed to accommodate the swelling, since its volume is greater in partial flexion than in extension.

Inspect the symmetry of the muscle contours above the knee for any visible muscular atrophy, particularly at the point where the muscles approach the knee. Note particularly the vastus medialis muscle, which often atrophies secondary to knee surgery.

To inspect the anterior aspect of the knee, have the patient stand straight, with knees extended fully; the patellas should be symmetrical and level. Normally, the tibia has a slight valgus angulation in comparison to the femur (Fig. 1). ("Valgus" refers to the bone distal to the joint, which in the knee is the tibia. To remember that valgus refers to lateral, associate the "l" in lateral with the "l" in valgus.) The valgus angle is usually more pronounced in females. Excessive valgus (knock-knees) or varus (bowlegs) are two of the more common deformities of the knee joint (Fig. 2).

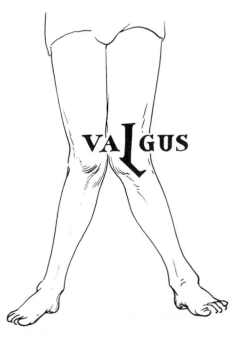

Fig. 1. Excessive valgus angulation.

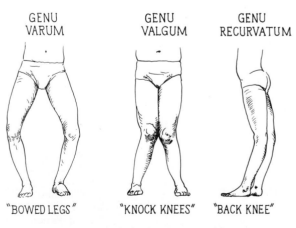

GENU VARUM   GENU VALGUM   GENU RECURVATUM

"BOWED LEGS"   "KNOCK KNEES"   "BACK KNEE"

Fig. 2. Common types of knee deformity.

From the side, note that the knee should be fully extended when the patient is standing. Knees which are slightly flexed indicate pathology if the patient cannot straighten them upon command, particularly if flexion is unilateral. Slight hyperextension is normal, provided that it is bilateral. The incidence of hyperextension of the knees is higher among females and among those individuals with "lax ligaments" (genu recurvatum) (Fig. 2).

BONY PALPATION

In preparation for palpation, have the patient sit on the edge of an examining table. The knee is more accessible if you are seated on an examination stool facing him. In this position, you can anchor his leg between yours, leaving both hands free for examination. A bed patient should be supine with his knees flexed to 90°.

Since some of the knee's contours disappear entirely in extension, the knee is easier to palpate when it is flexed, when the skin stretches tautly over the bones and makes the skeletal landmarks more distinct. In addition, the muscles, tendons, and ligaments around the joint become relaxed in the flexed, non-weight-bearing position, making it much easier to palpate the bony prominences and the joint margins.

Medial Aspect

To orient yourself for palpation, place your hands upon the knee joint so that your fingers curve around to the posterior popliteal area. Place your thumbs on the anterior portion of the knee and press into the soft tissue depressions on either side of the infrapatellar tendon (Figs. 3, 4). These depressions serve as central points of orientation for the palpation of the medial aspect of the knee joint. When you press into them, you are actually palpating a portion of the joint line between the femur and tibia.

Medial Tibial Plateau. Push your thumb inferiorly into the soft tissue depression until you can feel the sharp upper edge of the medial tibial plateau (Fig. 5). The upper, nonarticulating edge of the plateau is palpable posteriorly to the junction of the tibial plateau and the femoral condyle and anteriorly to the infrapatellar tendon. The plateau itself serves as one point of attachment for the medial meniscus (Fig. 6).

Tibial Tubercle. Follow the infrapatellar tendon distally to where it inserts into the tibial tubercle (Figs. 7, 8). Just medial to the tubercle lies the subcutaneous surface of the tibia, below the flare of the tibial plateau (Fig. 9). This area is of clinical significance because of the pes anserine insertion and bursa.

Medial Femoral Condyle. As you move your thumb upward, you will find the medial femoral condyle (Fig. 10), part of which is palpable immediately medial to the patella. More of the femoral condyle is accessible to palpation if the knee is flexed more than 90°. Occasionally, you may be able to feel a defect in the cartilaginous surface, secondary to osteochondral fragments or to osteoarthritis. The condyle is also palpable along its sharp medial edge, proximally as far as the superior portion of the patella and distally to the junction of the tibia and femur (Fig. 11). Small excrescences of bone (osteophytes) are often palpable in individuals with osteoarthritis of the knee.

Adductor Tubercle. Return to the medial surface of the medial femoral condyle (Fig. 12), and move further posteriorly until you locate the adductor tubercle in the distal end of the natural depression between the vastus medialis and hamstring muscles (Figs. 13, 14).

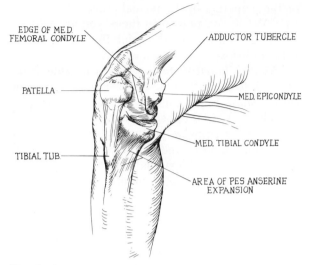

Fig. 3. Anatomy of the knee joint (anteromedial aspect).

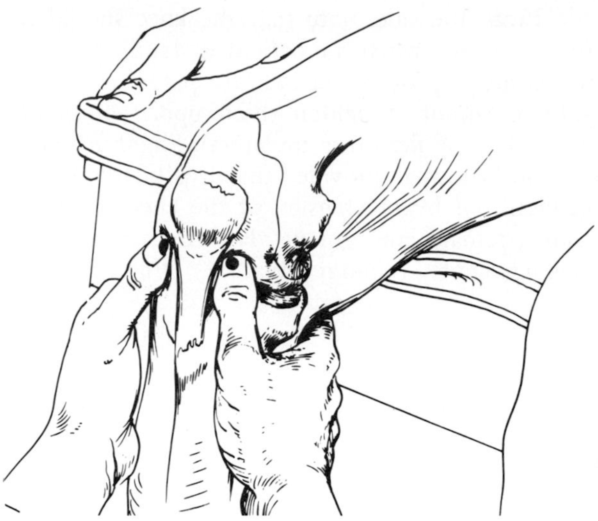

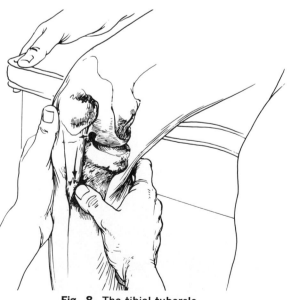

Fig. 4. Points of orientation for palpation of the knee.

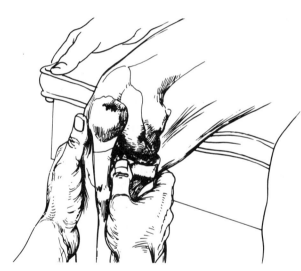

Fig. 5. The medial tibial plateau.

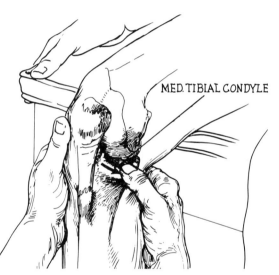

Fig. 6. The tibial plateau is a point of attachment for the medial meniscus.

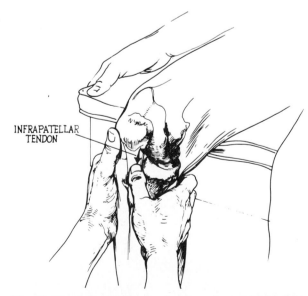

Fig. 7. The infrapatellar tendon is palpated toward its insertion.

Fig. 8. The tibial tubercle.

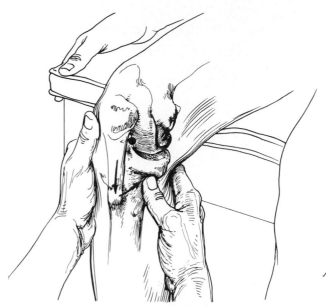

Fig. 9. The flare of the medial tibial plateau. The pes anserine insertion and bursa are located here.

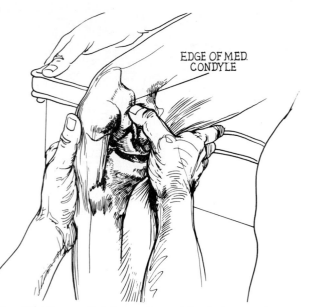

Fig. 10. The medial femoral condyle; it has a sharp medial edge.

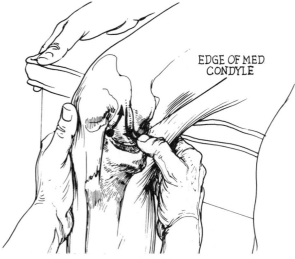

Fig. 11. The medial femoral condyle is palpable distally to the junction of the femur and tibia.

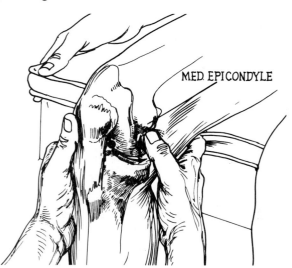

Fig. 12. The medial surface of the medial femoral condyle, the medial epicondyle.

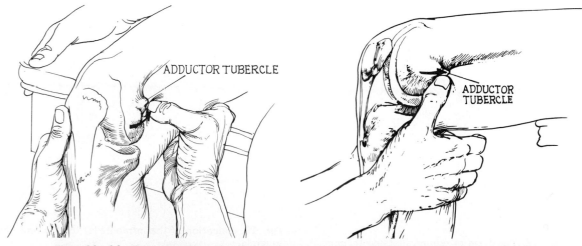

Figs. 13, 14. The adductor tubercle is located on the posterior medial portion of the medial femoral epicondyle.

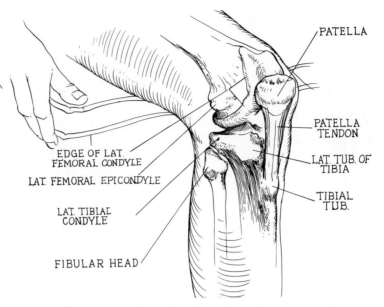

Fig. 15. Anatomy of the knee joint (anterolateral aspect).

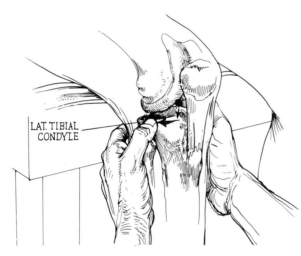

Fig. 16. The lateral tibial plateau.

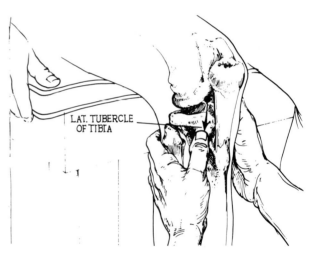

Fig. 17. Palpation of the lateral tibial tubercle.

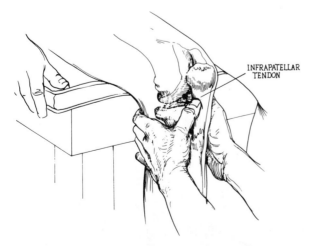

Fig. 18. Palpation of the infrapatellar tendon.

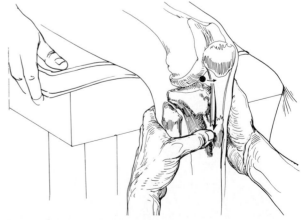

Fig. 19. Palpation of the infrapatellar tendon and tibial tubercle.

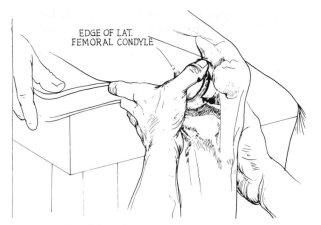

Fig. 20. The lateral femoral condyle.

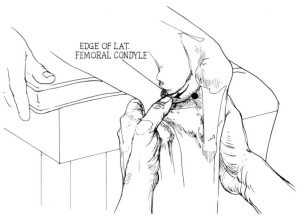

Fig. 21. The lateral femoral condyle is palpable distally to the tibia/femur juncture.

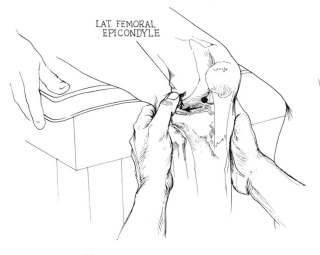

Fig. 22. The lateral femoral epicondyle.

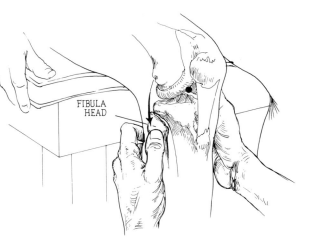

Fig. 23. The head of the fibula.

Lateral Aspect

The soft tissue depression just lateral to the infrapatellar tendon is the point of orientation for palpation of the bony prominences of the lateral aspect (Fig. 15).

Lateral Tibial Plateau.   Push down with your thumb into the soft tissue depression until you feel the upper edge of the lateral tibial plateau (Fig. 16). Palpate it along its sharp edge (lateral joint line) to the junction of the tibia and femur.

Lateral Tubercle.   The lateral tubercle is the large prominence of bone immediately below the lateral tibial plateau (Fig. 17). Palpate it as you again palpate the infrapatellar tendon and the tibial tubercle (Figs. 18, 19).

Lateral Femoral Condyle.   Return to the soft tissue depression and move upward and laterally onto the sharp edge of the lateral femoral condyle (Fig. 20). It is palpable along its smooth surface as far as the junction of the tibia and femur

(Fig. 21). Since much of it is covered by the patella, the lateral femoral condyle has less surface available for palpation than the medial femoral condyle. If the knee is flexed past 90°, however, more of the condylar articulating surface becomes palpable.

Lateral Femoral Epicondyle.   The lateral femoral epicondyle lies lateral to the lateral femoral condyle (Fig. 22).

Head of the Fibula.   From the lateral femoral epicondyle, move your thumb inferiorly and posteriorly across the joint line. The fibular head is situated at about the same level as the tibial tubercle (Fig. 23).

Trochlear Groove and Patella

The trochlear groove, the track in which the patella glides, is covered by articular cartilage but does not articulate with the tibia.

After placing your thumbs over the medial and lateral joint lines, move upward along the two

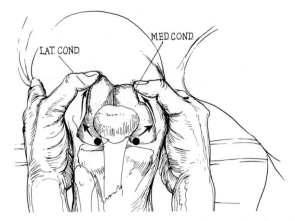

Fig. 24. Palpation of the medial and lateral walls of the trochlear groove. Notice that the lateral wall is higher.

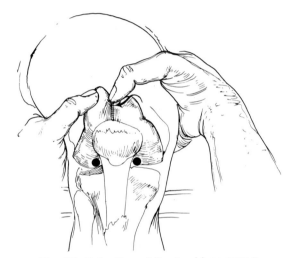

Fig. 25. Palpation of the trochlear groove.

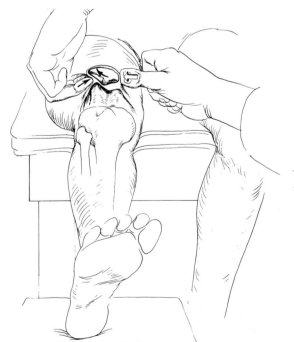

Fig. 26. Full knee extension permits palpation of the under surface of the patella.

femoral condyles to the highest point of the patella (Fig. 24). Then, above the patella, palpate toward the midline until you reach the depression of the trochlear groove (Fig. 25).

The patella is fixed in the trochlear groove in flexion and mobile in extension. Thus, the medial and lateral portions of the patella's undersurface are much more accessible to palpation when the knee is extended (Fig. 26). Note that it is easier to push the patella medially than laterally. Occasionally, you may find a cartilaginous defect under the patella or a roughened patellar border secondary to osteoarthritis.

SOFT TISSUE PALPATION

Soft tissue palpation is divided into four clinical zones: (1) the anterior aspect, (2) the medial aspect, (3) the lateral aspect, and (4) the posterior aspect.

To facilitate palpation of the soft tissue structures of the knee, have the patient sit on the end of the examining table, with his knees flexed to 90°. Then sit on a stool facing him.

Zone I—Anterior Aspect

Quadriceps. The quadriceps generally insert as a group into the superior and medial borders of the patella. The quadriceps tendon then crosses over the patella to form the infrapatellar tendon, which inserts into the tibial tubercle. Two of the quadriceps group, the vastus medialis and

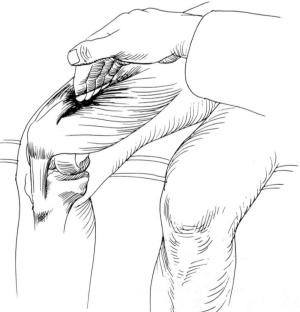

Fig. 27. A defect in the quadriceps muscle.

the vastus lateralis, form visible bulges on the medial and lateral sides of the knee and are easily palpable. They become more prominent upon isometric contraction. Notice that the muscle mass of the medialis extends further distally than the mass of the lateralis. Since the other quadriceps muscles are wrapped in a common fascial covering, it is difficult to palpate them; therefore, evaluate them as a unit. Palpate both thighs simultaneously, comparing the quadriceps for symmetry of definition and noting any defects such as ruptures and tears. Defects are most often found distally in the rectus femoris or the vastus intermedius just proximal to the patella (Fig. 27). They may present as transverse defects which feel softer than the normally firm quadriceps muscles. Look for any signs of atrophy, particularly in the vastus medialis, which frequently atrophies following knee joint effusion and knee surgery. Evaluate for atrophy of the quadriceps mechanism by using the edge of the tibial plateau as a fixed bony reference point and measuring the circumference of each thigh about three inches above the knee. Any difference in girth is significant (Fig. 28).

Infrapatellar Tendon. This tendon runs from the inferior border of the patella, and is palpable to its insertion into the tibial tubercle. This site of insertion is often tender in young individuals (Osgood-Schlatter's syndrome) (Fig. 29). The infrapatellar fat pad lies immediately posterior to the infrapatellar tendon at the level of the joint line, and tenderness elicited here may be evidence of hypertrophy or contusion of the fat pad. When the infrapatellar tendon has been avulsed from its insertion, it no longer feels rigid; instead, a palpable defect develops, along with extreme tenderness in the area of the tibial tubercle.

Since bursitis is a rather common ailment around the knee joint, the examiner should be familiar with the location of those clinically significant bursae in the area (Fig. 30). Most of these bursae are situated in the anterior clinical zone.

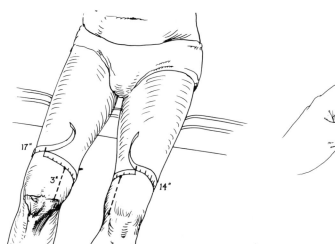

Fig. 28. The quadriceps may be evaluated for possible atrophy by measuring 3 inches up the thigh from the medial tibial plateau edge, and, at that point, measuring the thigh's circumference.

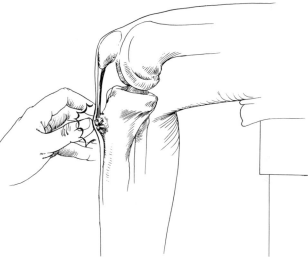

Fig. 29. Osgood-Schlatter syndrome—tenderness and swelling at the site of the infrapatellar tendon insertion into the tibial tubercle.

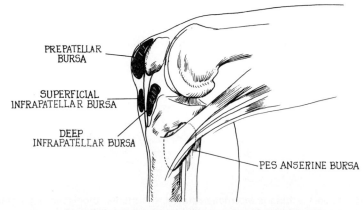

Fig. 30. Clinically significant bursae of the knee.

Superficial Infrapatellar Bursa. The superficial infrapatellar bursa lies in front of the infrapatellar tendon, and can become inflamed as a result of excessive kneeling.

Prepatellar Bursa. The prepatellar bursa overlies the anterior portion of the patella. It is subject to inflammation as a result of the combination of excessive kneeling and leaning forward (housemaid's knee). Note that, when the leg is extended, the skin over the patella can be picked up, much like the skin over the olecranon of the elbow. The prepatellar bursa aids in allowing the skin to glide freely over the patella, especially in flexion.

Pes Anserine Bursa. The pes anserine bursa is located between the tendons of the sartorius, gracilis, and semitendinosus muscles (pes anserine insertion) and the upper-medial aspect of the tibia, just medial to the tibial tubercle. It is not palpable. However, if it becomes inflamed, you may be able to feel some effusion and thickening.

Zone II— Medial Aspect

Beginning at the medial soft tissue depression, move your thumb medially and posteriorly along the upper edge of the tibial plateau, until you find the junction of the tibia and femur.

Medial Meniscus. The medial meniscus is attached to the upper edge of the plateau by small coronary ligaments. These ligaments are difficult to palpate; however, if the meniscus is detached (due

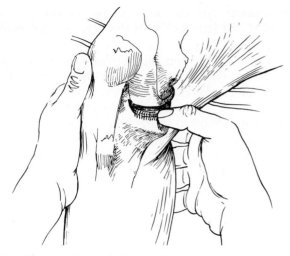

Fig. 31. Palpation of the medial meniscus (anterior portion and the coronary ligaments).

to tears in the coronary ligaments), tenderness may be elicited in the joint margin area. The anterior margin of the medial meniscus itself is just barely palpable deep within the joint space (Fig. 31). The meniscus is somewhat mobile, and when the tibia is internally rotated, its medial edge becomes more prominent and palpable. Conversely, upon external rotation of the tibia, the meniscus retracts and is not palpable (Fig. 32). When the meniscus has been torn, the area of the medial joint line becomes tender to palpation. Tears are much more common in the medial meniscus than they are in the lateral meniscus.

Medial Collateral Ligament. The medial

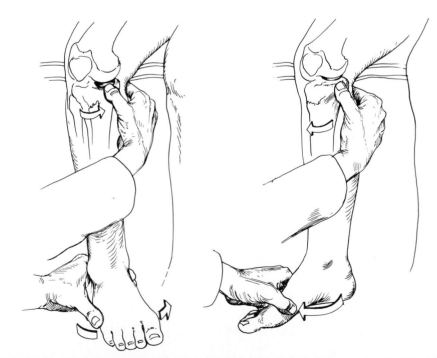

Fig. 32. Left. When the tibia is internally rotated, the medial meniscus is palpable. **Right.** When the tibia is externally rotated, the medial meniscus retracts.

collateral ligament, a broad, fan-shaped ligament, joins the medial femoral epicondyle and the tibia. The ligament has both a deep and a superficial portion. The deep portion inserts directly into the edge of the tibial plateau and meniscus, while the superficial portion inserts, more distally, onto the flare of the tibia. To palpate the anatomic region of the medial collateral ligament (the ligament itself is not distinctly palpable), first relocate the medial joint line. As you move medially and posteriorly along the joint line, the ligament lies directly under your fingertips. The medial collateral ligament is part of the joint capsule, and is frequently torn in valgus stress injuries, such as clipping injuries in football. Palpate the area of the ligament from origin to insertion for tenderness and interruption in continuity (Fig. 33). If it is avulsed from the medial epicondyle, the ligament may elevate a small bony fragment with it, in which case the point of origin becomes tender to palpation. If the ligament is torn at its midpoint, the tendon and

overlying soft tissue may be shredded. In that event, the defect becomes palpable and there is tenderness at the level of the medial joint line.

Sartorius, Gracilis, and Semitendinosus Muscles. On the posteromedial side of the knee, the tendons of these muscles form a visible ridge that crosses the knee joint before they insert into the lower portion of the medial tibial plateau (Fig. 34). They help support the knee's medial side, which is under considerable strain in gait due to the valgus angle between the femur and tibia.

To palpate these tendons, stabilize the patient's leg by holding it securely with your own legs. This frees your hands for palpation. In addition, you are in a position to offer resistance against knee flexion, which makes the tendons prominent. Cup your fingers around the knee and feel the tautness of the tendons (Fig. 35). Of this tendinous group, the semitendinosus is the most posterior and inferior tendon you can feel. The next tendon, the gracilis, lies slightly anterior and medial to the

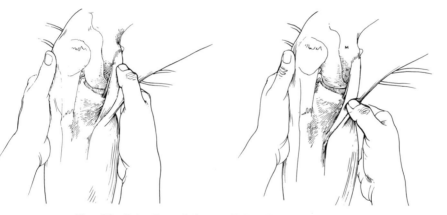

Fig. 33. Palpation of the medial collateral ligament.

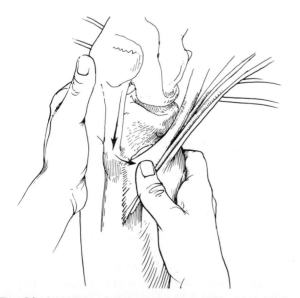

Fig. 34. Insertion of the sartorius, gracilis, and semitendinosus tendons.

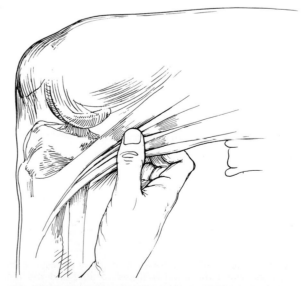

Fig. 35. Palpation of the sartorius, gracilis, and semitendinosus tendons.

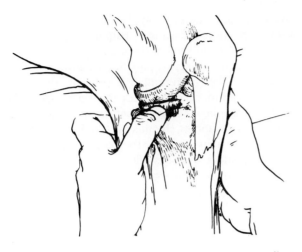

Fig. 36. The lateral meniscus and its coronary ligaments.

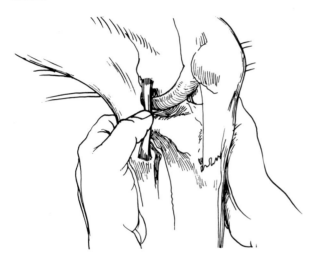

Fig. 37. The lateral collateral ligament.

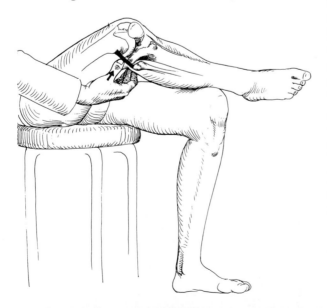

Fig. 38. The lateral collateral ligament is accessible to palpation when the knee is flexed to 90°, and the hip is abducted and externally rotated.

semitendinosus. The gracilis becomes even more prominent if you offer resistance to internal rotation of the leg. The tendons of the semitendinosus and gracilis muscles are round and should not be confused with the deeper semimembranosus tendon, which remains muscular to its insertion. The wide, thick band of the muscle just above the gracilis tendon is the sartorius. Since it is not as tendinous as the gracilis and the semitendinosus, the sartorius tendon is more difficult to palpate. The insertion of the semimembranosus muscle lies deep to this tendinous group on the posterior aspect of the tibia; you can palpate it by thrusting your fingers between the semitendinosus and the gracilis tendons. The semimembranosus is rarely pathologically involved except in cases of massive trauma to the knee. It is sometimes utilized as a muscle transplant to reinforce the knee's medial side. At the common insertion of these muscles lies the pes anserine bursa, which may become inflamed and cause pain during motion.

Zone III—Lateral Aspect

Lateral Meniscus. The lateral meniscus is best palpated when the patient's knee is in slight flexion, for it usually disappears within the joint upon full extension. The lateral meniscus is secured to the edge of the tibial plateau by coronary ligaments, which, when torn, can cause the meniscus to become detached. In such a case, the area is tender to palpation (Fig. 36).

If you probe firmly into the lateral joint space with your thumb, you may be able to feel the anterior margin of the lateral meniscus. The meniscus is attached to the popliteus muscle and not to the lateral collateral ligament. It is therefore more mobile than the medial meniscus. Perhaps because of its mobility, the lateral meniscus is seldom torn. When it is, the area of the lateral joint line becomes tender to palpation. Occasionally, a cyst of the lateral meniscus develops at the joint line. It is palpable as a firm, tender mass.

Lateral Collateral Ligament. The lateral collateral ligament is a stout cord that joins the lateral femoral epicondyle and the fibular head. It exists independently from the joint capsule (Fig. 37). To palpate it, have the patient cross his legs so that his ankle rests upon the opposite knee. When the knee is flexed to 90° and the hip is abducted and externally rotated, the iliotibial tract relaxes and makes the lateral collateral ligament easier to isolate. The ligament stands away from the joint itself, and lies laterally and posteriorly along the joint line (Fig. 38). The ligament may be torn in certain knee joint injuries, but the incidence of such tearing is not as high as for the medial collateral ligament. When it is torn, it becomes tender to palpation. Occasionally, the lateral collateral ligament is congenitally absent.

Anterior Superior Tibiofibular Ligament. This ligament lies in the crevice between the tibia and the fibular head. If you move anteriorly and medially from the head of the fibula, you can feel where the anterior superior tibiofibular ligament crosses the tibia/fibula articulation. Palpate the ligament for purposes of anatomic definition since it is rarely pathologically involved.

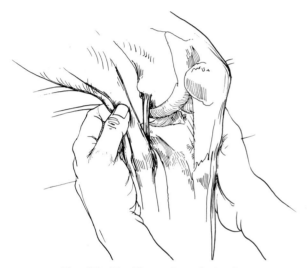

Fig. 39. The biceps femoris tendon.

Biceps Femoris Tendon. When the knee is flexed, the biceps femoris tendon becomes prominent where it crosses the knee joint before inserting into the fibular head (Fig. 39). It should be palpated near its insertion for any defects that may be present. The tendon is rarely torn, but can be avulsed from the fibula upon a severe trauma to the knee. The biceps femoris muscle and tendon should not be confused with the iliotibial tract.

Iliotibial Tract. The iliotibial tract is situated more anteriorly on the lateral aspect of the knee. It is palpable to the point where it inserts into the lateral tibial tubercle. The iliotibial tract is neither a muscle nor a tendon, but rather a long, thick band of fascia. The tract is more conveniently palpable when the knee is extended and the leg raised or when, against resistance, the knee is flexed. The anterior border immediately lateral to the superior pole of the patella is the portion most available for palpation (Fig. 40). Contractures in its substance are often a cause of knee deformity in paralytic cases such as poliomyelitis and meningomyelocele.

Common Peroneal Nerve. The common peroneal nerve is palpable where it crosses the neck of the fibula. The nerve can be rolled gently between the tip of your finger and the neck of the fibula, slightly inferior to the insertion of the biceps femoris muscle (Fig. 41). The common peroneal nerve must be palpated very carefully, since excessive pressure can injure it and cause foot drop.

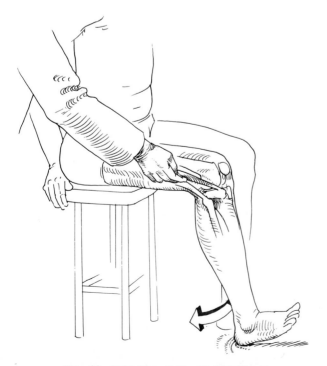

Fig. 40. Palpation of the iliotibial tract.

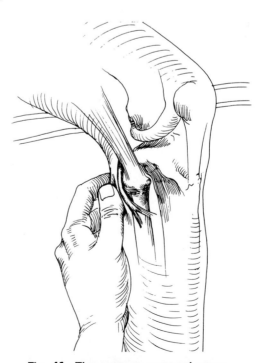

Fig. 41. The common peroneal nerve.

Zone IV—Posterior Aspect

Popliteal Fossa. The superior lateral border of the popliteal fossa is defined by the prominent biceps femoris tendon. The tendons of the semi-membranosus and the semitendinosus muscles form the superior medial border, while the inferior borders are formed by the two heads of the gastrocnemius muscles where they emerge from the fossa to enter the calf. A group of significant structures cross the popliteal area:

Posterior Tibial Nerve. The posterior tibial nerve, a branch of the sciatic nerve, is the most superficial structure crossing the popliteal area.

Popliteal Vein. The popliteal vein lies directly under the posterior tibial nerve.

Popliteal Artery. The popliteal artery, the deepest structure in the area, runs flush against the joint capsule.

When the knee is extended, the fascia covering the fossa is pulled tight and the structures underlying it are difficult to palpate. However, the fascia and muscles relax in flexion, and the deeper areas of the fossa become accessible to palpation (Fig. 42). Because the popliteal artery is covered by the fascia, the nerve, and the vein, it may be difficult to feel the popliteal pulse. Absence of this pulse may be due to vascular occlusive disease at a higher level in the extremity. A discrete swelling in the fossa may indicate a popliteal cyst, or Baker's cyst (commonly a distention of the gastrocnemius–semimembranosus bursa). This type of cyst is usually a painless, mobile swelling appearing on the medial side of the fossa, and is more readily palpable when the patient's knee is extended (Fig. 43).

Gastrocnemius Muscle. The two heads of this muscle are palpable at their origin on the posterior femoral surface just above the medial and lateral condyles when the patient flexes his knee against resistance. The gastroc heads are not as distinctly palpable as the hamstring muscle tendons just above them. If the gastroc is torn, you may be able to feel a small defect in the belly of the muscle; however, more often than not, palpation of the muscle reveals only slight tenderness.

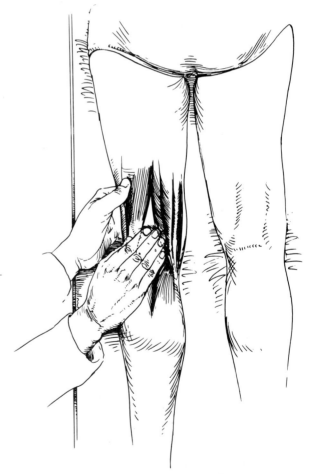

Fig. 43. Palpation of the popliteal fossa for Baker's cyst.

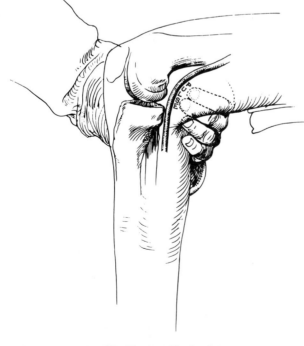

Fig. 42. The popliteal artery.

TESTS FOR JOINT STABILITY

The knee joint owes its stability to a strong and extensive joint capsule, collateral ligaments, cruciate ligaments, and surrounding muscles and tendons. The following tests evaluate the strength and integrity of those structures.

Collateral Ligaments

Ask the patient to lie supine on the table with one knee flexed just enough so that it unlocks from full extension. To test the medial collateral ligament, secure his ankle with one hand and place the other hand around the knee so that your thenar eminence is against the fibular head. Then, push medially against the knee and laterally against the ankle in an attempt to open the knee joint on the inside (valgus stress) (Fig. 44). Palpate the medial joint line for gapping, which may even be visible. If there is a gap, the medial collateral ligament is not supporting the knee prop-

erly. When stress on the injured joint is relieved, you can feel the tibia and femur "clunk" together as they close.

To test the lateral aspect of the knee for stability, reverse the position of your hands, and push laterally against the knee and medially against the ankle to open the knee joint on the lateral side (varus stress). Again, palpate the lateral joint line for any gapping (Fig. 45). As on the medial side, such a gap may be both palpable and visible. Upon the release of varus stress, the tibia and femur may clunk into position as they close.

If your fingers are too short to reach around the knee to palpate the joint lines, secure the patient's foot between your arm and body (in the axilla) so that your hands are free to palpate the joint line. In this way, your body acts as a lever on the foot and applies varus and valgus stress to the knee joint (Figs. 44, 45).

Since the medial collateral ligament is critical to stability, an isolated tear of this ligament leads to joint instability, whereas a similar defect in the lateral collateral ligament may have little effect either way. Most ligamentous injuries around the knee occur on the medial side.

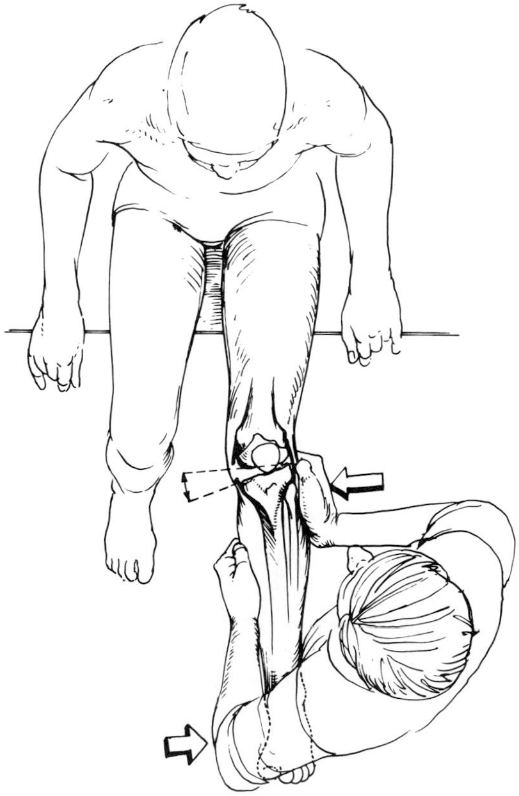

Fig. 44. To test the medial collateral ligament, apply valgus stress to open the knee joint on the medial side.

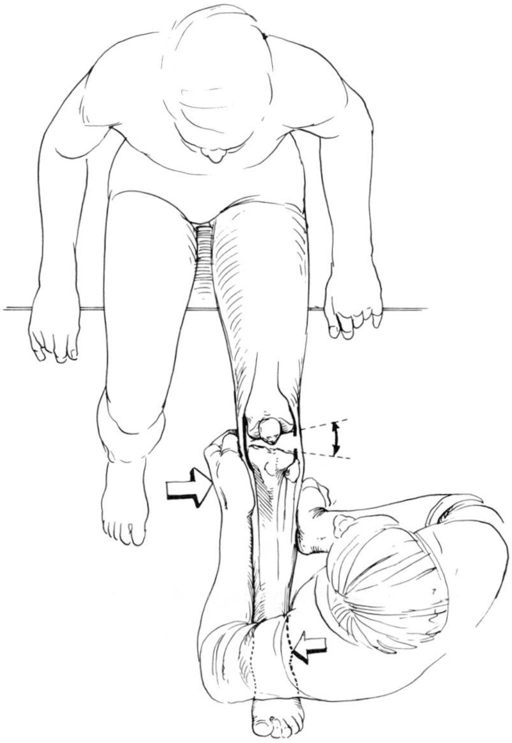

Fig. 45. To test the lateral knee for stability, apply varus stress to open the knee joint on the lateral side.

Cruciate Ligaments

The anterior and posterior cruciate ligaments are instrumental in preventing anterior and posterior dislocation of the tibia on the femur. These ligaments are intracapsular, originating on the tibia and inserting into the inner sides of the femoral condyles.

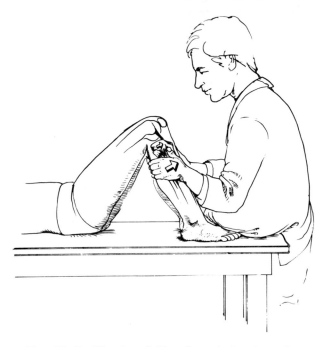

Fig. 46. Position for eliciting the anterior draw sign.

To test the integrity of the anterior cruciate ligament, have the patient lie supine on the examination table with his knees flexed to 90° and his feet flat on the table. Position yourself on the edge of the table so that you can stabilize his foot by sitting on it. Then cup your hands around his knee, with your fingers on the area of insertion of the medial and lateral hamstrings and your thumbs on the medial and lateral joint lines. Now, draw the tibia toward you (Fig. 46); if it slides forward from under the femur (positive anterior draw sign), the anterior cruciate ligament may be torn (Fig. 47). A few degrees of anterior draw are normal if an equal amount is present on the opposite side.

When you do find a positive anterior draw sign, it is important to repeat the maneuver with the patient's leg in internal and external rotation. External rotation of the leg tightens the posteromedial portion of the joint capsule; normally, there should then be reduced forward movement of the tibia on the femur, even if the anterior cruciate ligament is torn. Thus, if forward movement with the leg externally rotated is equal to forward movement with the leg in the neutral position, both the anterior cruciate ligament and the posteromedial portion of the joint capsule (and possibly the medial collateral ligament) may be damaged. Internal rotation tightens the structures on the posterolateral side of the knee. Normally, there should be reduced movement when the leg is pulled forward, even if the anterior cruciate ligament is torn. If the amount of forward movement

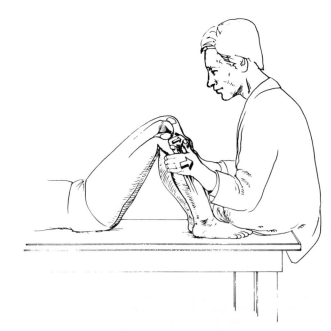

Fig. 47. A positive anterior draw sign: Torn anterior cruciate ligament.

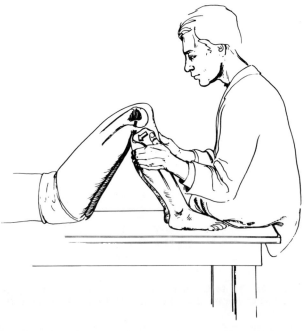

Fig. 48. A positive posterior draw sign: Torn posterior cruciate ligament.

of the tibia on the femur in internal rotation is equal to that in the neutral position, both the anterior cruciate ligament and the posterolateral portion of the joint capsule may be torn. The anterior cruciate ligament may be torn in association with tears of the medial collateral ligament.

Test the posterior cruciate ligament in a similar manner. Stay in the same position and push the tibia posteriorly (Fig. 48). If it moves backward on the femur, the posterior cruciate ligament is probably damaged (positive posterior draw sign). The anterior draw sign is more common than the posterior sign, since the incidence of damage to the anterior cruciate is much higher than to the posterior cruciate. In fact, an isolated tear of the posterior cruciate ligament is rare.

These tests for stability of the anterior and posterior cruciate ligaments are usually performed in one continuous motion and have been separated here mainly for the purpose of instruction. All procedures should be performed bilaterally, and all findings compared.

RANGE OF MOTION

There are three basic movements in the knee joint: (1) flexion (associated with glide), (2) extension (associated with glide), and (3) internal and external rotation.

Flexion and extension are primarily the result of movement between the femur and the tibia. Internal and external rotation involve displacement of the menisci on the tibia, as well as movement between the tibia and the femur. Extension is performed by the quadriceps, while flexion is performed by the hamstrings and gravity. Internal and external rotation (which take place when the knee

is slightly flexed) are performed by the reciprocal action of the semimembranosus, semitendinosus, gracilis, and sartorius on the medial side, and the biceps on the lateral side.

Active Range of Motion

The following quick tests determine whether or not there is any gross restriction in a patient's range of knee motion.

FLEXION. Ask the patient to squat in a deep knee bend. He should be able to flex both knees symmetrically.

EXTENSION. Instruct the patient to stand up from the squatting position, and take careful notice of whether he is able to stand straight, with knees in full extension, or whether one leg is relied upon more than the other during the procedure. You may also instruct him to sit on the edge of the examination table and to extend his knee fully (Fig. 49). The arc of motion from flexion to extension should be smooth. On occasion, a patient may be unable to extend the knee through the last 10° of motion and may be able to finish extension only haltingly, and with great effort. This is referred to as *extension lag* (Fig. 50). It frequently accompanies quadriceps weakness.

Note that the leg cannot be extended fully without some amount of external tibial rotation on the femur because of the physical configuration of the knee joint and its cruciate ligaments (A. Helfet's Helix). The medial femoral condyle is approximately a half-inch longer than the lateral femoral condyle. Therefore, as the tibia moves on the femoral condyles into full extension, it uses all available articulating surface on the lateral side,

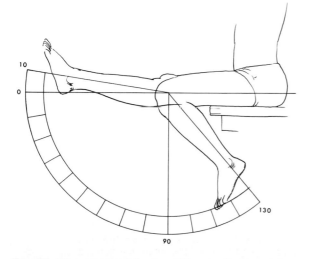

Fig. 49. The range of knee motion in flexion and extension.

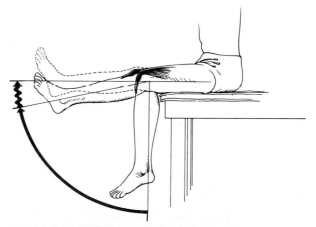

Fig. 50. Extension lag, when the last 10° or so of extension are performed haltingly and with difficulty.

while leaving about a half inch on the medial side. To use the remaining articular surface on the medial side and reach full extension, the medial side of the tibia must rotate laterally around the lateral femoral condyle. This lateral rotation allows the medial femoral condyle to complete its extension, and, in effect, "locks the knee joint home" in the full extension position (Fig. 51). The final locking movement (commonly called "screw home" motion) allows the patient to maintain the knee in extension over prolonged periods of standing without relying on his muscles.

Test screw home motion as follows: Draw one dot on the midpoint of the patella and another over the tibial tubercle while the patient's knee is flexed. The dot over the tibial tubercle should line up with the dot on the midpoint of the patella. Now, ask the patient to extend his leg fully. The tibial tubercle should rotate laterally from under its dot, indicating that the tibia has rotated externally on the femur. The tibial tubercle has also turned slightly lateral to the dot over the midpoint of the patella (Fig. 52). A torn meniscus may prevent screw home motion and block full extension of the knee.

INTERNAL AND EXTERNAL ROTATION.
Instruct your patient to rotate his foot medially and laterally, to test the knee's range of rotation. Under normal circumstances, he should be able to rotate the foot about 10° to either side.

Passive Range of Motion

FLEXION—135°. The patient may lie either prone or supine on an examining table, or he may sit on the very edge of the table with the popliteal fossa away from it and his legs dangling free. Grasp one leg at the ankle joint and place your other hand in the popliteal fossa to act as a fulcrum and to unlock the knee. Then, flex the leg as far as it will go, noting the distance between heel and buttock. With younger patients, it is relatively easy to flex the leg all the way so that the heel almost touches the buttock. The normal end point of knee flexion for adults is approximately 135° from an extended position. The same procedure should be repeated on the opposite leg and the ranges of knee flexion compared.

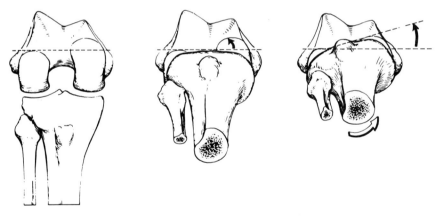

Fig. 51. Screw home motion of the knee with extension. In the non-weight-bearing position, the tibia externally rotates on the femur.

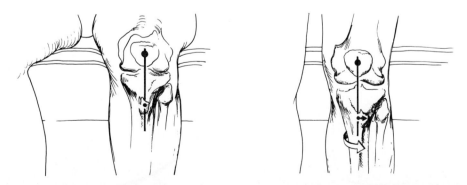

Fig. 52. Screw home motion test. **Left.** When the knee is flexed, place a dot on the midpoint of the patella and another over the tibial tubercle. **Right.** When the knee is extended, the tubercle rotates laterally from under the dot, indicating that the tibia has rotated externally on the femur.

EXTENSION—0°. Maintain your hands in position on the patient's ankle and knee and extend his knee. The arc of motion from flexion to extension should be smooth, and the knees should extend bilaterally to at least 0°, or beyond and into a few degrees of hyperextension.

INTERNAL ROTATION—10°
EXTERNAL ROTATION—10°

Place your hand on the patient's thigh just above the knee to stabilize the femur, grasp his heel with your free hand, and rotate the tibia. At the same time, palpate the tibial tubercle to ensure that it is moving. Perform the same test on the opposite leg and compare your findings. Normally, there should be approximately 10° of rotary motion to each side.

NEUROLOGIC EXAMINATION

Muscle Testing

EXTENSION

Primary Extensor
  Quadriceps
    Femoral nerve, L2, L3, L4

The extension of the knee was tested in part during the quick test for active range of motion (see page 187). Now, to perform the manual test, stabilize the thigh by placing one hand just above the knee. Then, instruct the patient to fully extend his knee. Once the knee is fully extended, offer resistance to extension just above the ankle joint. Palpate the quadriceps with your stabilizing hand during this test (Fig. 53).

FLEXION

Primary Flexor
  Hamstrings
    1) Semimembranosus
        tibial portion of sciatic nerve, L5
    2) Semitendinosus
        tibial portion of sciatic nerve, L5
    3) Biceps Femoris
        tibial portion of sciatic nerve, S1

To test the hamstrings as a group, have the patient lie supine on the examining table and stabilize his thigh just above the knee. Then instruct him to flex his knee while you resist his motion at the back of his ankle joint (Fig. 54). To bring the biceps femoris into greater activity, have the patient rotate his leg externally during the test. Similarly, to bring the semimembranosus and semitendinosus muscles into greater activity, instruct him to rotate his leg internally.

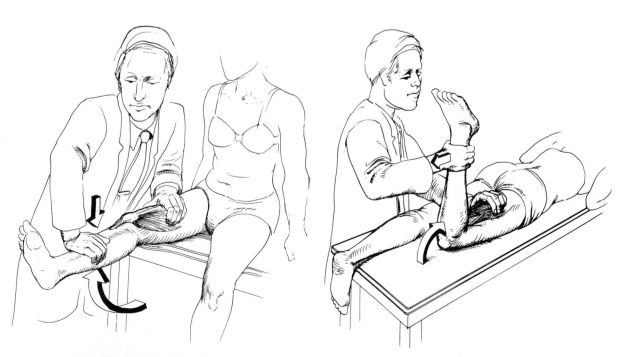

Fig. 53. Quadriceps muscle test.   **Fig. 54.** Hamstring muscle test.

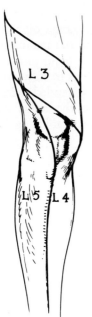
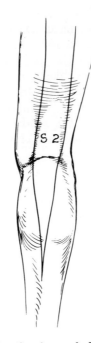

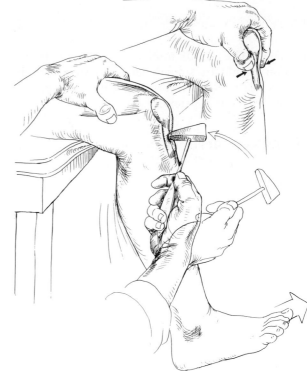

Fig. 55. Sensory distribution to the knee. **Left.** Anterior. **Right.** Posterior.

Fig. 56. The patellar reflex.

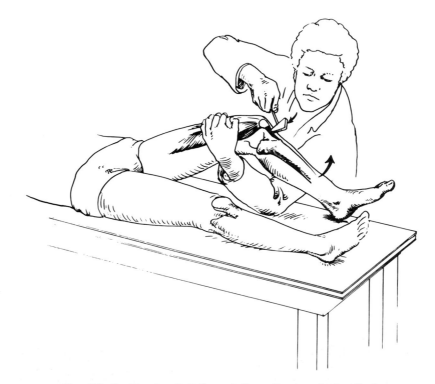

Fig. 57. Position to elicit the patellar reflex on a bed patient.

INTERNAL AND EXTERNAL ROTATION.

The muscles that allow internal and external rotation in the knee cannot be isolated for clinical testing. However, their strength has been tested earlier, in conjunction with the muscle tests for flexion and extension.

Sensation Testing

Those nerves taking origin from roots in the lumbar and sacral spines provide sensation to the skin over the knee and surrounding areas. The areas supplied by each particular neurologic level define broad bands, or dermatomes, which cover certain areas of the skin (Fig. 55).

Roughly, the sensory dermatomes of the knee region run in long, oblique bands as follows:

1) **L4** crosses the anterior portion of the knee, continuing down the medial side of the leg. The infrapatellar branch of the saphenous nerve supplies the skin over the area of the anteromedial flare of the tibial condyle. The saphenous nerve is the only sensory branch of the femoral nerve that continues into the leg. Its infrapatellar branch is often cut during knee surgery, particularly during the surgical removal of the medial meniscus.
2) **L3** spans the anterior thigh immediately at and above the knee joint. It is supplied by the femoral nerve.
3) **L2** crosses the anterior portion of the middle of the thigh and is supplied by the femoral nerve.
4) **S2** outlines a strip down the midline of the posterior thigh and the popliteal fossa. It is supplied by the posterior femoral cutaneous nerve of the thigh (Fig. 55).

Reflex Testing

PATELLAR REFLEX: L2, 3, 4. The patellar reflex, or knee jerk, is a deep tendon reflex, mediated through nerves emanating from the L2, 3, and 4 neurologic levels, but predominantly from **L4.** For clinical application, the patellar reflex is to be considered an **L4** reflex. However, even if the **L4** nerve root is pathologically involved, the reflex may still be present, since it is innervated by more than one neurologic level. While the patellar reflex may be significantly diminished, it is rarely totally absent.

To test this reflex, have your patient sit on the edge of the examining table with his legs dangling free (Fig. 56), or have him sit on a chair with one leg crossed over his knee. If he is a bed patient, support his knee in a few degrees of flexion (Fig. 57). In these positions, the infrapatellar tendon is stretched and primed. Then, to locate the tendon accurately, palpate the soft tissue depression on either side of the infrapatellar tendon. Elicit the reflex by tapping the tendon with a neurologic hammer at the level of the knee joint, using a short, smart wrist action. If the reflex is difficult to obtain, reinforce it by having the patient clasp his hands and attempt to pull them apart as you tap the tendon. The procedure should be repeated on the opposite leg, and the reflexes graded as normal, increased, decreased, or absent.

SPECIAL TESTS

McMURRAY TEST. During knee flexion and extension, a torn meniscus may produce a palpable or audible "clicking" in the region of the joint line. Tenderness elicited in palpation of the joint line on either side suggests the possibility of a torn meniscus. Posterior meniscal tears are difficult to identify, and the McMurray test was originally developed to assist in this difficult diagnosis.

Ask the patient to lie supine with his legs flat and in the neutral position. With one hand, take hold of his heel and flex his leg fully (Fig. 58). Then, place your free hand on the knee joint with your fingers touching the medial joint line and your thumb and thenar eminence against the lateral joint line, and rotate the leg internally and externally to loosen the knee joint (Fig. 59). Push on the lateral side to apply valgus stress to the medial side of the joint, while, at the same time, rotating the leg externally (Fig. 60). Maintain the valgus stress and external rotation, and extend the leg slowly as you palpate the medial joint line (Fig. 61). If this maneuver causes a palpable or audible "click" within the joint, there is a probable tear in the medial meniscus, most likely in its posterior half.

APLEY'S COMPRESSION AND DISTRACTION TESTS

Compression or Grinding Test. This is another procedure designed to aid in the diagnosis of a torn meniscus. Ask your patient to lie prone on the examining table with one leg flexed to 90°. Gently kneel on the back of his thigh to stabilize it

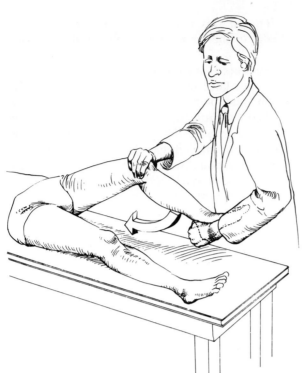

Fig. 58. The McMurray test for meniscal tears. Flex the knee.

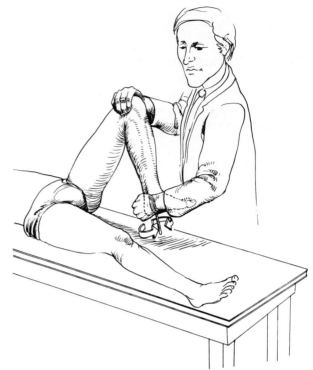

Fig. 59. With the knee flexed, internally and externally rotate the tibia on the femur.

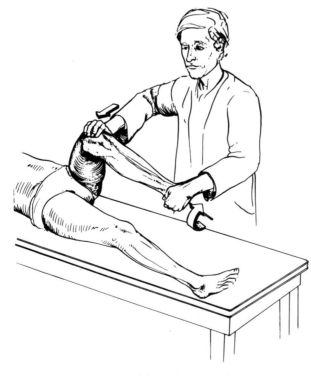

Fig. 60. With the leg externally rotated, place a valgus stress on the knee.

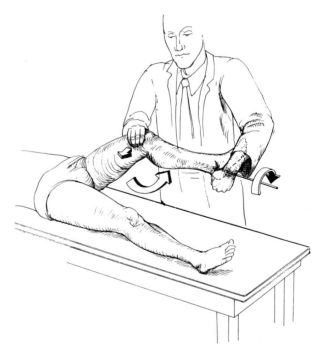

Fig. 61. With the leg externally rotated and in valgus, slowly extend the knee. If click is palpable or audible, the test is considered positive for a torn medial meniscus, usually in the posterior position.

while leaning hard on the heel to compress the medial and lateral menisci between the tibia and the femur (Fig. 62). Then, rotate the tibia internally and externally on the femur as you maintain firm compression. If this maneuver elicits pain, there is probably meniscal damage. Ask your patient to describe the location of his pain as accurately as possible. Pain on the medial side indicates a damaged medial meniscus; pain on the lateral side suggests a lateral meniscal tear.

Distraction Test. The distraction test helps to distinguish between meniscal and ligamentous problems of the knee joint. This test should follow the compression test in logical progression. Remain in the same position described for the compression test, and maintain your stabilization of the posterior thigh. Apply traction to the leg while rotating the tibia internally and externally on the femur (Fig. 63). This maneuver reduces pressure on the meniscus and puts strain upon the lateral and medial ligamentous structures. If the ligaments are damaged, the patient will complain of pain; if the meniscus alone is torn, the test should not be painful for him.

REDUCTION CLICK. This procedure is applicable to those patients having a locked knee due to a torn, dislocated, or "heaped up" meniscus. The positioning is the same as that for the McMurray test. (The patient lies supine on the table and the examiner holds his heel and foot with one hand and his knee with the other, so that thumb and fingers touch each side of the joint line). The object of the reduction click procedure is to reduce the displaced or torn portion of the meniscus by clicking it back into place. To do this, flex the knee while it is rotated both internally and externally. Then rotate and extend the leg until the meniscus slips back to its proper position and you hear a characteristic "click." This test will unlock a locked knee (caused by a torn meniscus) and permit full extension. The McMurray test can also unlock the knee joint and produce the reduction click.

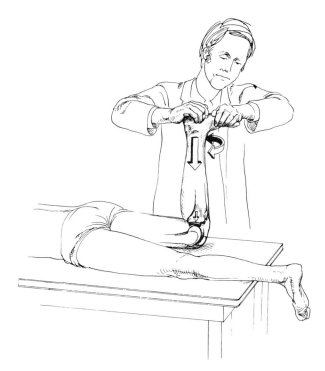

Fig. 62. Apley's compression test for meniscal tear.

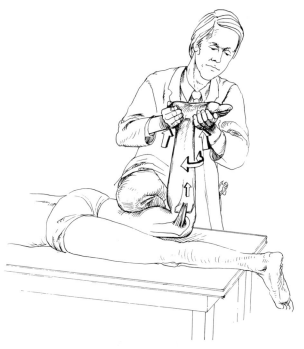

Fig. 63. Apley's distraction test for ligamentous damage.

"BOUNCE HOME" TEST. This test is designed to evaluate a lack of full knee extension, most often secondary to a torn meniscus, a loose body within the knee joint, or an intracapsular joint swelling. With the patient supine on the table, cup his heel in your palm and bend his knee into full flexion (Fig. 64). Now, passively allow the knee to extend (Fig. 65). The knee should extend completely, or "bounce home," into extension with a sharp end-point. However, if the knee falls short, offering a rubbery resistance to further extension, there is probably a torn meniscus or some other blockage (see range of motion tests), and bounce home motion cannot take place (Fig. 66).

PATELLA FEMORAL GRINDING TEST. This test is designed to determine the quality of the articulating surfaces of the patella and the trochlear groove of the femur. The patient should be supine on the examining table with his legs relaxed in the neutral position. First, push the patella distally in the trochlear groove (Fig. 67). Then instruct him to tighten his quadriceps and palpate and offer resistance to the patella as it moves under your fingers. The movement of the patella should be smooth and gliding; any roughness in its ar-

ticulating surfaces causes a palpable crepitation when the patella moves. If the test is positive, the patient usually complains of pain or discomfort. Clinically, patients most often complain of pain when they climb stairs or get up from a chair. These complaints are compatible with this condition, since, during those activities, the roughened undersurface of the patella is forced against the trochlear groove. In addition, chondromalacia patellae, osteochondral defects, or degenerative changes within the trochlear groove itself can precipitate symptoms of pain during such activity.

APPREHENSION TEST FOR PATELLAR DISLOCATION AND SUBLUXATION. This procedure is designed to determine whether or not the patella is prone to lateral dislocation. If you suspect that your patient has a recurrent dislocating patella, you should attempt to dislocate it manually while observing his face as he reacts to this test. Ask him to lie supine on the examining table, with his legs flat and the quadriceps relaxed. If you suspect that the patella may dislocate laterally, press against the medial border of the patella with your thumb. If everything is in order, this will produce little reaction; however, if the patella begins to dislocate, the expression on the patient's face will become one of apprehension and distress (Fig. 68).

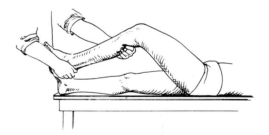

Fig. 64. The "Bounce Home" test. Flex the knee.

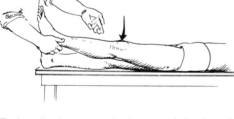

Fig. 65. Let the knee passively extend. It should fully "bounce home" into extension.

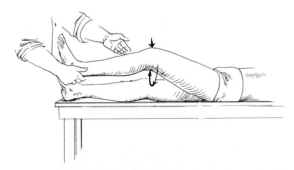

Fig. 66. Fluid in the knee joint prevents the knee joint from "bouncing home"; instead it may rebound.

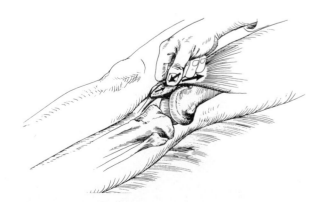

Fig. 67. The patellar femoral grinding test, to evaluate the quality of the patellar articulating surfaces.

TINEL SIGN. The Tinel test can refer either to the elicitation of pain from tapping for neuromata on the end of a cut nerve, or to the provocation of pain on the leading edge of a regenerating nerve. In the case of the knee, the testing concerns the area around the medial side of the tibial tubercle where the infrapatellar branch of the saphenous nerve runs. In knee surgery, this nerve is frequently cut, particularly during removal of the medial meniscus. If a neuroma has developed, tenderness can be elicited over the bulbous end of the severed nerve (Fig. 69).

KNEE JOINT EFFUSION TESTS

These tests are designed to document suspected effusion in the knee joint.

Test for Major Effusion. When the joint is distended by a large effusion, carefully extend the patient's knee and instruct him to relax the quadriceps muscles. Then, push the patella into the trochlear groove and quickly release it. The large amount of fluid lying under the patella is first forced to the sides of the joint, and then flows back to its former position, forcing the patella to rebound. This is referred to as a ballotable patella (Fig. 70).

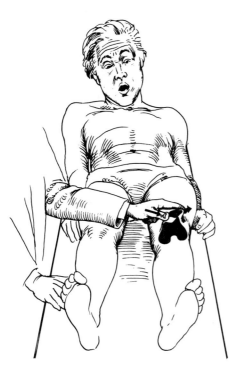

Fig. 68. The apprehension test for patellar dislocation.

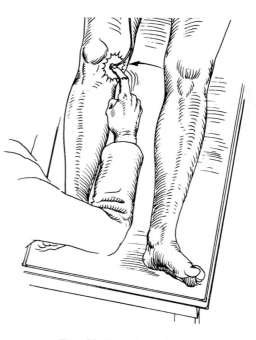

Fig. 69. The Tinel sign.

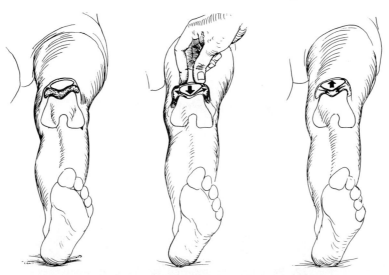

Fig. 70. Test for major effusion—a ballotable patella.

Test for Minor Effusion. In the case of minimal effusion in the knee joint, there is not enough fluid to ballot the patella. Therefore, to test for minimal effusion, keep your patient's knee in extension, and then "milk" the fluid from the suprapatellar pouch and lateral side into the medial side of the knee. When the fluid has been forced to the medial side, gently tap the joint over the fluid, which will traverse the knee to create a fullness on the lateral side (Fig. 71 A, B, C).

EXAMINATION OF RELATED AREAS

The joints both above and below the knee should be examined in a truly comprehensive examination of the knee joint. A herniated disc in the lumbar spine or osteoarthritis of the hip both can refer pain to the knee. Less often, foot problems such as ligamentous sprains or infections may occasionally manifest in the knee (Fig. 72).

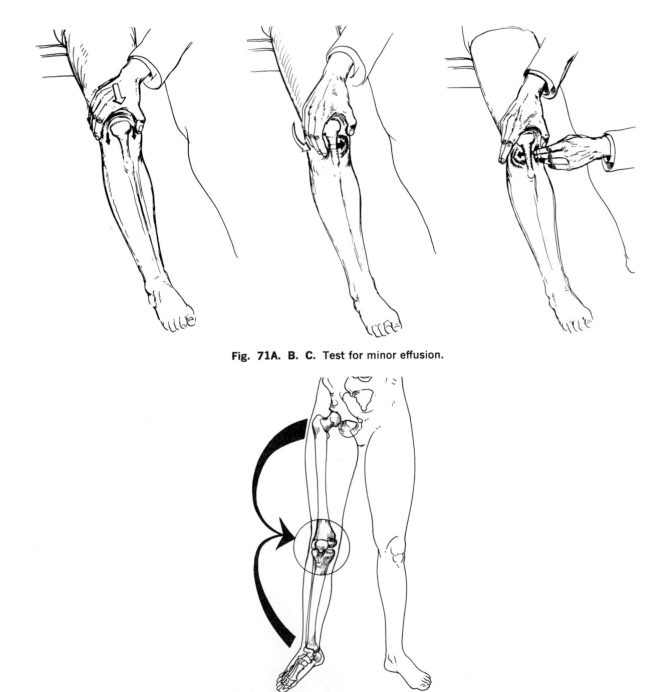

Fig. 71A. B. C. Test for minor effusion.

Fig. 72. Pain may be referred to the knee from the hip, the lumbar spine, and from the foot and ankle.

8

Physical Examination of the Foot and Ankle

INSPECTION
BONY PALPATION
  Medial Aspect
    First Metatarsocuneiform
    Navicular Tubercle
    Head of the Talus
    Medial Malleolus
    Sustentaculum Tali
    Medial Tubercle of the Talus
  Lateral Aspect
    Fifth Metatarsal Bone
    Fifth Metatarsophalangeal Joint
    Calcaneus
    Peroneus Tubercle
    Lateral Malleolus
  Sinus Tarsi Area
    Dome of the Talus
    Inferior Tibiofibular Joint
  Area of the Hindfoot
    Dome of the Calcaneus
    Medial Tubercle
  Plantar Surface
    Sesamoid Bones
    Metatarsal Heads
SOFT TISSUE PALPATION
  Zone I   — Head of the First Metatarsal Bone
  Zone II   — Navicular Tubercle and Talar Head
  Zone III — Medial Malleolus
  Zone IV — Dorsum of the Foot between the
                Malleoli
  Zone V   — Lateral Malleolus
  Zone VI — Sinus Tarsi
  Zone VII — Head of the Fifth Metatarsal
  Zone VIII — Calcaneus
  Zone IX — Plantar Surface of the Foot
  Zone X   — Toes

TESTS FOR ANKLE JOINT STABILITY
RANGE OF MOTION
  Active Range of Motion
  Passive Range of Motion
    Ankle Dorsiflexion _____ 20°
    Ankle Plantar Flexion __ 50°
    Subtalar Inversion _____ 5°
    Subtalar Eversion _____ 5°
    Forefoot Adduction ____ 20°
    Forefoot Abduction ____ 10°
  First Metatarsophalangeal Joint
    Flexion _____ 45°
    Extension _____ 70°–90°
  Motion of the Lesser Toes
NEUROLOGIC EXAMINATION
  Muscle Testing
    Dorsiflexors
    Plantar Flexors
  Sensation Tests
  Reflex Tests
    Achilles Tendon Reflex (S1)
SPECIAL TESTS
    Tests for Rigid or Supple Flat Feet
    Tibial Torsion Test
    Forefoot Adduction Correction Test
    Ankle Dorsiflexion Test
    Homans' Sign
EXAMINATION OF RELATED AREAS

The foot and ankle are the focal points to which the total body weight is transmitted in ambulation, and they are well tailored to that function. The thick heel and toe pads perform as shock absorbers in the acts of walking and running, and the joints are capable of the adjustments necessary for fine balance on a variety of terrain.

Because of this concentrated stress, the foot and ankle are often involved in static deformities not ordinarily affecting other parts of the body. Moreover, the foot is subject to a high incidence of general systemic conditions, such as rheumatoid arthritis and diabetes.

Since the foot brings man into immediate and direct physical contact with his environment, its constant exposure and susceptibility to injury more or less necessitate an artificial encasement, the shoe, which in itself can cause and compound many foot problems. Therefore, the judicious examination of the foot and ankle includes a careful scrutiny of the patient's footwear.

INSPECTION

When the patient enters the examination room, inspect the external appearance of the shoe and foot. A deformed foot can deform any good shoe; in fact, in many cases, the shoe is a literal showcase for certain disorders. For example, the shoes of an individual with flat feet usually have broken medial counters due to the prominence of the talar head (Fig. 36); the shoes of an individual with a drop foot display scuffed toes from scraping the floor in swing phase (Fig. 16, Gait Chapter); and the shoes of patients who toe-in show excessive wear on the lateral border of the sole. Creases of the forepart of the shoe may also reflect foot pathology; creases that are markedly oblique, rather than transverse, indicate possible hallux rigidus, since toe-off then occurs on the lateral side of the foot (Fig. 78). The absence of creases indicates no toe-off. Of course, foot trouble may also stem from objects protruding inside the shoe, such as nails and rivets, or from rough stitching or a wrinkled shoe lining.

Since a comprehensive examination of the foot and ankle includes an inspection of the entire lower extremity as well as the lumbar spine, have the patient remove his clothing from the waist down. As he undresses, observe his foot and ankle as they bear weight, for it is in the weight-bearing position that most abnormal conditions manifest themselves.

To begin inspection, count the toes to make certain that there are the customary five, for oc-

casionally you may find a supernumary digit, a congenital anomaly. The toes should appear straight, flat, and in proportion to each other as well as to those of the other foot. A disproportionately large toe may be either swollen or a congenital anomaly. Overlapping toes may or may not be an adaptation to a bunion; they are not usually painful in themselves.

Ask the patient to be seated to determine whether his feet at rest assume the normal few degrees of plantar flexion and inversion rather than dorsi flexion and eversion (spastic flat feet). Then evaluate the general shape of the foot. Normally, the dorsum of the foot is domed due to the medial longitudinal arch (Fig. 1), which extends between the first metatarsal head and the calcaneus. The arch is more prominent in the non-weight-bearing position; occasionally, it may be abnormally high (pes cavus) (Fig. 2) or absent (pes planus). Additionally, in children, you may find the forefoot inclined medially on the hindfoot (forefoot adductus) (Fig. 93), or the hindfoot in excessive valgus or varus (Fig. 37).

Note that the foot changes color in the weight-bearing and non-weight-bearing positions. Normally, it takes a few seconds for the color to change from a dark to a lighter pink when the foot becomes non-weight-bearing. If the foot is a light pink when elevated but becomes beet red when lowered (dependent rubor), there may be small-vessel vascular disease or arterial insufficiency.

The skin of the foot is extremely thick at the normal weight-bearing areas: The heel, the lateral

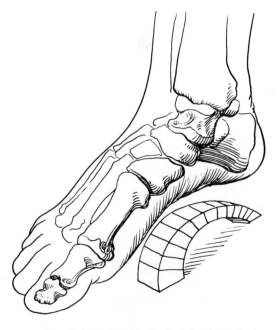

Fig. 1. The longitudinal arch of the foot.

border, and the first and fifth metatarsal heads. A pathologic increase in this skin thickness (callosity) is caused by these areas bearing abnormal amounts of weight. This condition most often manifests itself over the metatarsal heads (Fig. 29).

Finally, inspect the foot and ankle for obvious unilateral or bilateral swelling. Unilateral swelling usually indicates a residual edema secondary to trauma (fractured ankle, for example); bilateral swelling may be evidence of cardiac or lymphatic problems, or of pelvic obstruction to venous return. Swelling may also be local or generalized. Local swelling commonly occurs around the malleoli secondary to a sprain; generalized swelling is secondary to massive trauma, and involves the entire foot, occasionally extending up the tibial shaft.

BONY PALPATION

To palpate the foot and ankle, have the patient sit on the edge of the examining table with his legs dangling free, while you sit on a stool facing him. Stabilize the foot and lower leg with one hand by holding the foot around the calcaneus. In this position, it is relatively easy to manipulate the foot into the various postures for palpation. Since the bones of the foot are, in most instances, subcutaneous, their prominences present the most practical reference points (Fig. 3).

Medial Aspect

Head of the First Metatarsal Bone and the Metatarsophalangeal Joint. The head of the first metatarsal bone and the metatarsophalangeal joint are palpable at the ball of the foot. Note any associated bony excrescences involving the head of the metatarsal (Fig. 4). The metatarsophalangeal joint is the joint most frequently involved in gout and bunions. From the joint, probe proximally along the medial shaft of the first metatarsal bone.

First Metatarsocuneiform. The metatarsal flares slightly at its base, and meets the first cuneiform bone to form the first metatarsocuneiform joint (Fig. 5). The first cuneiform bone projects distally nearly half an inch further than the other cuneiform bones. It articulates with the base of the first metatarsal in a simple plane joint, providing gliding movement.

Navicular Tubercle. As you continue moving proximally along the medial border of the foot, the next large bony prominence you encounter is the navicular tubercle (Fig. 6). The navicular articulates with five other bones: Proximally with the talar head, distally with the three cuneiforms, and laterally with the cuboid bone. Aseptic necrosis of the navicular, characterized by local tenderness and a limping gait, is sometimes found in children. Further, if the tubercle is too prominent, it may press against the medial counter of the shoe and become painful.

Head of the Talus. The medial side of the talar head is immediately proximal to the navicular. You can find it by inverting and everting the forefoot; the resultant motion between the talus and navicular is palpable. Eversion causes the head to become more prominent as it juts out from under the navicular. If the talar head is difficult to find, draw a line between the medial malleolus and the navicular tubercle, bisect the line, and probe that area. The head of the talus lies directly under your fingers; when the foot is in the neutral position, it feels like a slight depression (Figs. 7, 8). In pes planus, the head becomes prominent on the medial side.

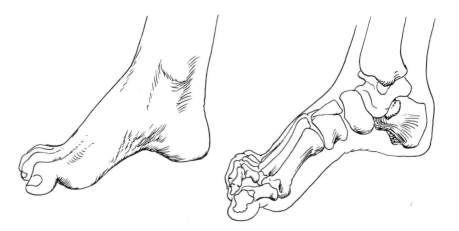

Fig. 2. An abnormally high arch (pes cavus).

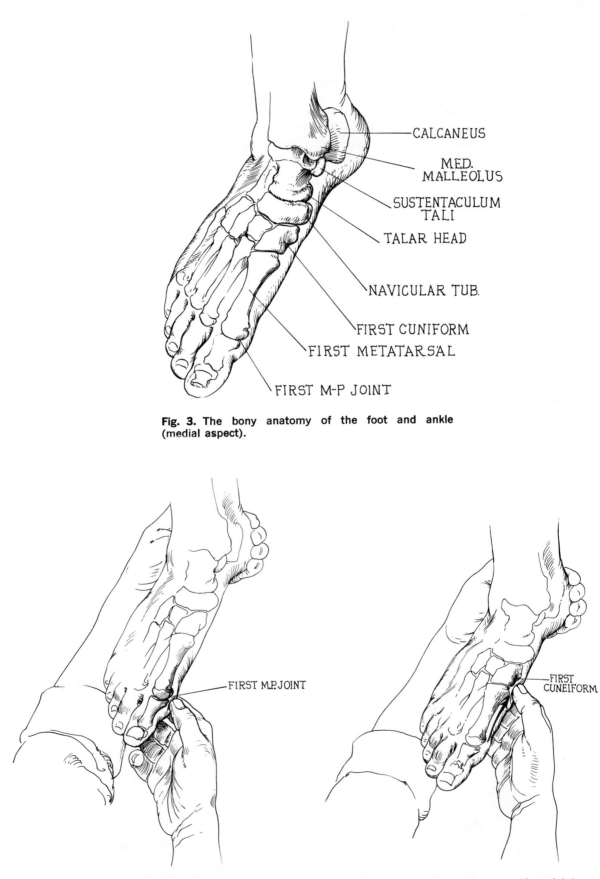

CALCANEUS

MED. MALLEOLUS

SUSTENTACULUM TALI

TALAR HEAD

NAVICULAR TUB.

FIRST CUNIFORM

FIRST METATARSAL

FIRST M-P JOINT

Fig. 3. The bony anatomy of the foot and ankle (medial aspect).

FIRST M.P.JOINT

FIRST CUNEIFORM

Fig. 4. The first metatarsophalangeal joint.   **Fig. 5.** The first metatarsocuneiform joint.

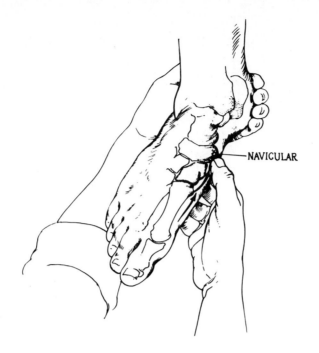

Fig. 6. The navicular tubercle.

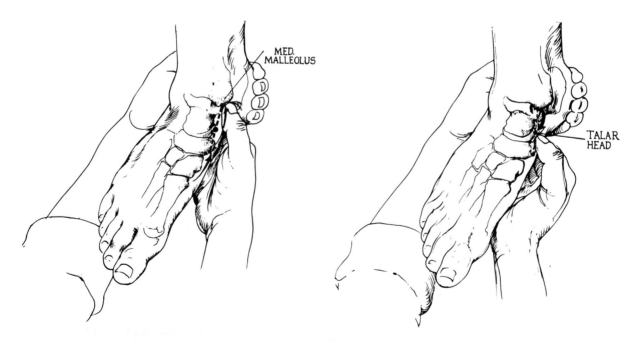

Figs. 7, 8. The head of the talus may be located by drawing a line between the medial malleolus and the navicular tubercle; the talar head lies under the point of bisection.

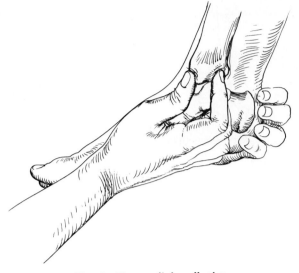

Fig. 9. The medial malleolus.

Medial Malleolus. From the head of the talus, probe proximally until you come to the prominent medial malleolus (the distal end of the tibia). The malleolus embraces the medial aspect of the talus, adding bony stability to the ankle joint. It articulates with one-third of the medial side of the talus (Fig. 9).

Sustentaculum Tali. Move plantarward approximately a finger's breadth from the distal end of the malleolus until you find the sustentaculum tali (Fig. 10). The sustentaculum tali is small, and may not be palpable at all, but it has anatomic significance. Clinically, it supports the talus and serves as an attachment for the spring ligament; problems within this anatomic alignment may well lead to pes planus.

Medial Tubercle of the Talus. The medial tubercle of the talus, which is small and barely palpable, lies immediately posterior to the distal end of the medial malleolus. It is the point of insertion for the posterior aspect of the ankle's medial collateral ligament (Fig. 11).

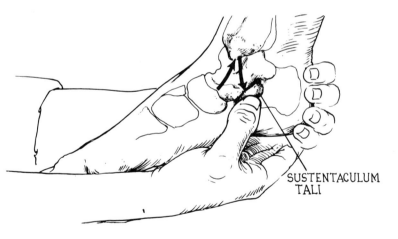

SUSTENTACULUM TALI

Fig. 10. The sustentaculum tali—the large medial extension of the calcaneus.

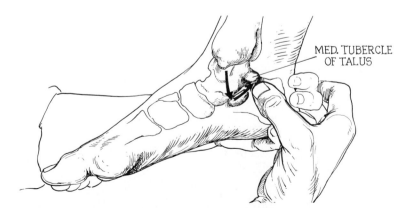

MED. TUBERCLE OF TALUS

Fig. 11. The medial tubercle of the talus.

Lateral Aspect

To palpate the lateral aspect of the foot, continue your present stabilization of the patient's foot (Fig. 12).

Fifth Metatarsal Bone; Fifth Metatarsophalangeal Joint. These are situated at the lateral side of the ball of the foot (Fig. 13). Note that the first and fifth metatarsal heads are normally the most prominent. Probe proximally along the lateral shaft of the fifth metatarsal to its flared base, the styloid process (Fig. 14). Notice that the peroneus brevis inserts into the process. Directly behind the flare of the process and in front of the cuboid lies a depression, which is further accentuated by the groove in the cuboid itself. This groove is created by the peroneus longus muscle tendon as it runs to the medial plantar surface of the foot (Fig. 15).

Calcaneus. Move proximally along the foot's lateral border to the calcaneus, which is subcutaneous and easily palpable (Fig. 16).

Peroneal Tubercle. The peroneal tubercle lies on the calcaneus, distal to the lateral malleolus (Fig. 17). Normally, it is about a quarter of an inch in length; however, its size may vary somewhat in different patients. The tubercle is a significant landmark because it separates the peroneus brevis and longus tendons at the point where they pass around the lateral calcaneus.

Lateral Malleolus. The lateral malleolus, located at the distal end of the fibula (Fig. 18), extends further distally and is more posterior than the medial malleolus. Its configuration permits the ankle mortise to point 15° laterally, and its additional distal extension acts as a deterrent to eversion ankle sprains. The medial malleolus, having less distal extension, does not enjoy this mechanical advantage, and is less effective in preventing the inversion type of sprain that is so commonly seen. These differences in length and position of the malleoli can be more readily appreciated if you place your fingers on the anterior portion of both malleoli (Fig. 19). The incidence of malleolar fracture due to trauma is relatively high.

If you place your thumb on the most anterior portion of the lateral malleolus (Fig. 20) and plantar flex your patient's foot, the anterolateral portion of the talar dome becomes palpable as it rotates out from under the ankle mortise (Fig. 21).

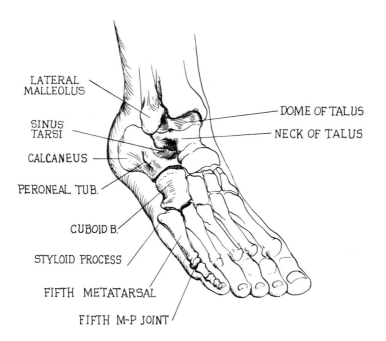

LATERAL MALLEOLUS

SINUS TARSI

CALCANEUS

PERONEAL TUB.

CUBOID B.

STYLOID PROCESS

FIFTH METATARSAL

FIFTH M-P JOINT

DOME OF TALUS

NECK OF TALUS

Fig. 12. The bony anatomy of the foot and ankle (lateral aspect).

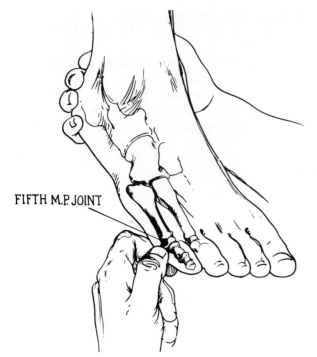

FIFTH M.P. JOINT

Fig. 13. The fifth metatarsophalangeal joint.

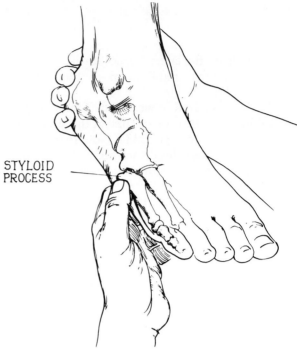

STYLOID PROCESS

Fig. 14. The styloid process of the fifth metatarsal.

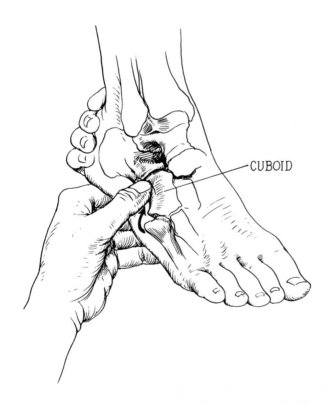

CUBOID

Fig. 15. The groove in the cuboid bone created by the peroneus longus muscle tendon.

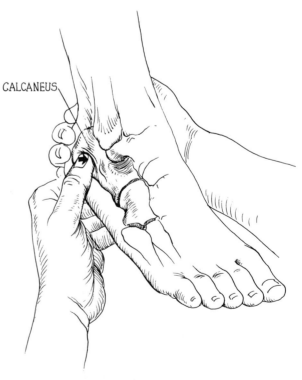

CALCANEUS

Fig. 16. The calcaneus.

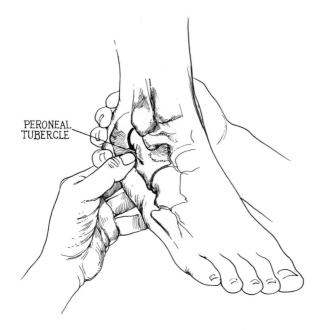

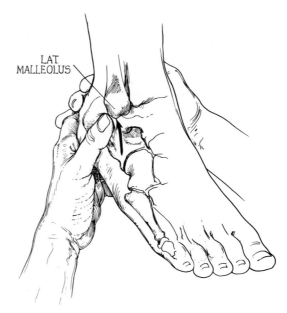

Fig. 17. The peroneal tubercle—a small lateral extension of the calcaneus.

Fig. 18. The lateral malleolus.

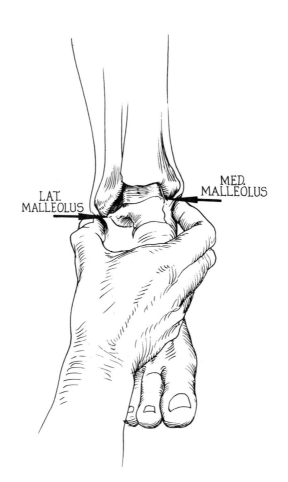

Fig. 19. The lateral malleolus extends further distally than the medial malleolus.

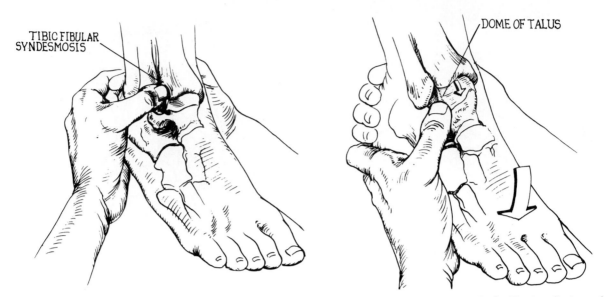

Figs. 20, 21. Palpation of the lateral edge of the dome of the talus (anterolateral portion). Plantar flexion of the foot exposes a larger surface of the talar dome.

Sinus Tarsi Area

Stabilize the patient's foot at the calcaneus with one hand and place the thumb of your free hand into the soft tissue depression just anterior to the lateral malleolus (Fig. 22). The depression lies directly over the sinus tarsi, which is filled by the extensor digitorum brevis muscle and an overlying pad of fat. However, you can palpate the superior dorsal aspect of the calcaneus near its articulation with the cuboid bone through these soft tissues. If you then invert the foot; you may be able to palpate the lateral side of the talar neck by pushing your finger deeper into the sinus. It is

directly through this area that a subtalar arthrodesis is performed.

Dome of the Talus. Keep the patient's foot in inversion and plantar flex it. A small portion of the dome of the talus becomes palpable; a greater portion of its surface is palpable on its lateral side than on the medial side adjacent to the medial malleolus. Occasionally, a defect is palpable in the articulating surface of the dome.

Inferior Tibiofibular Joint. This joint lies immediately proximal to the talus. Since the anterior inferior tibiofibular ligament overlies this joint, clear palpation of the joint itself is impossible; however, you can feel a slight depression directly over it (Fig. 20). The bones of the joint may separate (diastasis) following injury to the ankle.

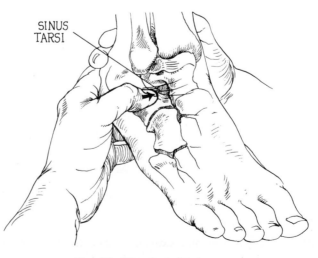

Fig. 22. The sinus tarsi.

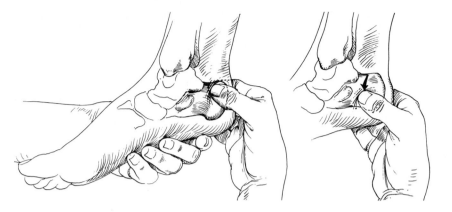

Fig. 23. The dome of the calcaneus: The bare posterior one-third of the calcaneus.

Area of the Hindfoot

Have the patient relax his foot; take hold of the hindfoot, and place your thumb and fingers in the soft tissue depressions on either side of the Achilles tendon.

Dome of the Calcaneus. The bare posterior third of the dome protrudes sharply from behind the ankle joint. As you move plantarward along the walls of the calcaneus, notice that the bone flares outward at its plantar base (Fig. 23). This flair may become excessive following a compression fracture of the posterior third of the os calcis.

Medial Tubercle. The medial tubercle lies on the medial plantar surface of the calcaneus (Fig. 24). It is rather broad and large, and gives attachment to the abductor hallucis muscle medially and to the flexor digitorum brevis muscle and the plantar aponeurosis anteriorly. The medial tubercle is not really sharp and distinct unless it is associated with a heel spur, when it becomes tender to palpation. The medial tubercle is weight bearing, whereas the lateral tubercle of the calcaneus is not. In children, pain over the posterior aspect of the os calcis (due to epiphysitis) is not uncommon. Because of this pain, these patients may avoid heel strike altogether during gait (Gait Chapter, Fig. 8).

Plantar Surface

In general, palpation of the bony prominences on the plantar surface is difficult because of the overlying fascial bands, the pads of fat, and large callosities. To examine the plantar surface, have the patient extend his leg with the sole of his foot facing you, and stabilize the lower limb by holding his leg posterior to the ankle joint.

Sesamoid Bones. From the medial tubercle of the calcaneus, palpate distally along the medial longitudinal arch past the base of the first metatarsal bone to the first metatarsophalangeal joint. If you press firmly on the first metatarsal, you can feel the two small sesamoid bones that lie (Fig. 25) within the flexor hallucis brevis tendon. The head of the first metatarsal bears a large part of the body's weight, and the sesamoids distribute some of the weight-bearing pressure. They also provide a mechanical advantage for the flexor tendon of the great toe, especially at toe-off. If they become inflamed (sesamoiditis), they may become tender.

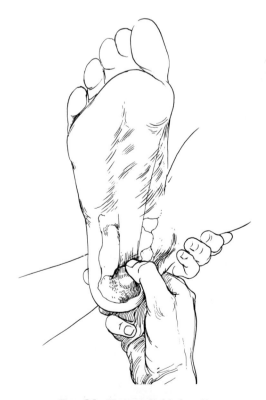

Fig. 24. The medial tubercle.

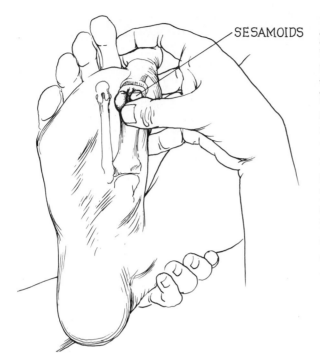

SESAMOIDS

Fig. 25. The sesamoid bones within the flexor hallucis brevis tendon.

Metatarsal Heads. Move laterally and palpate each metatarsal head by placing your thumb upon the plantar surface and your index finger upon the dorsal surface (Figs. 26, 27). The transverse arch of the forefoot is located immediately behind the metatarsal heads (Fig. 28); it is this arch that makes the first and fifth metatarsal heads most prominent. As you palpate the heads, try to determine if any one is disproportionately prominent. If one is, it must bear an unaccustomed amount of weight and is subject to a variety of problems. This pathology occurs most often to the second metatarsal head; callosities that have formed because of the increased pressure may obscure the head completely (Fig. 29). Occasionally, the fifth metatarsal head exhibits excessive callosity. Pain in the second, third, or fourth metatarsal heads may be secondary to aseptic necrosis (lack of blood supply) which, in turn, creates an antalgic gait.

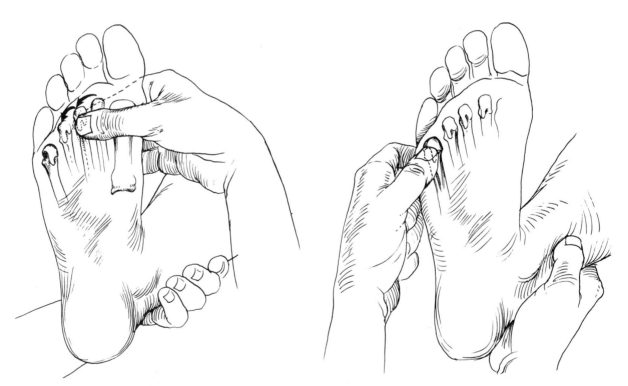

Figs. 26, 27. The metatarsal heads should be palpated with the thumb on the plantar surface and the forefinger on the dorsal surface. Palpate each head individually.

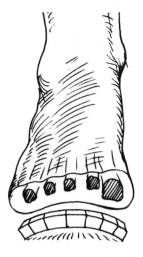

Fig. 28. The transverse arch of the foot is located immediately behind the metatarsal heads.

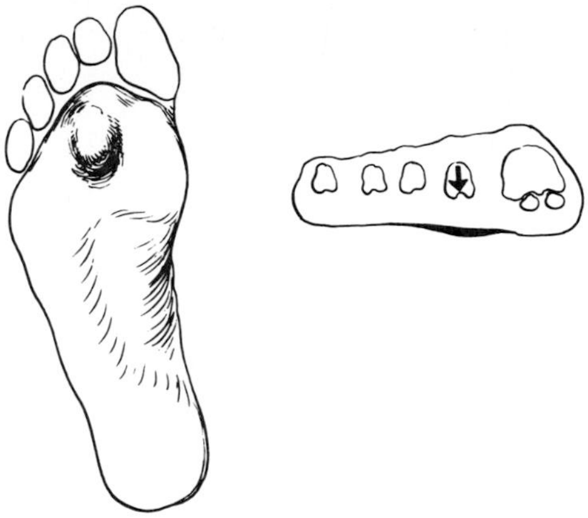

Fig. 29. Left. Callosities commonly develop under the metatarsal heads. **Right.** A dropped second metatarsal head with associated plantar callus formation.

SOFT TISSUE PALPATION

Zone I—Head of the First Metatarsal Bone

The area surrounding the prominent head of the first metatarsal bone and the first metatarsophalangeal joint is the site of that common pathologic condition, hallux valgus (Fig. 30).

Hallux valgus is a deformity characterized by lateral deviation of the great toe. In many cases, the deviation is so excessive that it causes the big toe to overlap the second toe (Fig. 31). The first metatarsal shaft may be medially angulated (metatarsus primus varus) as well. Under such circumstances, an excrescence of bone may grow over the medial aspect of the first metatarsal head and cause the surrounding soft tissue to swell. The resultant increased pressure and friction against the shoe can cause the development of a bursa, which frequently becomes tender and inflamed. Characteristically, the surrounding area appears reddened (bunion formation) (Fig. 32).

The medial aspect of the first metatarsal head is also a common site for gout. Tophi (deposits of urate crystals in the tissues about the joints) often develop at the first metatarsophalangeal joint and cause pain as well as deformity. Take care not to confuse such tophi deposits with the bunion formation associated with hallux valgus.

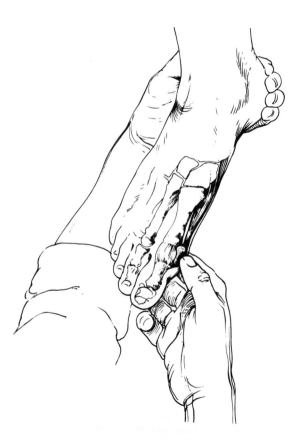

Fig. 30. A bursal formation over the head of the first metatarsal and the metatarsophalangeal joint.

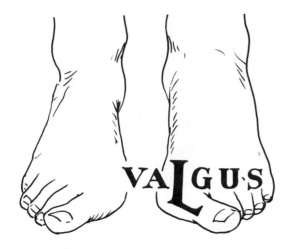

Fig. 31. Hallux valgus. The "L" in valgus refers to the lateral deviation of the phalanx.

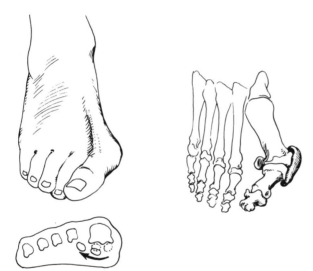

Fig. 32. Hallux valgus with bunion formation.

Zone II—Navicular Tubercle and the Talar Head

As has been stated previously, the plantar portion of the talar head articulates with the sustentaculum tali and the anterior portion with the posterior aspect of the navicular. The talar head lacks bony support between these two articulations. This gap is supported by the tibialis posterior tendon and the spring ligament, which runs from the sustentaculum tali to the navicular (Figs. 33, 34). In pes planus (flat feet), the talar head displaces medially and plantarward from under cover of the navicular and stretches the spring ligament and the tibialis posterior, resulting in the loss of the medial longitudinal arch (Fig. 35). A callosity may develop over the now prominent talar head at the point where the skin presses against the shoe's medial counter. Because of the callosity, the stretched soft tissue structures (Fig. 36), and the valgus angle of the os calcis (when viewed from the posterior aspect of the foot) (Fig. 37), the area may be exceedingly tender to palpation.

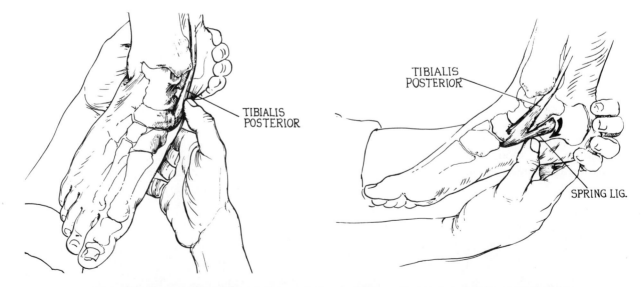

Figs. 33, 34. The gap between the navicular and the sustentaculum tali is supported by the tibialis posterior tendon and the spring ligament.

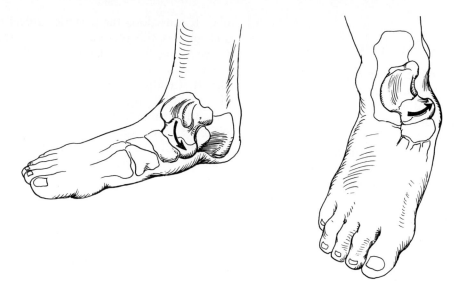

Fig. 35. Pes planus—the talar head displaces medially and plantarward.

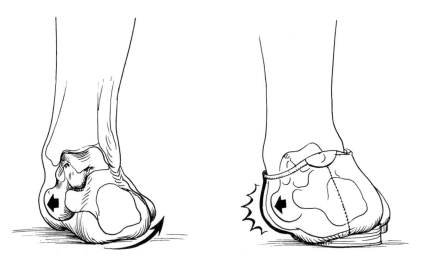

Fig. 36. Left. Medial prominence of the head of the talus in pes planus. **Right.** Callosity development over the head of the talus in association with shoe-wearing.

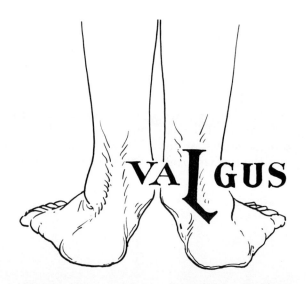

Fig. 37. The os calcis in valgus and in pes planus.

Zone III—Medial Malleolus

Deltoid Ligament. The medial collateral ligament of the ankle joint is palpable just inferior to the medial malleolus (Fig. 38). A broad, strong ligament, the deltoid's size and strength compensate for the comparatively short length of the medial malleolus. While the deltoid ligament is more massive than the lateral ankle ligament, it is not as easy to palpate. Tenderness or pain elicited during its palpation may indicate a tear from an eversion ankle sprain (Fig. 39).

Return to the medial malleolus to palpate the soft tissue depression between its posterior aspect and the Achilles tendon. Within this depression lie several important soft tissue structures. From anterior to posterior they are:

1) tibialis posterior tendon;
2) flexor digitorum longus tendon;
3) posterior tibial artery and tibial nerve;
4) flexor hallucis longus tendon (Fig. 38).

(The order of these structures can be remembered by the mnemonic "Tom, Dick, an' Harry": Tibialis posterior, flexor Digitorum longus, Artery, Nerve, flexor Hallucis longus.)

Tibialis Posterior Tendon. This tendon is most prominent when the patient inverts and plantar flexes his foot. It is both palpable and visible where it passes immediately behind and inferior to the medial malleolus. If spasticity, meningomyelocele, or poliomyelitis have weakened the other muscles around the ankle, the relatively strong tibialis posterior may, as a consequence, cause plantar flexion and an inversion deformity of the foot.

Flexor Digitorum Longus Tendon. This muscle lies just behind the tibialis posterior tendon. To palpate it, have the patient flex his toes while you resist his motion. Although the muscle's tendon does not become very prominent, you should be able to feel its motion immediately behind the tibialis posterior, just above the medial malleolus.

Flexor Hallucis Longus Tendon. This tendon actually lies on the posterior aspect of the ankle joint, rather than around the medial malleolus. It runs along the posterior aspect of the tibia and grooves the posterior aspect of the talus between its medial and lateral tubercles as it crosses the ankle joint. Because it is deep to other muscles, the tendon of the flexor hallucis longus muscle cannot be palpated.

All of these tendons pass so closely around the posterior aspect of the medial malleolus (particularly the tibialis posterior) that they groove the bone and must be protected by a synovial lining. When this lining becomes inflamed (synovitis), the patient complains of pain behind the medial malleolus and the area is tender to palpation.

Posterior Tibial Artery. The posterior tibial artery lies between the tendons of the flexor digitorum longus and the flexor hallucis longus muscles (Fig. 40). Its pulse is not always easy to find. However, it is easier to palpate when the foot is relaxed in a non-weight-bearing position and the tendons in the area are slack. You may feel the pulse by pressing gently into the soft tissue space behind the tibialis posterior and the flexor digitorum longus tendons. After you have felt it, compare it to the opposite side. A diminution of this pulse may indicate arterial occlusion. The posterior tibial artery has clinical significance because it provides the main blood supply to the foot.

Tibial Nerve. The tibial nerve is located immediately posterior and lateral to the posterior tibial artery, and follows the artery's course into the foot. The nerve is difficult to palpate as an isolated structure, but, since it is the main nerve supply to the sole of the foot, its anatomic position should be noted. The neurovascular bundle is bound to the tibia by a ligament, creating a *tarsal tunnel* which, if it is too small or too tight, can cause neurovascular problems in the foot. Although its incidence is less frequent, this syndrome is similar to that of the carpal tunnel syndrome in the hand.

Long Saphenous Vein. Return to the medial malleolus and palpate the long saphenous vein, which is often visible immediately anterior to the medial malleolus. When veins in the upper extremity cannot be located, this vein is almost always an accessible site for intravenous infusion. Varicosity in the lower extremity frequently involves the long saphenous vein.

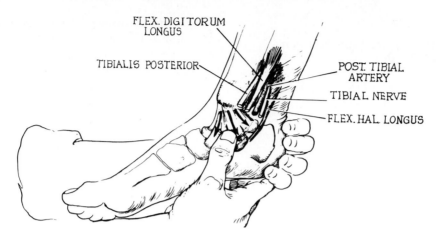

Fig. 38. The deltoid ligament.

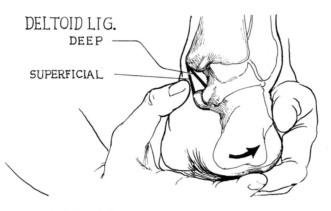

Fig. 39. Pain elicited upon eversion may be due to a sprain of the deltoid ligament.

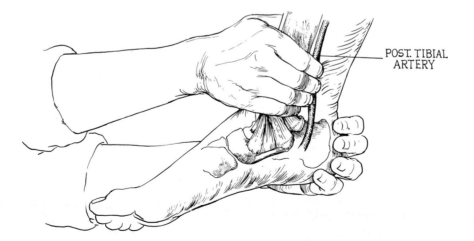

Fig. 40. Palpation of the posterior tibial artery, the main blood supply to the foot.

Zone IV—Dorsum of the Foot between the Malleoli

There are three important tendons and one vessel that pass between the malleoli. From medial to lateral they are:

1) tibialis anterior tendon;
2) extensor hallucis longus tendon;
3) dorsal pedal artery;
4) extensor digitorum longus tendon.

The tibialis anterior, the extensor hallucis longus, and the extensor digitorum longus muscles are the main dorsiflexors of the foot. If they are not functioning, the patient exhibits "drop-foot," or steppage gait.

Tibialis Anterior Tendon. This tendon is the most prominent, as well as the most medial, of the three tendons. It is also the strongest dorsiflexor and inverter of the foot, and its loss alone can result in a drop-foot. To make palpation of the tibialis anterior easier, instruct the patient to dorsiflex and invert his foot. The tendon should then become quite prominent where it crosses the ankle joint. Palpate it distally to its insertion onto the medial aspect of the base of the first metatarsal and the first cuneiform bones (Fig. 41) and proximally along the tendon to the muscle belly on the lateral side of the tibial shaft.

Extensor Hallucis Longus Tendon. This tendon is situated immediately lateral to the tibialis anterior tendon and becomes most prominent when the big toe is actively extended. It stands out immediately lateral to the tibialis anterior tendon at the level of the ankle joint: Palpate it along the dorsum of the foot to its insertion into the base of the distal phalanx of the big toe (Fig. 42). The insertion of the extensor hallucis longus may be surgically transferred from the toe to the dorsum of the foot, to assist in dorsiflexion for patients who have foot drop.

Extensor Digitorum Longus Tendon. This tendon lies lateral to the extensor hallucis longus. Palpate it first where it crosses the ankle joint. Distal to the ankle, the tendon divides into four parts, each of which inserts into the dorsal base of the distal phalanx of the four lesser toes. The tendons become prominent for palpation when the toes are extended.

Dorsal Pedal Artery. The dorsal pedal artery lies between the extensor hallucis longus and the extensor digitorum longus tendons on the dorsum of the foot. It is absent approximately 12 to 15 percent of the time (Fig. 43). Since the pedal

artery is subcutaneous, its pulse is easier to detect than that of the posterior tibial artery. This artery provides a secondary blood supply to the foot, augmenting that provided by the posterior tibial artery. In some instances, the pulse of the dorsal pedal artery may be reduced, usually as a result of vascular disease.

The tibialis anterior, the extensor hallucis longus, and the extensor digitorum longus muscles take origin from the anterior compartment on the leg's anterolateral side, between the tibia and the fibula. This anterior compartment is a tight, fibro-osseous area, and the strong anterior fascia, the posterior tibia, the fibula, and the interosseous ligament render it inflexible and unyielding. Because of its inability to expand, fractures of the tibia, hematomas within the muscles, or any other pathology that may cause swelling within the anterior compartment can result in necrosis of the muscles, nerves, and vessels, which in turn can create a foot drop or a deformed foot (anterior compartment syndrome). In the armed forces, this syndrome is quite often seen after a prolonged march. Normally, the structures of the anterior compartment should feel soft and yielding. If they are tight and intractable, and if palpation elicits tenderness, there is evidence of an anterior compartment syndrome.

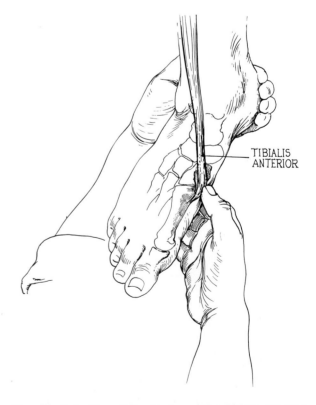

TIBIALIS ANTERIOR

Fig. 41. Palpation of the tendon of the tibialis anterior muscle.

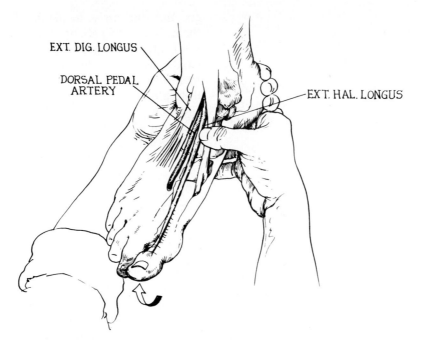

Fig. 42. Palpation of the tendon of the extensor hallucis longus muscle.

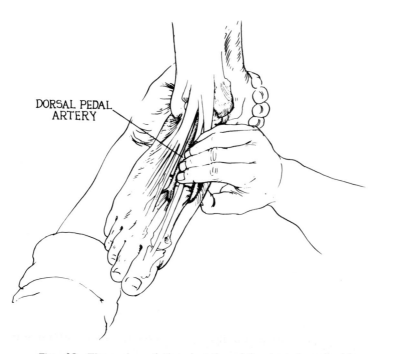

Fig. 43. The pulse of the dorsal pedal artery is palpable.

Zone V—Lateral Malleolus

There are three clinically important ligaments which comprise the lateral collateral ligaments of the ankle joint (Fig. 44). From anterior to posterior, they are:

1) anterior talofibular ligament,
2) calcaneofibular ligament,
3) posterior talofibular ligament.

None of these ligaments is as broad or as strong as is the deltoid ligament on the medial side. Although they are not distinctly palpable, it is important to know their anatomical locations because of their repeated involvement in sprains of the ankle (inversion plantar injury).

Anterior Talofibular Ligament. This ligament has a high incidence of sprain because it is the first of the three lateral collateral ligaments to undergo stress when the ankle is inverted and plantar flexed. It runs from the anterior portion of the lateral malleolus to the lateral aspect of the talar neck. The area of the tendon is most easily palpated in the sinus tarsi. The ligament itself is not a distinctly palpable structure. If the ligament is sprained, there is generally a palpable swelling and tenderness. However, a defect in the ligament itself does not become palpable.

Calcaneofibular Ligament. The calcaneofibular ligament stretches plantarward to its insertion into the lateral wall of the calcaneus. It actually attaches to a small tubercle on the calcaneus, slightly posterior to the peroneal tubercle. In severe ankle sprains, the ligament may be torn, but only after the anterior talofibular ligament has also been torn. The loss of function of both ligaments results in ankle instability.

Posterior Talofibular Ligament. This ligament takes origin from the posterior edge of the lateral malleolus and passes posteriorly to the small lateral tubercle on the posterior aspect of the talus. It is stronger than the two other collateral ligaments, and its primary function is to prevent forward slippage of the fibula onto the talus. Because of its strength and location, it is involved in only the most severe injuries to the ankle (dislocations).

Peroneus Longus and Brevis Tendons. These tendons pass immediately behind the lateral malleolus as they cross the ankle joint (Fig. 45). The brevis is closer to the malleolus, grooving the bone as it passes, while the longus lies just posterior to the brevis. The peronei are the primary foot everters, and they assist in plantar flexion. To palpate them, have the patient actively evert and plantar flex his foot. Occasionally, the retinaculum (fascial band) which holds the tendons to the lateral malleolus may be incomplete, and the tendons may dislocate from behind the lateral malleolus. This situation produces the snapping tendon syndrome; the snap of the dislocating tendons may be both audible and palpable.

As they pass the calcaneus, the peronei tendons are separated by the peroneal tubercle (Fig. 45). They are held to the tubercle by a retinaculum and are surrounded by synovium. They are, therefore, subject to tenosynovitis. In addition, the tunnel through which they run may narrow, causing stenosing tenosynovitis. In that event, the area of the peroneal tubercle feels thick and is tender to palpation. Palpate the peroneus brevis to its insertion into the styloid process (Fig. 46). Tenderness in this area may be due to an avulsion or a fracture of the tip of the styloid process in association with an ankle sprain, or to an inflamed bursa over the process itself.

Zone VI—Sinus Tarsi

The sinus tarsi (just anterior to the lateral malleolus) is commonly affected by ankle sprains. Its normal concavity may be filled with edema, and the course of the anterior talofibular ligament becomes tender from the anterior portion of the lateral malleolus to the talar neck (Fig. 47). Deep tenderness within the sinus tarsi is evidence of some problem in the subtalar complex and is usually indicative of fracture, rheumatoid arthritis, or spastic foot syndrome.

Extensor Digitorum Brevis Muscle. When the patient extends his toes, the muscle belly of the extensor digitorum brevis bulges out of the sinus tarsi and is easily palpable.

Zone VII—Head of the Fifth Metatarsal

Overlying the lateral side of the head of the fifth metatarsal bone, there is a bursa which is subject to inflammation. Excessive friction or pressure upon this bursa can cause both bursitis and the development of an associated excrescence of bone over its lateral aspect with subsequent redness, swelling, and tenderness. This condition is known as "tailor's bunion." (Traditionally, tailors crossed their legs and held their feet in such a way that the lateral aspect of the fifth metatarsal head rested against the floor) (Fig. 48).

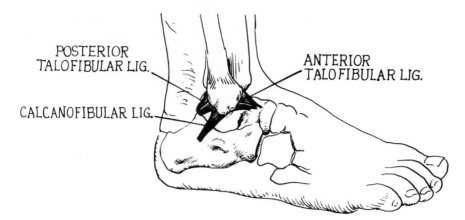

POSTERIOR TALOFIBULAR LIG.

ANTERIOR TALOFIBULAR LIG.

CALCANOFIBULAR LIG.

Fig. 44. Three important ligaments of the lateral aspect of the ankle.

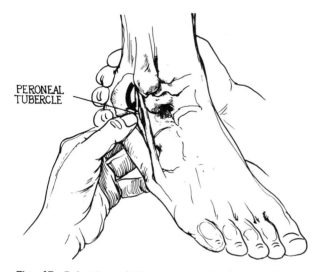

PERONEAL TUBERCLE

Fig. 45. Palpation of the peroneus longus and brevis muscle tendons as they cross the peroneal tubercle.

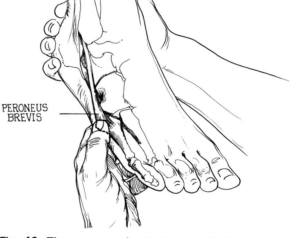

PERONEUS BREVIS

Fig. 46. The peroneus brevis is palpable to its insertion into the styloid process.

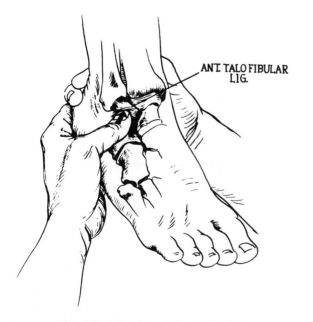

ANT. TALO FIBULAR LIG.

Fig. 47. Palpation of the sinus tarsi.

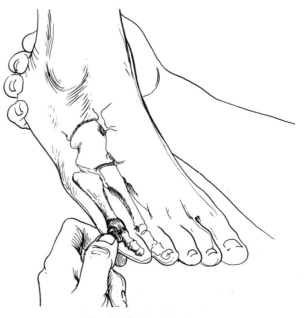

Fig. 48. Tailor's bunion.

Zone VIII—*Calcaneus*

The gastrocnemius and the soleus muscles form a common tendon, the tendon of Achilles, which inserts into the calcaneus. The Achilles tendon is the thickest and strongest tendon in the body. It is palpable from about the lower one-third of the calf to the calcaneus. It can be ruptured from a sharp blow or from an abrupt strain caused by a moment of sudden excess activity. A sharp blow may produce a transverse laceration, whereas a sudden strain may cause a shredding of the tendon.

Should the tendon be ruptured, the resulting defect is palpable, although it may have become obscured by swelling in the period between injury and presentation. Initially, the area is quite painful and tender, and powerful plantar flexion of the foot is usually impossible. If the patient can still walk, he will exhibit accompanying gait abnormalities, such as absence of "toe-off" (push-off) from the stance phase and a flat-footed gait.

To test the continuity of the gastrocnemius and soleus muscles, have the patient lie prone on the examination table, and squeeze the calf of his leg to determine if there is any resultant plantar flexion of the foot. Normally, there is such motion (Fig. 49). However, if the Achilles tendon is ruptured, the motion is markedly decreased or absent (Fig. 50). The tendon may also develop tenosynovitis, and palpation may elicit tenderness and crepitation upon motion.

Retrocalcaneal Bursa. The retrocalcaneal bursa lies between the anterior surface of the tendon of Achilles and the bare posterior superior angle of the calcaneus.

Calcaneal Bursa. This bursa lies between the insertion of the Achilles tendon and the overlying skin.

These two bursae can become inflamed as a result of either damage to the tendon or excessive pressure upon the area. The calcaneal bursa is more commonly enlarged, a condition usually due to oversized or tight shoes and particularly to high heels.

Locate the retrocalcaneal bursa by pinching the soft tissue, anterior to the tendon of Achilles; locate the calcaneal bursa by lifting the skin posterior to the tendon—the bursa lies directly between your fingers (Fig. 51). Any palpable thickening or tenderness in either area suggests the presence of bursitis.

Zone IX—*Plantar Surface of the Foot*

The central bony prominence in the area of the hindfoot is the broad medial tubercle of the calcaneus. Most of the muscles of the plantar surface of the foot originate from this bone. Their origins are not palpable because of the thick pad of fat covering the bone; however, the area should be palpated because of the possibility of a heel spur protruding from the medial tubercle and its attendant bursa, both of which cause tenderness and affect the heel strike phase of gait (Fig. 52).

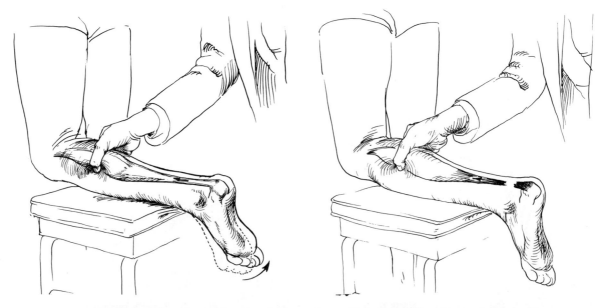

Figs. 49, 50. A test for continuity of the gastrocsoleus muscles' common tendon. Absence of foot-plantar flexion motion indicates a ruptured Achilles tendon.

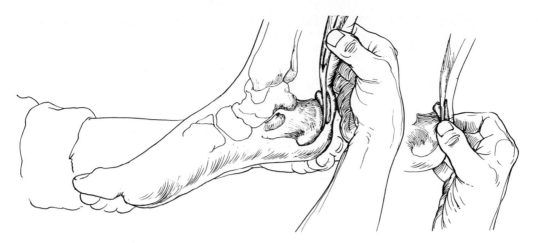

Fig. 51. The Achilles tendon, or calcaneal, bursa.

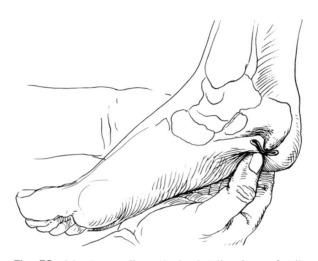

Fig. 52. A heel spur affects the heel strike phase of gait.

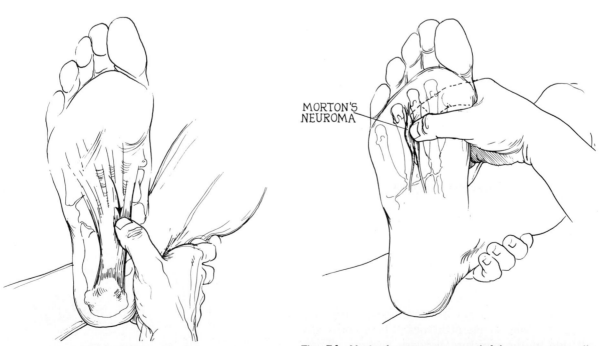

MORTON'S
NEUROMA

Fig. 53. The plantar aponeurosis.

Fig. 54. Morton's neuroma—a painful neuroma usually located between the 3rd and 4th metatarsal heads.

Plantar Aponeurosis (or Plantar Fascia). These strong bands of fascia originate at the medial tuberosity of the calcaneus, splay out over the sole, and insert into ligamentous structures near the metatarsal heads in the forefoot (Fig. 53). The plantar aponeurosis covers all the soft tissue structures of the foot, and acts as a virtual tie-beam for the support of the medial longitudinal arch.

Palpate the plantar surface of the foot. It should feel smooth, nontender, and nonnodular. Point tenderness may indicate plantar fasciitis, while discrete palpable nodules in the fascia indicate Duputyren's contracture. Most often, nodules found on the skin of the sole (particularly on the ball of the foot) are plantar warts, which are more tender when pinched than when under direct pressure.

Palpate the soft tissues between each of the metatarsal heads for tenderness and swelling. It is not uncommon to find painful neuromas in the space between the third and fourth metatarsal heads (Morton's neuroma) (Fig. 54). Callosities on the plantar surface, unlike warts, are tender to pressure but not to pinching.

Zone X—Toes

Normally, the toes lie flat and straight on the floor as they bear weight. But there are several pathologic conditions indigenous to them.

Claw Toes. Claw toes are characterized by hyperextension of the metatarsophalangeal joints and flexion of the proximal and distal interphalangeal joints. The condition generally involves all of the toes and is often associated with pes cavus (Fig. 55). Callosities are likely to develop over the dorsal surface of the toes due to the constricting pressure of the shoes upon the flexed interphalangeal joint. Also, callosities may develop on the plantar surface of the metatarsal heads and the tips of the toes (especially on the second toe), since they are forced to bear excessive amounts of weight (Fig. 56).

Hammer Toes. Hammer toes are typified by hyperextension of the metatarsophalangeal and distal interphalangeal joint and flexion of the proximal interphalangeal joint. In most cases, only one toe is involved (usually the second toe) (Fig. 57), and frequently a callosity, caused by shoe pressure, develops over the proximal interphalangeal joint of the affected toe.

Corns. The soft tissue variety is more commonly found between the toes, particularly between the fourth and fifth toes. These corns are soft due to the moisture between the toes. They

should be palpated gently, for they are frequently tender (Fig. 58). Hard corns are most often situated in areas of excessive pressure, such as on the dorsum of flexed interphalangeal joints, especially on the fifth toe. Hard corns, too, may be tender to direct pressure (Fig. 59).

Ingrown Toenails. Ingrown toenails involve the medial and lateral aspects of the great toe. The anterior corners of the nail dig into the surrounding skin, causing swelling and infection of the adjacent soft tissue. The area of involvement feels warm and boggy and is tender to palpation (Fig. 60).

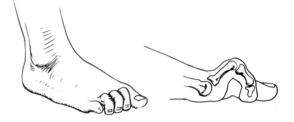

Fig. 55. Claw toes.

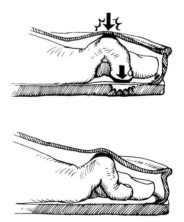

Fig. 56. Top. Callosity formation caused by claw toes. **Bottom.** Callosity formation caused by hammer toes.

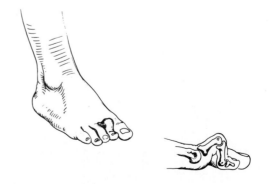

Fig. 57. Hammer toes.

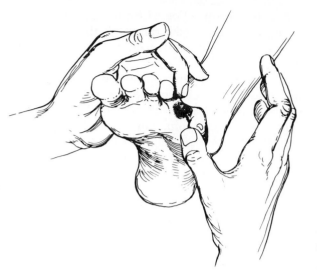

Fig. 58. Soft corns.

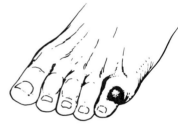

Fig. 59. Hard corns.

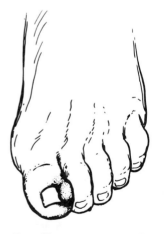

Fig. 60. Ingrown toenail.

TESTS FOR ANKLE JOINT STABILITY

Since the ankle joint bears weight and is important for walking, it must be both stable and mobile. Inversion or eversion sprains can stretch or tear the joint's supporting ligaments and produce instability. Excessive inversion stress is the most common cause of ankle injury for two anatomic reasons: (1) the medial malleolus is shorter than the lateral malleolus, and the talus can thus be forced to invert farther than it can evert; and (2) the ligamentous thickenings on the lateral side of the joint are separate, and are therefore not as strong as the massive deltoid ligament on the medial side.

The anterior talofibular ligament is the ligament most often involved in ankle sprains, and tenderness elicited along its course may indicate such damage. To test the ligament, turn the patient's foot into plantar flexion and inversion. If inversion stress increases his pain, there is a distinct possibility that the ligament is sprained or torn.

While inversion stress may indicate the condition of the ligament, it cannot give evidence of ankle joint instability if only the anterior talofibular ligament is torn. However, such a tear would allow the talus to slide forward on the tibia, since the anterior talofibular ligament is the only structure preventing forward subluxation of the talus. Therefore, you should test for anterior instability between the tibia and talus (the anterior draw sign). For the anterior draw sign test, the patient should sit on the edge of the examining table, with his legs dangling and his feet in a few degrees of plantar flexion. Place one hand on the anterior aspect of the lower tibia and grip the calcaneus in the palm of your other hand. Then, draw the calcaneus (and talus) anteriorly, while pushing the tibia posteriorly. Normally, the anterior talofibular ligament is tight in all positions of the ankle joint, and there should be no forward movement of the talus on the tibia (Fig. 61). Under abnormal conditions, however, the talus slides anteriorly from under the cover of the ankle mortise (positive draw sign); you may even feel a "clunk" as it moves (Fig. 62).

The anterior talofibular and the calcaneofibular ligaments must both be torn to produce gross lateral ankle instability. To check the integrity of these ligaments, invert the calcaneus; if the talus gaps and rocks in the ankle mortise, the anterior talofibular and calcaneofibular ligaments are damaged with resultant lateral ankle instability (Figs. 63, 64).

The posterior talofibular ligament can be torn only in conjunction with the other lateral ligaments; it takes a massive trauma to the ankle joint, such as dislocation, to damage the talofibular ligament.

To test the stability of the deltoid ligament on the medial side, stabilize the patient's leg around the tibia and calcaneus and evert his foot. If the deltoid ligament is torn, you may feel a gross gapping at the ankle mortise.

After you complete the test on the involved foot, test the normal one as a means of comparison to determine the extent of abnormal gapping. A stress x-ray is the best way to confirm these physical findings.

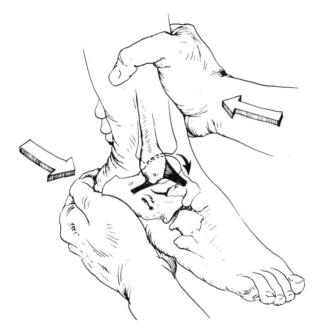

Fig. 61. The anterior draw sign test to evaluate the intactness of the anterior talofibular ligament.

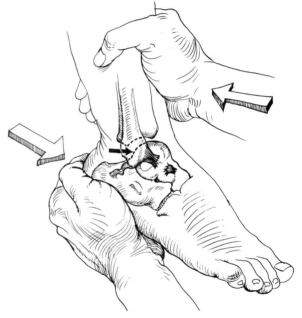

Fig. 62. A positive anterior draw sign.

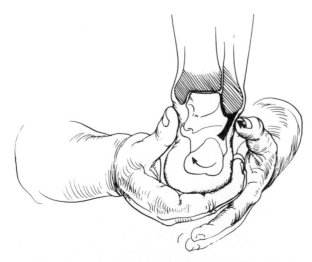

Fig. 63. A test to evaluate the stability of the anterior talofibular and the calcaneofibular ligaments.

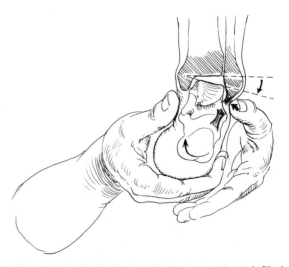

Fig. 64. The ankle is unstable if the anterior talofibular and calcaneofibular ligaments are torn.

RANGE OF MOTION

Movements of the foot and ankle almost invariably involve more than a single joint. The basic ankle and foot motions are:

1) Ankle Motion
   Dorsiflexion
   Plantar flexion
2) Subtalar Motion
   Inversion
   Eversion
3) Midtarsal Motion
   Forefoot adduction
   Forefoot abduction
4) Toe Motion
   Flexion
   Extension

Note that the patient may be able to move his foot considerably even if his ankle joint is fused; therefore, it is important to distinguish between ankle and subtalar or midtarsal movement.

Active Range of Motion

There are several quick tests which, while they are not pure active tests, nevertheless help to determine whether or not there is any gross restriction in a patient's range of ankle and foot motion.

To test plantar flexion and toe motion, ask the patient to walk on his toes; to test dorsiflexion,

instruct him to walk on his heels. To test inversion, have him walk on the lateral borders of his feet; to test eversion, instruct him to walk on the medial borders of his feet (Fig. 65). Although these quick tests can satisfactorily indicate functional abnormality, they do not permit precise measurement or evaluation of separate motion.

If your patient is unable to perform any of these procedures, you should conduct passive testing to determine the cause of his limited range of motion.

Passive Range of Motion

ANKLE DORSIFLEXION   —20°
ANKLE PLANTAR FLEXION—50°

Dorsiflexion and plantar flexion take place between the talus and the tibia and fibula within the ankle mortise. A line drawn between the midpoints of the medial and lateral malleoli approximates the axis of ankle joint motion.

Instruct the patient to sit on the edge of the examining table and to let his legs dangle. Since his knees are bent, the gastrocnemius is relaxed (its origin and insertion are brought closer together) and is eliminated as a possible restriction of dorsiflexion. Stabilize the subtalar joint by holding the calcaneus. Then, to ensure that ankle motion alone takes place and that there is no substitution of forefoot motion, invert the forefoot to lock it onto the hindfoot. Now, as you grip the forefoot, push the foot as one unit into dorsiflexion and plantar flexion (Figs. 66, 67).

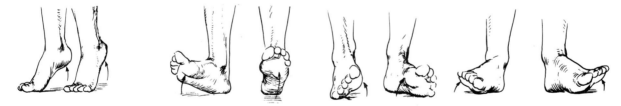

Fig. 65. Quick tests for foot and ankle range of motion.

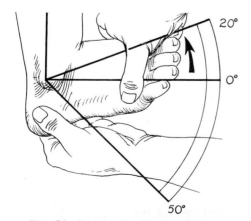

Fig. 66. Range of ankle dorsiflexion.

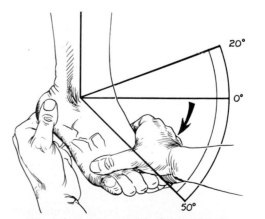

Fig. 67. Range of ankle plantar flexion.

When the foot is plantar flexed, there is normally a slight degree of lateral talar mobility between the malleoli. While this motion is difficult to record, it should be noted. The dorsum of the talus fits into a socket, or mortise, formed by the tibia or fibula, and both its socket and the talus are wider anteriorly. When the ankle is dorsiflexed, the talus is held tightly between the two malleoli. But when the ankle is plantar flexed, the narrower posterior portion lies between the malleoli, and there is a slight degree lateral mobility. If the intermalleolar distance has narrowed secondary to trauma, or if the foot and ankle have been cast in a position of equinus for a prolonged period (contracting the intermalleolar distance), the wider anterior portion of the talar dome may no longer fit easily into the mortise, and dorsiflexion could be restricted (Fig. 68).

Restricted ankle movement may also be caused by extra-articular swelling (edema secondary to sprain or to cardiac failure); such swelling can constrict the ankle almost as if it were bandaged or placed in a cast. Intra-articular swelling also reduces ankle motion (Fig. 69), as does a fusion of the ankle joint or a contracted joint capsule (Figs. 70, 71).

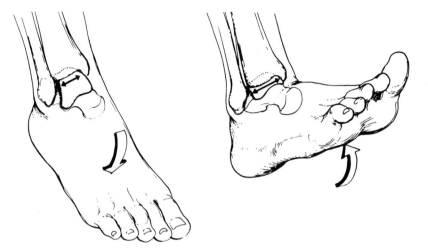

Fig. 68. If intermalleolar distance has narrowed, dorsiflexion is limited. The wider anterior portion of the talar dome may no longer fit easily into the mortise.

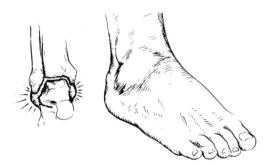

Fig. 69. Swelling can restrict range of motion.

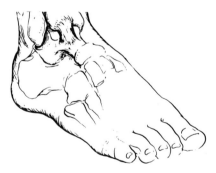

Fig. 70. Range of motion may be limited by fusion of a joint.

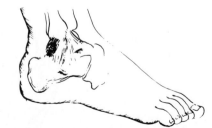

Fig. 71. A contracture of the joint capsule can limit the range of motion.

SUBTALAR INVERSION—5°
SUBTALAR EVERSION —5°

These motions adjust the foot so that it can function on uneven surfaces. The motions take place primarily at the talocalcaneal, talonavicular, and calcanecuboid joints. To test inversion and eversion, have the patient remain seated on the edge of the examining table and stabilize his tibia by holding it around its distal end. Then, grip the calcaneus, and alternately invert and evert the heel (Figs. 72, 73). A patient who has subtalar arthritis (secondary, perhaps, to a calcaneal fracture extending to the subtalar joint) may complain of pain during this motion. There is a distinct and obvious difference between the subtalar motions of younger and older patients.

FOREFOOT ADDUCTION—20°
FOREFOOT ABDUCTION—10°

The motions of forefoot adduction and abduction take place primarily at the midtarsal joint (the talonavicular and calcaneocuboid joints). To test these motions, hold the patient's foot at the calcaneus with one hand to stabilize the heel in the neutral position during the test, and move the forefoot medially and laterally with your free hand. This range of motion is difficult to measure accurately, but it can be felt (Figs. 74, 75).

Although the motions of inversion and eversion may be tested independently from those of abduction and adduction, under normal circumstances the four movements are combined, with inversion almost invariably accompanied by adduction (called "supination"), and eversion by abduction (called "pronation").

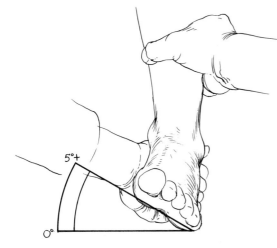

Fig. 72. Foot inversion test.

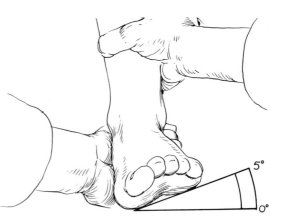

Fig. 73. Foot eversion test.

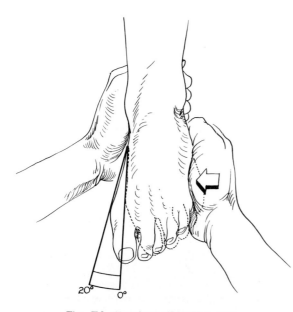

Fig. 74. Forefoot adduction test.

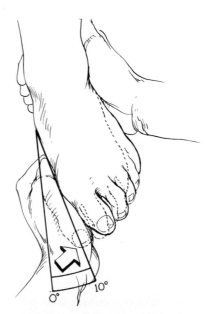

Fig. 75. Forefoot abduction test.

First Metatarsophalangeal Joint

FLEXION   —45°
EXTENSION—70°–90°

Since it is principally involved with the toe-off phase of gait, the first metatarsophalangeal joint is crucial to normal ambulation. To test it, stabilize the patient's foot and move his great toe through flexion and extension at the metatarsophalangeal joint (Fig. 76). Normal toe-off requires a minimum of 35° to 40° of extension.

If motion is markedly reduced in the first metatarsophalangeal joint or if the joint is fused or partially fused (hallux rigidus), the patient may walk with a protective gait, shortening the toe-off (push-off) phase, stepping with an oblique bend to the foot, and avoiding motion or pressure on the first metatarsophalangeal joint. In that event, toe-off is then carried out by the four lateral toes (Fig. 77), and walking becomes unnatural and painful. Additionally, the patient's shoes may show oblique, rather than the normal transverse creases over

the toes (Fig. 78). In the case of hallux rigidus, any attempt to extend the toe may produce minimal motion while causing severe pain. Flexion, however, may be almost normal.

The proximal interphalangeal joint of the great toe is capable only of flexion (approximately 90°).

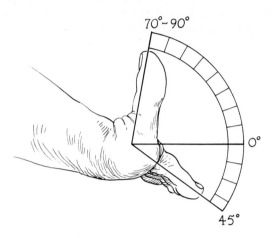

Fig. 76. The normal flexion/extension range of the first metatarsophalangeal joint.

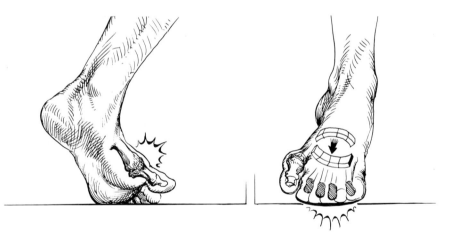

Fig. 77. Abnormal foot position due to hallux rigidus. Toe-off is carried out by the lateral four toes in hallux rigidus.

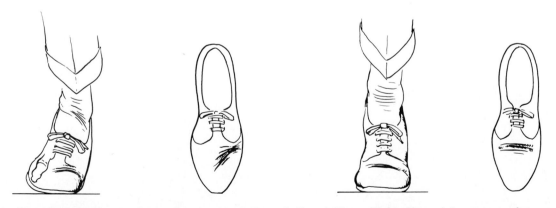

Fig. 78. Left. Abnormal oblique shoe creases indicate hallux rigidus. **Right.** Normal transverse shoe creases.

MOTION OF THE LESSER TOES. Although active flexion in the lesser toes takes place at the distal and proximal interphalangeal joints, active extension normally takes place only at the metatarsophalangeal joints. Thus, all four of the lesser toes should be extended and flexed passively, both at the metatarsophalangeal and at the proximal and distal interphalangeal joints. Normally, individuals flex their toes to grasp the ground or their shoes to gain extra stability during the stance phase of gait.

Claw toes restrict extension in the proximal and distal interphalangeal joints and flexion in the metatarsophalangeal joint, while hammer toes restrict flexion in the distal interphalangeal joint, extension in the proximal interphalangeal joint, and flexion at the metatarsophalangeal joint.

NEUROLOGIC EXAMINATION

Muscle Testing

The muscles of the foot fall into two main functional categories: the dorsiflexors and the plantar flexors. According to the location of their insertions on the foot, many of these muscles have the additional function of performing inversion or eversion. In general, the tendons in front of the malleoli dorsiflex the foot, and those behind the malleoli plantar flex it. In this neurologic examination, first the dorsiflexors and then the plantar flexors will be tested, both from lateral to medial.

Dorsiflexors

1) Tibialis Anterior
deep peroneal nerve, L4, (L5)
2) Extensor Hallucis Longus
deep peroneal nerve, L5
3) Extensor Digitorum Longus
deep peroneal nerve, L5

The primary dorsiflexors of the foot lie in the anterior tibial compartment. Since they share common innervation (the deep peroneal nerve), any pathology which prevents the nerve from functioning results in foot drop.

TIBIALIS ANTERIOR. This muscle is predominantly innervated by L4, but also receives some L5 innervation. To test the muscle in function, ask the patient to walk on his heels with his feet inverted. The tendon of the tibialis anterior muscle can be seen where it crosses the anteromedial portion of the ankle joint; it is quite prominent distally toward its insertion. Individuals having weak tibialis anterior muscles are unable to perform this functional dorsiflexion–inversion test, and may exhibit "drop-foot" or steppage gait.

For the manual test of the tibialis anterior muscle the patient should sit on the edge of the examination table. Support his lower leg, and place your thumb near the dorsum of his foot in such a position that he must dorsiflex and invert his foot to reach it. Then try to force his foot into plantar flexion and eversion by pushing against the first metatarsal head and shaft. Palpate the tibialis anterior muscle as you perform the test (Fig. 79).

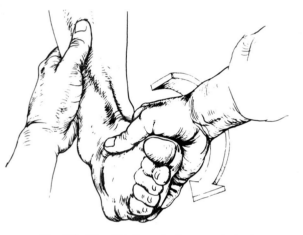

Fig. 79. The tibialis anterior muscle test.

EXTENSOR HALLUCIS LONGUS. The extensor hallucis longus can be functionally tested by having the patient walk on his heel, with his foot neither inverted or everted. The tendon should stand out clearly all the way to its insertion at the proximal end of the distal phalanx of the great toe.

For the manual test of the extensor hallucis longus, the patient should sit on the edge of the table. Support his foot with one hand around the calcaneus and again place your thumb in such a position that he must dorsiflex his great toe to reach it. Oppose his dorsiflexion by placing your thumb on the nail bed of the great toe and your fingers on the ball of the foot and push down on the toe (Fig. 80). If your thumb is placed across the interphalangeal joint, you are also testing the extensor hallucis brevis. Therefore, to test only the extensor hallucis longus, make certain that your resistance is distal to the interphalangeal joint.

EXTENSOR DIGITORUM LONGUS. The tendon of this muscle is the third most prominent of the dorsiflexors. To test it in function, instruct the patient to walk on his heel as he did for the extensor hallucis longus muscle test. The tendon should stand out on the dorsum of the foot, crossing in front of the ankle mortise and fanning out to insert, by slips, into the dorsal surfaces of the middle and distal phalanges of the four lateral toes.

For the manual test, the patient should sit on the edge of the table. Secure his foot around the calcaneus and place the thumb of your free hand in such a position that he must extend his toes to reach it. Then, oppose his motion by pressing on the dorsum of the toes and by attempting to bend them plantarward (Fig. 81). The toes should be virtually unyielding.

EXTENSOR DIGITORUM BREVIS. The tests for this muscle are the same as those for the longus. The muscle belly of the brevis can be palpated for consistency where it bulges out from the sinus tarsi. However, it cannot be isolated for muscle testing.

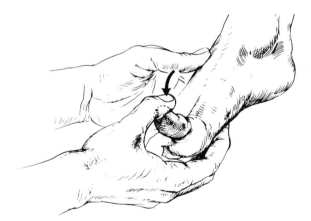

Fig. 80. The extensor hallucis longus muscle test.

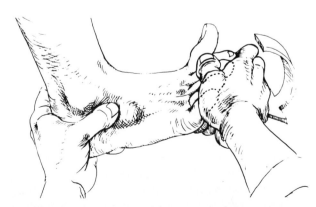

Fig. 81. Testing the strength of the digitorum longus muscle.

Plantar Flexors

1) Peroneus Longus and Brevis
   superficial peroneal nerve, S1
2) Gastrocnemius and Soleus
   tibial nerve, S1, S2
3) Flexor Hallucis Longus
   tibial nerve, L5
4) Flexor Digitorum Longus
   tibial nerve, L5
5) Tibialis Posterior
   tibial nerve, L5

PERONEUS LONGUS AND BREVIS. The tendons of these muscles are the first two tendons posterior to the lateral malleolus. They should be tested in function simultaneously. Since they are the evertors of the foot and ankle, ask the patient to walk on the medial borders of his feet. As he does so, the tendons of the peronei should become prominent where they turn around the lateral malleolus, pass on either side of the peroneal tubercle (the brevis above, the longus below), and run to their respective insertions.

For the manual test of the peronei, the patient should sit on the edge of the table. Secure his ankle by stabilizing the calcaneus and place your other hand in a position that forces him to plantar flex and evert his foot to reach it with his small toe. Then, oppose his plantar flexion and eversion by pushing against the fifth metatarsal head and shaft with the palm of your hand (Fig. 82). (Avoid applying pressure to the toes, since they may move.)

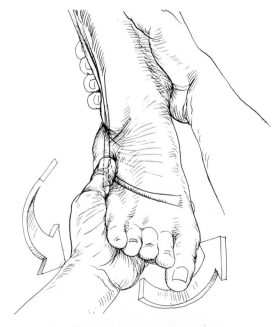

Fig. 82. The peronei muscle test.

GASTROCNEMIUS AND SOLEUS. The common tendon of insertion for the gastrocnemius and soleus muscles is the most prominent tendon behind the malleoli. Because the gastrocsoleus unit is stronger than all the other leg muscles combined, it is difficult to detect existing weakness by manual muscle testing. Therefore, observe these muscles in function. First, ask the patient to walk on his toes, an act he will be unable to perform if there is gross muscle weakness. Then instruct him to jump up and down on the balls of his feet, one at a time, to force the calf muscles to support almost two and one-half times the body's weight. If he lands flat-footed or is otherwise incapable of performing this test, there is probably at least minimal weakness in the calf muscle (Fig. 83). Elderly individuals or patients with backaches should not be expected to perform this functional test.

FLEXOR HALLUCIS LONGUS. This muscle lies medial to the Achilles tendon. To evaluate its function, simply observe the patient's gait. The muscle's action is integral to the smooth toe-off phase of gait. There is no other functional method that tests this muscle.

For the manual test of the flexor hallucis longus, have the patient sit on the edge of the table, and support his foot by stabilizing the calcaneus. Then instruct him to bend or curl his great toe, and oppose this plantar flexion. Repeat the procedure on the opposite foot and compare the relative strengths of the two muscles.

FLEXOR DIGITORUM LONGUS. This tendon lies immediately medial to the flexor hallucis longus tendon. There is no accurate method by which to test it in function. Test it manually by stabilizing the calcaneus and having the patient bend or curl his toes. Oppose this flexion by trying to bend the toes into dorsiflexion. Again, the toes should be unyielding.

TIBIALIS POSTERIOR. This tendon lies just posterior to the medial malleolus. While the muscle is difficult to isolate for testing in function, its tendon is palpable as it comes around the medial malleolus and inserts into the navicular tubercle. A combination of plantar flexion and inversion makes the tendon stand out quite clearly.

For the manual test of the tibialis posterior, have the patient sit on the examination table and stabilize his foot. Then, have him plantar flex and invert his foot while you resist his motion. If the tibialis posterior is stronger than the other tendons around the ankle, it can deform the foot, especially in children.

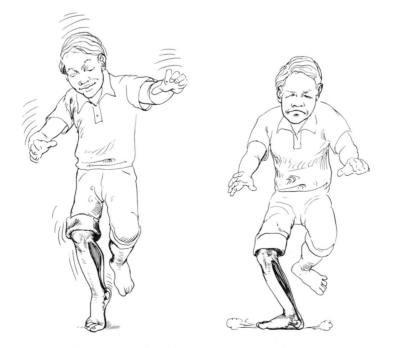

Fig. 83. Left. To test the gastrocsoleus unit, have the patient hop up and down on the ball of his foot. **Right.** If he lands flat-footed, there is probable weakness in the calf muscle.

Sensation Tests

Sensation to the skin over the lower leg and foot is supplied by nerves emanating from the lumbar and sacral regions. The areas which are supplied by each particular neurologic level can be broadly defined as bands, or dermatomes, that cover certain areas of the skin. The **L4** dermatome crosses the knee joint and covers the medial side of the leg (medial to the crest of the tibia, the medial malleolus, and the medial side of the foot). The **L5** dermatome covers the lateral side of the leg (lateral to the crest of the tibia) and the dorsum of the foot. The **S1** dermatome covers the lateral side of the foot (Fig. 84).

The sensation of each peripheral nerve should be tested as it innervates the dorsum of the foot. The medial side of the foot is supplied by the saphenous nerve, the dorsum by the peroneal nerve, and the lateral side by the sural nerve (Fig. 85).

Reflex Tests

ACHILLES TENDON REFLEX (S1). The Achilles tendon reflex is a deep tendon reflex, mediated through the gastrocnemius-soleus muscles. It is supplied predominantly by nerves emanating from the S1 cord level. If the S1 root is cut or compressed, the Achilles tendon reflex is virtually absent.

To test the Achilles tendon reflex, ask the patient to sit on the edge of the examining table with his legs dangling, and put the tendon into slight stretch by gently dorsiflexing the foot. Then, to locate the tendon accurately, place your thumb and fingers into the soft tissue depressions on either side of it. Tap the tendon with the flat end of a neurologic hammer, using a wrist-flexing action to induce a sudden, involuntary plantar flexion of the foot (Fig. 86). It is sometimes helpful to reinforce the reflex by having the patient attempt to pull his clasped hands apart (or push them together) just as the tendon is struck.

There are several alternative methods of testing the Achilles tendon reflex, some of which are described below. The selection of an appropriate method depends, of course, upon the patient's condition.

If he is bedridden, cross his leg over his opposite knee so that the ankle joint is free. Prime the tendon by slightly dorsiflexing the foot. Then strike the tendon of Achilles using the flat end of the neurologic hammer. The reflex may be reinforced, if necessary.

If the patient is lying prone in bed, ask him to flex his knee to 90° and prime the tendon by slightly dorsiflexing the foot. Then strike the Achilles tendon.

If the ankle joint is swollen, or if it would be prohibitively painful to tap the Achilles tendon directly, test the ankle reflex by having the patient lie prone with his ankle over the edge of the bed or examination table. Press against the ball of your patient's foot with your fingers to dorsiflex it, and strike your fingers with the neurologic hammer. The reflex should be detectable through your hand (Fig. 87).

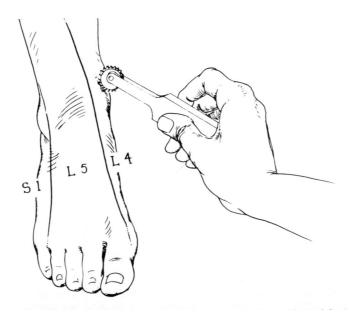

Fig. 84. Testing the sensory distribution to the ankle and foot.

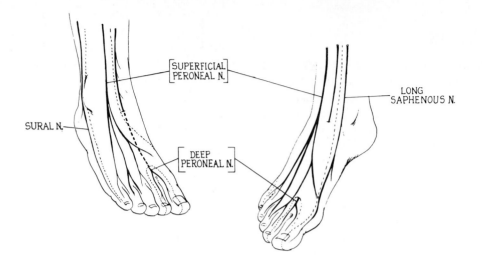

Fig. 85. Sensory distribution to the foot and ankle.

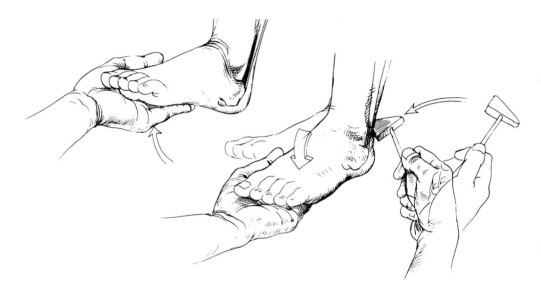

Fig. 86. Testing the Achilles tendon reflex.

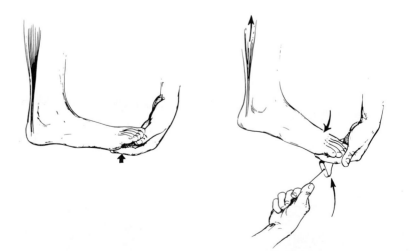

Fig. 87. An alternate method for testing the Achilles tendon reflex.

SPECIAL TESTS

TEST FOR RIGID OR SUPPLE FLAT FEET.
Observe the patient's feet as he stands on his toes and while he is seated. If the medial longitudinal arch is absent in all positions, the patient has rigid flat feet. If the arch is present while he is on his toes or sitting and absent only when he stands, his flat feet are supple and are correctable with longitudinal arch supports (Figs. 88, 89).

TIBIAL TORSION TEST.
In children, toeing-in may be caused by excessive internal rotation of the tibia. If you suspect tibial torsion, you must first locate the fixed bony points at either end of the tibia: the tibial tubercle below the knee and the two malleoli at the ankle. Normally, a line drawn between the malleoli is rotated externally 15° from a perpendicular line drawn from the tibial tubercle to the ankle. If there is internal tibial torsion, the malleolar line may face directly anteriorly, close to the perpendicular line (Figs. 90, 91, 92).

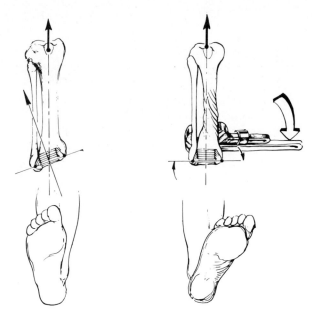

Fig. 90. Toeing-in may be caused by **excessive internal rotation of the tibia.**

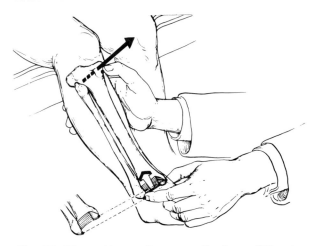

Fig. 91. The ankle mortise normally faces 15° externally.

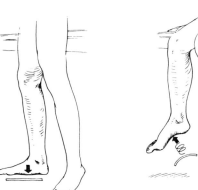

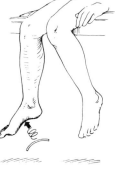

Fig. 88. Supple flat feet present a visible longitudinal arch in positions other than standing.

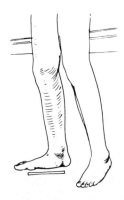

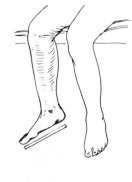

Fig. 89. Rigid flat feet remain flat in any position.

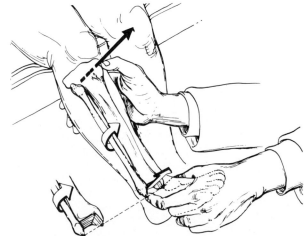

Fig. 92. The ankle mortise in internal tibial torsion faces anteriorly or internally.

FOREFOOT ADDUCTION CORRECTION TEST. Forefoot adduction in children may or may not need correction (Fig. 93). If you can manually correct the adduction and abduct the forefoot beyond the neutral position, no treatment will be necessary since the foot will ultimately correct itself (Fig. 94). If, however, you can only partially correct the forefoot to the neutral position or less, the foot will probably not correct itself, and cast correction is necessary (Figs. 95, 96).

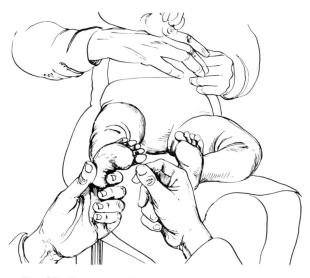

Fig. 93. Forefoot adduction is common in children.

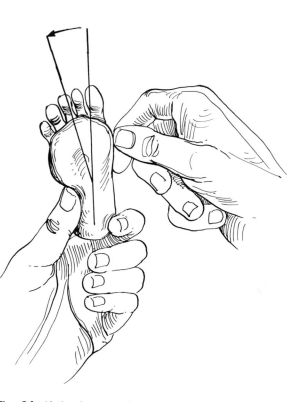

Fig. 94. If the foot can be abducted manually beyond the neutral position, no correction is necessary.

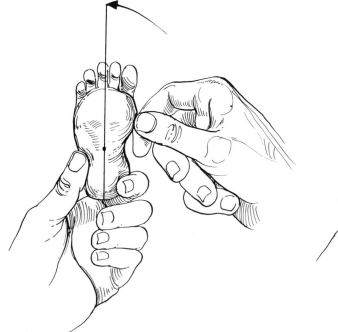

Fig. 95. This foot does not abduct beyond the neutral position.

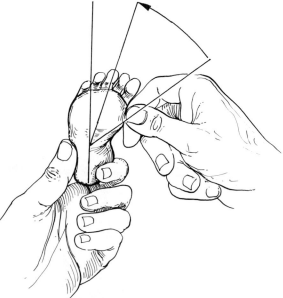

Fig. 96. Cast correction is necessary for this forefoot adduction, which cannot be corrected even to the neutral position.

ANKLE DORSIFLEXION TEST. When the ankle cannot be dorsiflexed or brought to the plantar grade position with the knee extended, and when you know the limitation of motion to be caused by either the gastrocnemius or the soleus muscles, you may determine which muscle is causing the limitation by means of the following test. First, flex the knee joint. If you are able to achieve ankle dorsiflexion when the knee is flexed, the gastroc muscle is the cause of the limitation, since flexion of the knee slackens the gastroc (a two-joint muscle) by bringing its origin closer to its insertion (Figs. 97, 98). Since the soleus is a one-joint muscle, it is not affected by flexion of the knee; if the soleus is responsible for the limited motion, the limitation will be the same whether or not the knee is flexed.

HOMANS' SIGN. To test for deep vein thrombophlebits, forcibly dorsiflex the patient's ankle when his leg is extended. Pain in the calf resulting from this maneuver indicates a positive Homans' sign. Tenderness elicited upon deep palpation of the calf muscle is further evidence of deep vein thrombophlebitis (Figs. 99, 100).

EXAMINATION OF RELATED AREAS

All the other joints in the lower extremity should be examined in conjunction with a complete examination of the foot and ankle, since it is possible for pathology in the knee, hip, or lumbar region to refer pain to the foot and ankle (Fig. 101).

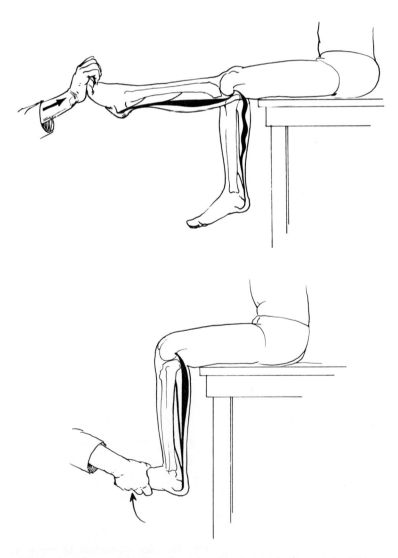

Figs. 97, 98. Special test to distinguish between gastrocnemius and soleus muscle tightness.

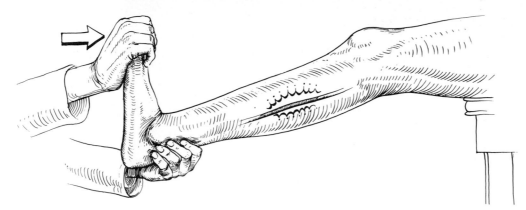

Fig. 99. Homans' Sign for deep vein thrombophlebitis.

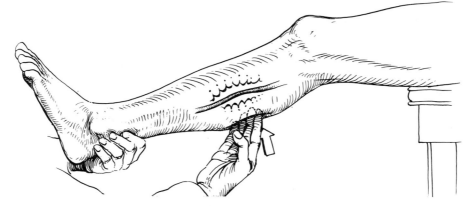
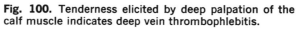

Fig. 100. Tenderness elicited by deep palpation of the calf muscle indicates deep vein thrombophlebitis.

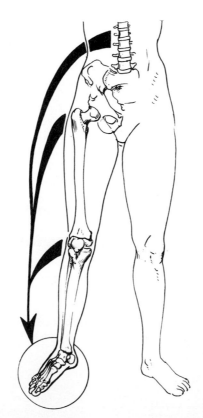

Fig. 101. Pathology in the lumbar spine, the hip, or the knee can refer pain to the foot and ankle.

9

Physical Examination of the Lumbar Spine

INSPECTION
BONY PALPATION
  Posterior Aspect
  Anterior Aspect
    Sacral Promontory
SOFT TISSUE PALPATION
  Zone I — Midline Raphe
  Zone II — Iliac Crest
  Zone III — Posterior Superior Iliac Spines
  Zone IV — Sciatic Area
  Zone V — Anterior Abdominal Wall and
             Inguinal Area
RANGE OF MOTION
  Flexion
  Extension
  Lateral Bending
  Rotation
NEUROLOGIC EXAMINATION
  Superficial Reflexes
    Superficial Abdominal Reflex
    Superficial Cremasteric Reflex
    Superficial Anal Reflex
  Pathologic Reflexes
    Babinski Test
    Oppenheim Test
SPECIAL TESTS
  Tests to Stretch the Spinal Cord or Sciatic Nerve
    Straight Leg Raising Test
    Well Leg Straight Leg Raising Test
    Hoover Test
    Kernig Test
  Tests of Increased Intrathecal Pressure
    Milgram Test
    Naphziger Test
    Valsalva Maneuver
  Tests to Rock the Sacroiliac Joint
    Pelvic Rock Test
    Gaenslin Test
    Patrick or Fabere Test
  Neurologic Segmental Innervation Test
    Beevor's Sign
EXAMINATION OF RELATED AREAS

The lumbar spine transports the cauda equina to the lower extremity and provides mobility for the back. It also furnishes support for the upper portion of the body and transmits weight to the pelvis and lower extremity. Since there are no ribs attached to it, the lumbar spine has a relatively wide range of motion.

INSPECTION

To more thoroughly examine the lumbar spine, have the patient disrobe completely. As he disrobes, observe the fluidity of his movement. A patient with back trouble may splint his spine rigidly in the process of undressing to avoid bending, twisting, or other motions that could be painful for him. Any awkward or unnatural movement of the spine could also be a sign of some existing pathology.

To begin inspection, check the back for areas of redness and unusual skin markings. A patchy, reddened coloration may indicate either infection or the long-term use of a heating element, which results in a mottling of the skin. Skin markings such as lipomata, hairy patches, café-au-lait spots, or birth marks often denote underlying neurologic or bone pathology.

Soft, doughy lipomata (fatty masses) appearing as lumps in the area of the low back may be a sign of spina bifida (nonunion of the vertebral arch at the spinous process), or of dumbbell-shaped lipomas extending into the cauda equina through a bony defect (Fig. 21).

An unusual patch of hair on the back may be evidence of some bony defect in the spine, such as diastematomyelia (a congenital bony bar, separating the lateral halves of the spinal cord). A hairy patch (faun's beard), in conjunction with a lipoma, gives a reinforced indication of underlying bony pathology (Fig. 1).

Skin tags, or pedunculated tumors, indicate the presence of neurofibromatosis and are often accompanied by secondary skin markings (café-au-lait spots) (Fig. 1). Neurofibromatosis tumors, like those of lipomata, may impinge upon the spinal cord and the nerve roots.

Birth marks or excessive port wine marks should be carefully investigated, since they also suggest underlying bony pathology (spina bifida).

Posture can give a graphic representation of many spinal disorders and should be thoroughly analyzed. The shoulders and pelvis should appear level, and the bony, as well as the soft tissue, structures on both sides of the midline should be symmetrical. When the patient is standing, an obvious inclination or listing to one side or the other may be a sign of a possible sciatic scoliosis, secondary to a herniated disc. From the side view, a gentle lumbar lordotic curve is normal (Fig. 2). However, it is not uncommon to find the normal lumbar lordosis entirely absent (paravertebral muscle spasm) (Fig. 3). On occasion, an extremely sharp kyphosis (Gibbus deformity) may be present (Fig. 4). In addition, abnormally exaggerated lumbar lordosis is a common characteristic of a weakened anterior abdominal wall.

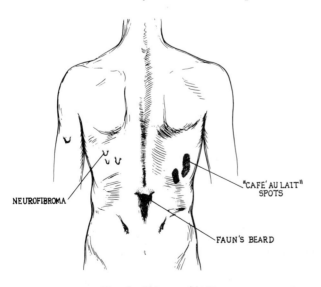

Fig. 1. Skin markings.

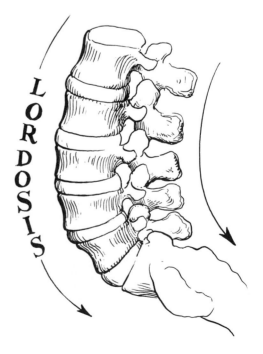

Fig. 2. Normal lumbar lordosis.

BONY PALPATION

To palpate the lumbar spine, sit on a stool behind the standing patient (Fig. 5). Then place your fingers on the tops of the iliac crests and your thumbs on the midline of the back at the L4/L5 junction (the same level as the tops of the iliac crests) and palpate the interspace between the vertebrae (Fig. 6). The spinous processes of L4 and L5 lie above and below the interspace. Since these two processes do not overlap each other, they mark the actual levels of the vertebral bodies and are an excellent reference point from which to identify the other vertebrae.

Posterior Aspect

Spinous Processes. After locating the L4/L5 interspace, move superiorly to palpate the individual spinous processes of the other lumbar vertebrae (Fig. 7). Then, after returning to L4/L5, palpate inferiorly for the smaller spinous processes; locate the S2 spinous process by drawing a line between the posterior superior iliac crests. Pain referred from the spine may be reproduced in the back or the legs during this palpation (Fig. 8).

In the area of the sacral triangle, gaps between the small spinous processes or the absence of any of the sacral or lumbar processes suggest a spina bifida (Fig. 9). A visible or palpable "step-off" from one process to another may be an indication of spondylolisthesis (forward slippage of one vertebra on another, most often L5 on S1, or L4 on L5) (Fig. 10), secondary to a bony defect (spondylolysis) in the posterior elements of the spine (pars interarticularis). This condition commonly causes the backache so often reported by teenagers. In conjunction with this defect, there is the possibility that a nerve root has been stretched or a disc herniated, with accompanying pain down the legs.

Posterior Aspect of the Coccyx (Fig. 11). A painful coccyx (coccydynia) is usually the result of a direct blow. The only way to fully palpate the coccyx is through a rectal examination. (See page 169).

To complete palpation of the lumbar spine's posterior aspect, examine the posterior superior iliac spines, the iliac crests, the greater trochanters, and the ischial tuberosities, as described in the Hip Chapter, pages 146 to 149 (Figs. 12 to 15).

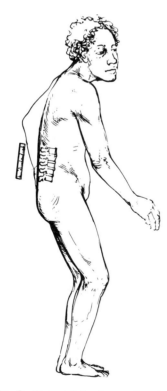

Fig. 3. Paravertebral muscle spasm.

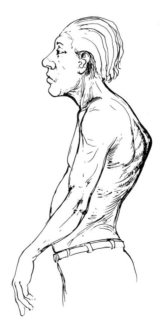

Fig. 4. Gibbus deformity.

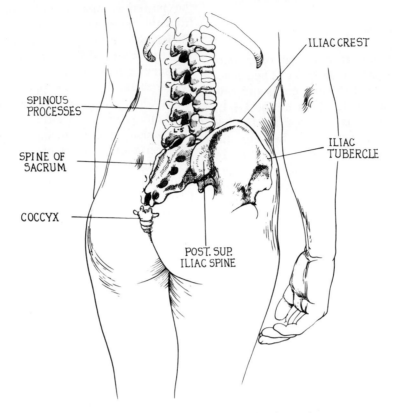

Fig. 5. The anatomy of the posterior lumbar spine.

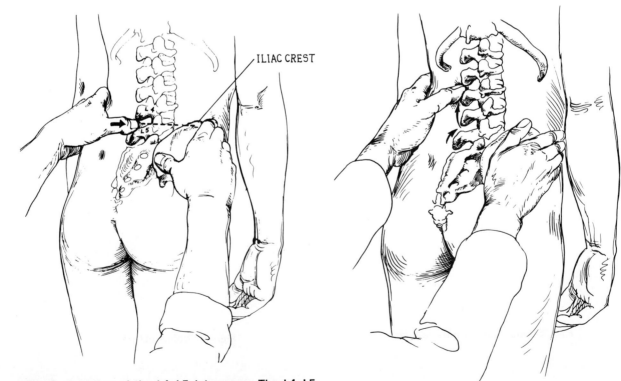

Fig. 6. Palpation of the L4—L5 interspace. The L4—L5 interspace lies at the same level as the tops of the iliac crests.

Fig. 7. Palpation of the spinous processes.

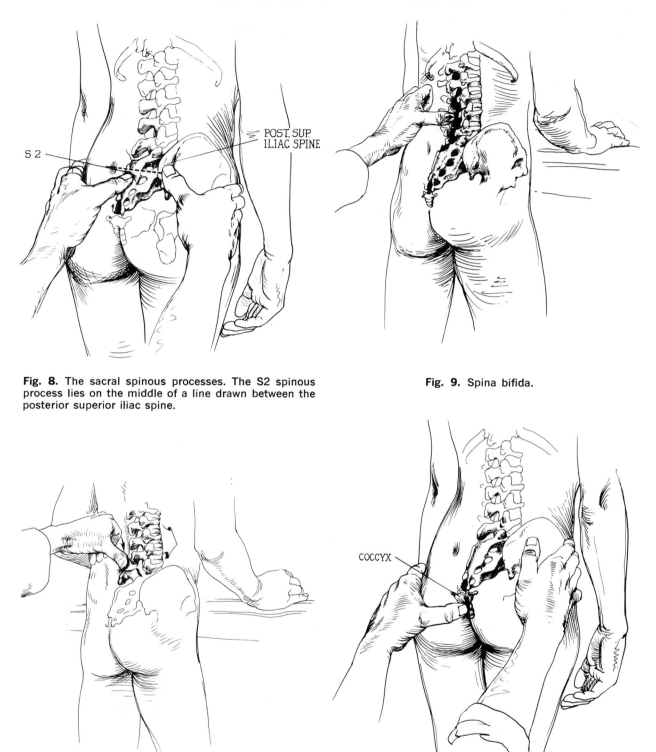

Fig. 8. The sacral spinous processes. The S2 spinous process lies on the middle of a line drawn between the posterior superior iliac spine.

Fig. 9. Spina bifida.

Fig. 10. Spondylolisthesis.

Fig. 11. The coccyx.

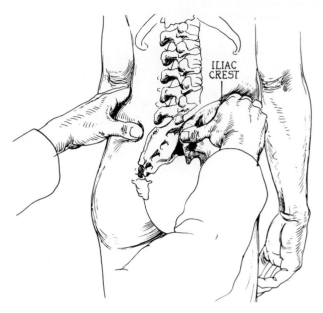

Fig. 12. The starting position for palpation of the posterior superior iliac spines and iliac crest.

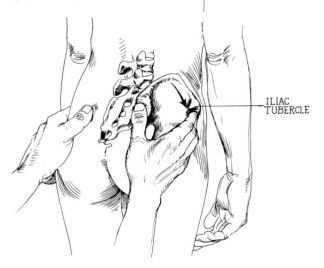

Fig. 13. The posterior iliac crests and iliac tubercles.

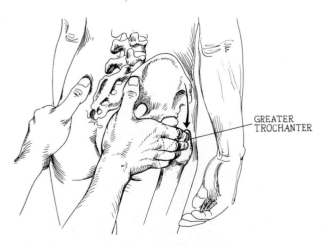

Fig. 14. The greater trochanters.

Anterior Aspect

To examine the anterior aspect of the spine, have the patient lie supine on an examination table, with his knees bent to relax the abdominal muscles.

The umbilicus lies at the L3–L4 disc space, the point at which the aorta divides into the common iliacs; anterior portions of the L4, L5, and S1 bodies and discs are palpable below the artery's division. The anterior portions of these vertebral bodies are covered by anterior longitudinal ligaments (Fig. 16).

Sacral Promontory. The L5–S1 articulation is the most prominent anterior portion of the spine in this area. If you place your fingers just below the umbilicus, and gently, but with increasing pressure, push into the abdomen through the linea alba while encouraging the patient to relax, you can, with some difficulty, feel the bony surface of the L5 and S1 vertebral bodies (Fig. 17).

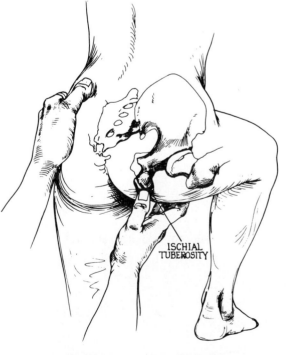

Fig. 15. The ischial tuberosities.

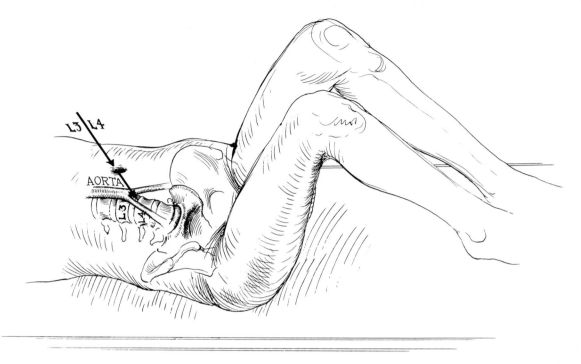

Fig. 16. The anterior aspect of the lumbar spine. The umbilicus lies at the L3–L4 disc space level.

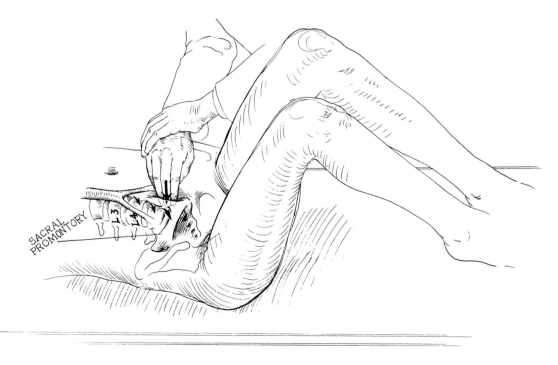

Fig. 17. The sacral promontory.

SOFT TISSUE PALPATION

The examination of the soft tissues of the lumbar spine is divided into five clinical zones:

1) the midline raphe
2) the iliac crest
3) the posterior superior iliac spines
4) the sciatic area
5) the anterior abdominal wall and the inguinal area

Zone I—Midline Raphe

Supraspinous and Interspinous Ligaments (Fig. 18). These ligaments joint the spinous processes of the lumbar and sacral vertebrae posteriorly. The supraspinous ligament, a strong, fibrous cord, connects the spinous processes from the seventh cervical vertebra to the sacrum. It is broadest in the lumbar region, where its thickness is palpable over the vertebrae. The interspinous ligaments are short and strong, and connect the adjoining spinous processes. Because they lie between the processes and not over them, they are not palpable. Palpate down the line of spinous processes; if either the supraspinous or interspinous ligaments are ruptured, the area may be tender and a defect may be palpable between the spinous processes (Fig. 19).

Paraspinal Muscles. The paraspinal muscles are composed of three layers of muscles, of which only the superficial layer (the sacrospinalis system —composed of the spinalis, the longissimus, and the iliocostalis) is palpable.

To palpate these muscles, position yourself behind the patient and ask him to put his head back so that the fascia covering the muscles relaxes.

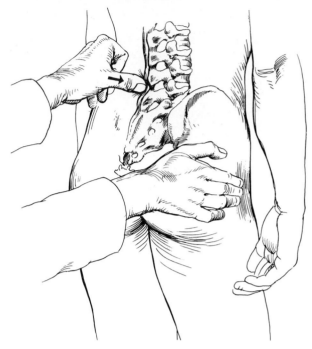

Fig. 18. The supraspinous and the interspinous ligaments.

It is not possible to differentiate between the three components of the sacrospinalis system, and they should be palpated as a unit on either side of the midline raphe. As you palpate, knead them between your fingers, noting any tenderness, spasm, defects, or dissimilarity in size and consistency. Under abnormal circumstances, the paraspinal muscles on one side may seem prominent and feel more rigid (secondary to spasm), perhaps causing the patient to list to one side. If the muscles are in spasm on both sides, they may stand out in prominent, almost steel-hard ridges, completely obliterating the normal lumbar lordosis. Because of their segmental innervation, the paraspinal

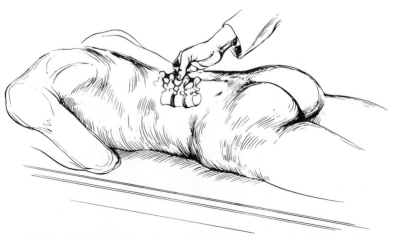

Fig. 19. A defect in the supraspinous and interspinous ligaments.

muscles are also subject to local atrophy (Fig. 20). Occasionally, a lipomata may be palpable in the midline or on either side of it (Fig. 21). The lipomata has clinical significance since it may impinge upon the spinal cord or indicate spina bifida.

Zone II—Iliac Crest

The gluteal muscles originate from various portions of the iliac blade, just below the crest. Their origins are palpable just under the lip of the posterior iliac crest, from the posterior to the anterior iliac spines. For a complete description of the palpation of the gluteal muscles, see the Hip and Pelvis Chapter, page 154.

As you probe the area of the gluteal origins, check for fibrofatty nodules, which are sometimes found lodged just under the lip of the iliac crest's posterior portion (Fig. 22). They may be tender to palpation and can cause localized low back pain. Neuromata of the cluneal nerves are also tender to palpation (Fig. 23).

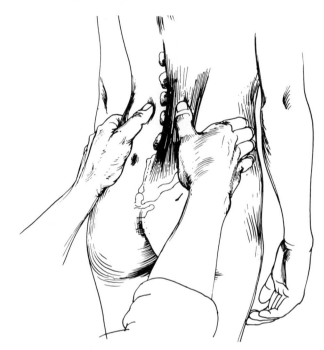

Fig. 20. Palpation of the paraspinal muscles.

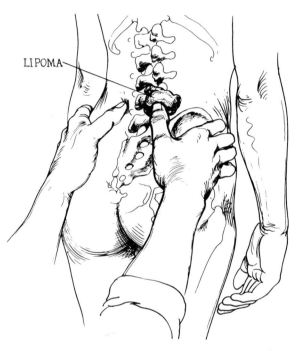

Fig. 21. A lipomata may impinge upon the spinal cord or signal spina bifida.

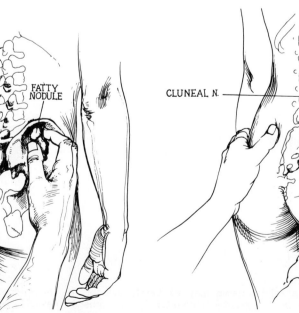

Fig. 22. Fibro-fatty nodules are sometimes found lodged under the lip of the posterior iliac crest.

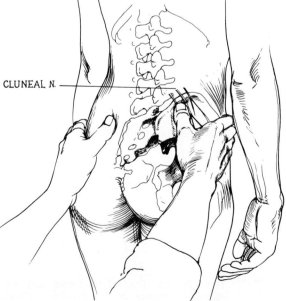

Fig. 23. The neuromata of the cluneal nerves.

Zone III—Posterior Superior Iliac Spines

The sacral triangle is formed by the two posterior superior iliac spines and the top of the gluteal cleft. Palpate carefully within the triangle, for it is a common area of pain due to low back sprains or the avulsion of a tendon from the posterior superior iliac spines. The posterior superior iliac spines are points of attachment for the sacrotuberous ligaments, which, together with the sacrospinous ligaments, connect the sacrum and the ischium and provide stability for the sacroiliac joint.

Zone IV—Sciatic Area

Sciatic Nerve. The sciatic nerve, the largest nerve in the body, runs vertically down the midline of the posterior thigh, gives off branches to the hamstring muscles, and then divides into two terminal branches, the tibial and the peroneal divisions. The sciatic nerve is fairly easy to locate as it exits the pelvis through the greater sciatic foramen under cover of the piriformis muscle and passes midway between the greater trochanter and the ischial tuberosity.

To palpate the sciatic nerve, have the patient flex his hip, and locate the midpoint between the ischial tuberosity and the greater trochanter. Press firmly at that midpoint to palpate the nerve; it is usually barely palpable (Figs. 24, 25). A herniated disc or a space-occupying lesion which bears down upon the contributing nerve roots can cause the nerve to be tender to palpation.

Zone V—Anterior Abdominal Wall and Inguinal Area

Anterior Abdominal Muscles. These muscles are a key factor in normal lumbar spine support; weakness results in an abnormal increase in lumbar lordosis, and the resultant change in posture generates low back pain (Fig. 26).

The anterior abdominal muscles are segmental, and receive segmental innervation in the same manner as the paraspinal muscles. To palpate the abdominals, have the patient cross his arms on his chest and do a quarter sit-up. Then palpate each segment of the rectus abdominus, and note any muscle weakness or deficit.

Inguinal Area. The inguinal area should be examined for a possible abscess within the psoas muscle, which can manifest as a draining sinus, a swelling, or a pointing abscess. Since the psoas muscle takes origin from the anterior portion of the T12–L5 vertebral bodies and discs, pain from a psoas abscess increases when the hip is actively flexed. Pain in the inguinal area usually indicates pathology in the hip joint.

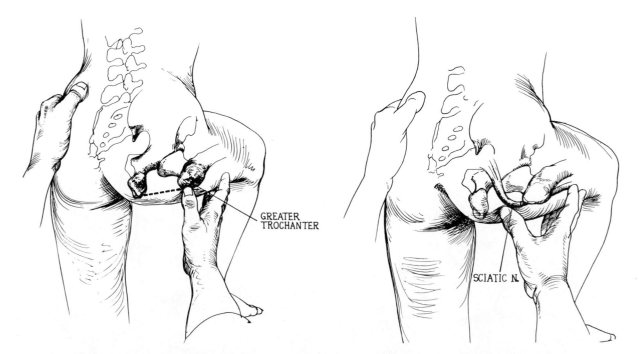

GREATER TROCHANTER

SCIATIC N.

Figs. 24, 25. The sciatic nerve may be barely palpable at the midpoint between the ischial tuberosity and the greater trochanter. The hip must be flexed to palpate the nerve.

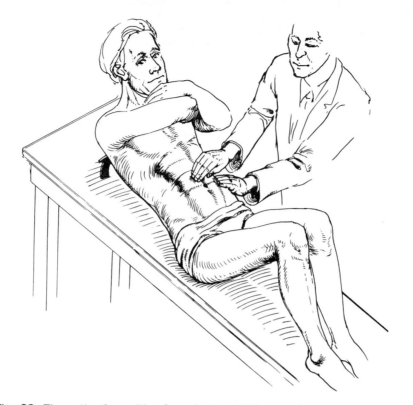

Fig. 26. The patient's position for palpation of the anterior abdominal muscles.

RANGE OF MOTION

The bodies of the lumbar vertebrae are separated by elastic segmental intervertebral discs which are composed of an annulus fibrosus and a nucleus pulposus. The range of motion between vertebrae is determined partly by the discs' resistance to distortion and partly by the angle and size of the articular surfaces between the processes. Vertebral motion is greatest where the discs are thickest and the joint surfaces largest. Both of these conditions exist in the lower lumbar region (L4, L5, S1), and motion taking place between L5–S1 is greater than that between L1–L2. Where there is more motion, however, there is more chance of breakdown, and herniated discs and osteoarthritis are found in the lower spine much more often than in the upper lumbar spine.

The movements of the lumbar spine are (1) flexion, (2) extension, (3) lateral bending, and (4) rotation.

Since there are no restraining ribs in the lumbar spine, more flexion and extension can take place than in the thoracic spine. For the same reason, a relatively large amount of rotation is theoretically possible. However, the interlocking articular

surfaces and the tightening effect of the surrounding ligaments and the annulus fibrosus check these movements in the lumbar spine and reduce its range of motion.

In comparison to the joints of the extremities, there is relatively little motion in the individual facet joints of the lumbar spine. Major motion, such as flexion, primarily involves motion in the hip; only an insignificant amount of movement actually takes place in the spine itself. This has been demonstrated by the fact that spinal fusion does not affect a patient's mobility to any great degree. The tests presented here to evaluate range of motion in the lower back are designed chiefly to detect a gross restriction in movement.

Flexion

Flexion in the lumbar spine involves relaxation of the anterior longitudinal ligament and stretching of the supraspinal and interspinal ligaments, the ligamentum flavum, and the posterior longitudinal ligament. Flexion is limited by the size of the vertebral bodies.

To test flexion, instruct the patient to bend as far forward as he can with his knees straight, and to try to touch his toes. If he cannot, measure the distance from his fingertips to the floor (Fig.

27). It is interesting to note that there is no reversal of the normal lumbar lordosis during flexion and that, at most, the low back merely flattens out. Flexion in the low back does not produce kyphosis as it does in the cervical spine. Patients whose paraspinal muscles are in spasm may refuse to perform this range of motion test. Lumbar pain not associated with muscle spasm usually decreases the range of motion since any attempt at full motion would increase the pain.

Extension

Extension in the lumbar spine stretches the anterior longitudinal ligament and relaxes the posterior ligaments. Extension is motored by the intrinsic muscles of the back; the increase in lumbar lordosis is resisted by the rectus abdominis muscles.

To test extension, stand beside the patient and place one hand on his back so that your palm

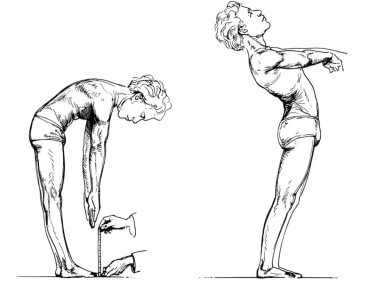

Fig. 27. Left. Range of flexion in the lumbar spine. **Right.** Range of extension in the lumbar spine.

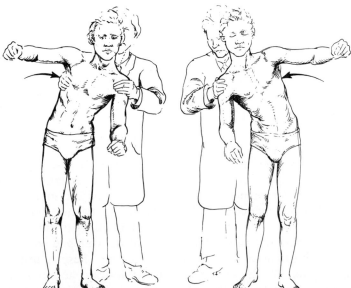

Fig. 28. Range of lateral bending in the lumbar spine should be equal on both sides.

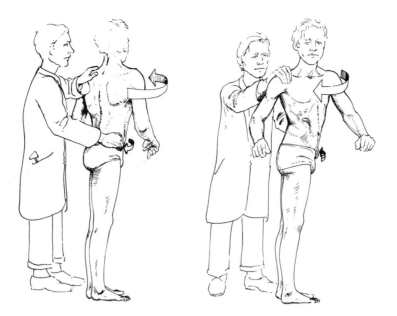

Fig. 29. Range of rotation in the lumbar spine.

rests on his posterior superior iliac spine and your fingers extend toward the midline. Then, instruct him to bend backward as far as he can, using your hand as a fulcrum for his motion (Fig. 27). You may assist the patient manually by pushing gently on his chest.

The range of extension achieved should be estimated and recorded. Spondylolisthesis causes increased back pain upon extension; patients with this condition may find some relief in flexion.

Lateral Bending

Lateral bending in the lumbar spine is not a pure motion, for it must occur in conjunction with elements of spinal rotation. Its range is limited by the surrounding ligaments.

To test lateral bending, first stabilize the iliac crest and ask the patient to lean to the left, and then to the right, as far as he can. Note how far he can bend to each side and compare the ranges of motion. To conduct the passive test for lateral bending, stabilize the patient's pelvis, grip his shoulder, and lean him to each side (Fig. 28). Any discrepancy in the ranges of active and passive lateral bending of the low back should be noted.

Rotation

To test rotation in the lumbar spine, position yourself behind the patient and stabilize his pelvis

by placing one hand on his iliac crest and the other on his opposite shoulder. Then turn the trunk by rotating the pelvis and the shoulder posteriorly. Repeat the same procedure for the opposite hip and shoulder and compare the ranges of rotation (Fig. 29).

NEUROLOGIC EXAMINATION

The neurologic examination of the lumbar spine includes an examination of the entire lower extremity, since spinal cord or cauda equina pathology, such as herniated discs, tumors, and avulsed nerve roots, is frequently manifested in the extremity itself in the form of altered reflexes, sensation, and muscle strength. Therefore, this examination describes the clinical relationship between the various muscles, reflexes, and sensory areas in the lower extremity and their particular cord levels, so that detection and location of spinal cord problems can be accomplished with relative accuracy and ease.

To clarify this clinical relationship, the examination will be conducted along neurologic lines, rather than by regions. Thus, for each neurologic level, we shall test the muscles, reflexes, and sensory areas that most clearly receive innervation from that level.

Note that there is no real neurologic examination of the lumbar spine itself. Since only gross differences can be discerned, much of this testing has taken place in tests for range of motion.

NEUROLOGIC LEVELS T12, L1, L2, L3

Since there are no individual reflexes for the T12, L1, L2, and L3 levels, their integrity can only be evaluated through muscle and sensory tests.

Muscle Testing

Iliopsoas: nerves emanating from T12, L1, L2, L3

The iliopsoas is the main flexor of the hip. To test it, have the patient sit on the edge of the examining table with his legs dangling. First, stabilize his pelvis by placing your hand over his iliac crest and ask him to actively raise his thigh from the table. Now, place your other hand over the distal femoral portion of his knee and ask him to raise his thigh further while you resist his motion. After determining the maximum resistance he can overcome, repeat the test for the opposite iliopsoas muscle and compare their relative strengths. For details of testing, see page 160.

Sensation Testing

The nerves emanating from L1, L2, and L3 provide sensation over the general area of the anterior thigh between the inguinal ligament and the knee joint. The L1 dermatome runs in an oblique band on the upper anterior portion of the thigh, immediately below the inguinal ligament; the L3 dermatome runs in an oblique band on the anterior thigh, immediately above the knee cap; and the L2 dermatome lies between these two bands, on the anterior aspect of the midthigh.

NEUROLOGIC LEVELS L2, L3, L4

L2, L3, and L4 are best evaluated by muscle and sensory tests; the patellar reflex, although supplied by L2, L3, and L4, is essentially an L4 reflex and will be tested as such.

Muscle Testing

Quadriceps: L2, L3, L4, Femoral Nerve

For this test, the patient should sit on the edge of the examining table. Stabilize the distal end of his thigh and instruct him to extend his knee, while you offer resistance to his motion. For further details, see page 189.

Hip Adductor Group: L2, L3, L4, Obturator Nerve

The hip adductors, like the quadriceps, can be tested in a massive grouping. For the test, the patient should be either seated or supine. Instruct him to abduct his legs; after placing your hands on the medial sides of both knees, ask him to adduct his legs against your resistance. See page 163 for further details.

NEUROLOGIC LEVEL L4

Muscle Testing

Tibialis Anterior: L4, deep peroneal nerve

To test the tibialis anterior, offer resistance to dorsiflexion and inversion by pushing against the dorsal and medial aspects of the head of the first metatarsal bone. See page 227 for further details (Fig. 79, Foot and Ankle Chapter).

Reflex Testing

Patellar Reflex

The patellar reflex is a deep tendon reflex, mediated through nerves emanating from the L2, L3, and L4 nerve roots, but predominantly from L4. For clinical application, the patellar reflex is considered an L4 reflex; however, even if the L4 nerve root is totally cut, the reflex is still present in significantly diminished form, since it receives innervation from sources other than L4. For details on how to elicit the reflex, see page 191.

Sensation Testing

The L4 dermatome covers the medial side of the leg. The knee represents the division between the L3 dermatome (above) and the L4 dermatome (below). On the leg, the sharp crest of the tibia is the dividing line between the L4 dermatome on the medial side and the L5 dermatome on the lateral side (Fig. 30).

L4
NEUROLOGIC LEVEL

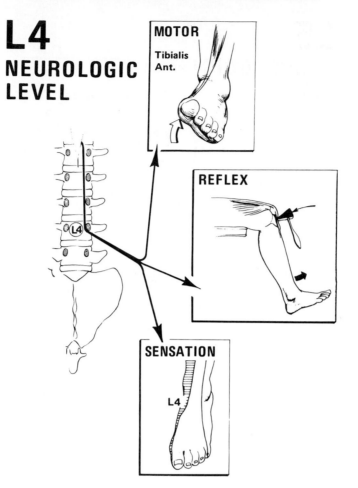

Fig. 30. Neurologic level L4.

NEUROLOGIC LEVEL L5

Muscle Testing

Extensor Hallucis Longus: L5, Deep Peroneal
Nerve

To test the strength of the extensor hallucis longus, place your thumb on the dorsal surface of the patient's foot so that he must dorsiflex his great toe to reach for it. Oppose this motion by pushing on the nail bed of the great toe (Foot and Ankle Chapter, Fig. 80). For details see page 227.

Gluteus Medius: L5, Superior Gluteal Nerve

To test the strength of the gluteus medius muscle, have the patient lie on his side as you stabilize his pelvis with one hand. Then instruct him to abduct his leg. After he has attained full abduction, resist his motion by pushing against the lateral side of the thigh at the level of the knee joint. Further details of this test are on page 162.

Extensor Digitorum Longus and Brevis:
L5, Deep Peroneal Nerve

For this test, the patient should sit on the edge of the examining table. First, secure the cal-

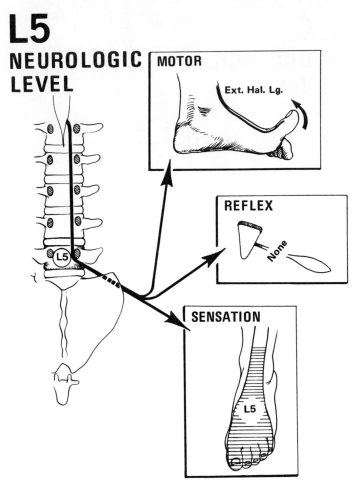

Fig. 31. Neurologic level L5.

caneus, and place the thumb of your free hand in a position that forces him to dorsiflex his toes to reach for it. Then try to oppose this extension. The toes should be virtually unyielding. Details of this test are given on page 228 (Fig. 81, Foot and Ankle Chapter).

Reflex Testing

There is no easily elicited reflex supplied by the L5 neurologic level. Although the tibialis posterior muscle provides an L5 reflex, it is difficult to obtain and very slight. If, after having performed the sensory and motor tests, the integrity of the L5 level is still uncertain, test the tibialis posterior reflex as follows: Hold the forefoot in a few degrees of eversion and dorsiflexion and tap the tendon of the tibialis posterior muscle on the medial side of the foot just before it inserts into the navicular tuberosity. Normally, this should evoke a small plantar inversion response.

Sensation

The L5 dermatome covers the lateral leg and dorsum of the foot. The crest of the tibia represents the dividing line between the L5 and L4 dermatomes (Fig. 31).

NEUROLOGIC LEVEL S1

Muscle Testing

Peroneus Longus and Brevis: S1, Superficial Peroneal Nerve

To test the peronei, secure the patient's ankle, have him plantar flex and evert his foot, and oppose his motion by pushing against the head of the

S1
NEUROLOGIC LEVEL

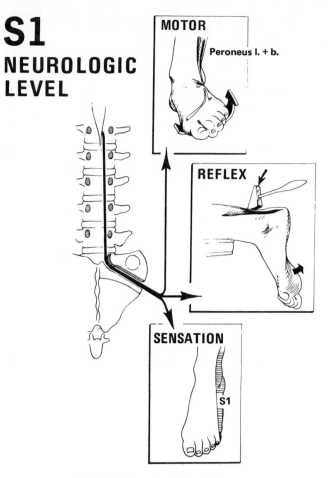

MOTOR

Peroneus l. + b.

REFLEX

SENSATION

S1

Fig. 32. Neurologic level S1.

fifth metatarsal with the palm of your hand. Details of this test are given on page 228 (Fig. 82, Foot and Ankle Chapter).

Gastrocnemius–Soleus Muscles: S1, S2, Tibial Nerve

The gastrocsoleus group is so strong that there is no legitimate manual test for it. For details of the functional testing of the group, see page 229.

Gluteus Maximus: S1, Inferior Gluteal Nerve

To test the strength of the gluteus maximus muscle, have the patient lie prone on the examining table with his knees flexed and his hip extended. Resist hip extension and palpate the gluteus maximus for tone. Details are on page 161 (Fig. 50, Hip and Pelvis Chapter).

Reflex Testing

Achilles Tendon Reflex

The Achilles tendon reflex is a deep tendon reflex, mediated through the gastrocnemius muscle. To test it, put the Achilles tendon into slight stretch by gently dorsiflexing the foot. Then strike the tendon to induce a sudden, involuntary plantar flexion of the foot. For a more complete description of this test, and for alternate methods of eliciting the reflex, see page 230 (Foot and Ankle Chapter).

Sensation Testing

The S1 dermatome covers the lateral malleolus and the lateral side and plantar surface of the foot (Fig. 32).

NEUROLOGIC LEVEL S2, S3, and S4

The nerves which emanate from the S2, S3, and S4 neurologic levels are the principal nerve supply for the bladder. S2, S3, and S4 also supply the intrinsic muscles of the foot. Although the bladder muscles cannot be isolated for testing, neurologic problems which affect the bladder may also have a visible effect on the intrinsic muscles of the toes; therefore, the toes should be inspected for any obvious deformity. There is no deep reflex supplied by S2, S3, and S4.

Sensation Testing

The dermatomes around the anus are arranged in three concentric rings and receive innervation from S2 (outermost ring), S3 (middle ring), and S4–S5 (innermost ring). A sharp instrument traced gently over the skin in these three areas determines whether sensation is normal or paresthetic.

The following table delineates applicable tests for those clinically relevant neurologic levels. It applies specifically to examination of herniated lumbar discs (Table 1).

Superficial Reflexes

The abdominal, cremasteric, and anal reflexes are superficial, or upper motor neuron, reflexes requiring skin stimulation and are mediated through the central nervous system (cerebral cortex). The patellar and Achilles tendon reflexes, on the other hand, are deep tendon or lower motor neuron reflexes and require tendon stimulation; they are mediated through the anterior horn cell. The absence of any superficial reflex may indicate an upper motor neuron lesion, an absence which has increased significance if it is associated with exaggerated deep tendon reflexes. Deep tendon reflexes are prevented from excessive reaction by the inhibitory properties of the cerebral centers; therefore, an exaggerated deep tendon reflex in combination with the loss of a superficial reflex is a double indication of cerebral or upper motor neuron pathology.

SUPERFICIAL ABDOMINAL REFLEX. To test the superficial abdominal reflex, have the patient lie supine on the examining table. Using the sharp end of a neurologic hammer, stroke each quadrant of the abdomen, noting whether the umbilicus moves toward the point being stroked (Fig. 33). The lack of an abdominal reflex indicates an upper motor neuron lesion. The abdominal muscles are innervated segmentally, the upper muscles from T7 to T10, the lower muscles from T10 to L1. Therefore, pinpointing the involved quadrant gives an indication of the level of the lesion if a lower motor lesion exists.

SUPERFICIAL CREMASTERIC REFLEX. The superficial cremasteric reflex may be elicited by stroking the inner side of the upper thigh with the sharp end of a neurologic hammer (Fig. 34). If the reflex is intact, the scrotal sac on that side is pulled upward as the cremaster muscle (T12) contracts. Absence or reduction of both cremasteric reflexes indicates an upper motor neuron lesion, while a unilateral absence suggests a probable lower motor neuron lesion between L1 and L2.

SUPERFICIAL ANAL REFLEX. To test this reflex, simply touch the perianal skin. The external and anal sphincter muscles (S2, S3, S4) should contract in response.

Pathologic Reflexes

Pathologic reflexes are also superficial reflexes in that they, too, are mediated through the central nervous system (cerebral cortex). However, the significance of their presence or absence is the reverse of that of the normal superficial reflexes: The presence of a pathologic reflex indicates an upper motor neuron lesion and its absence reflects integrity, whereas for the normal superficial reflexes, the presence of the reflex indicates integrity and its absence an upper motor neuron lesion.

Table 1. Neurology of the Lower Extremity

Disc	Root	Reflex	Muscles	Sensation
L3–L4	L4	Patellar reflex	Anterior tibialis	Medial leg and medial foot
L4–L5	L5	None	Extensor hallucis longus	Lateral leg & dorsum of foot
L5–S1	S1	Achilles reflex	Peroneus longus & brevis	Lateral foot

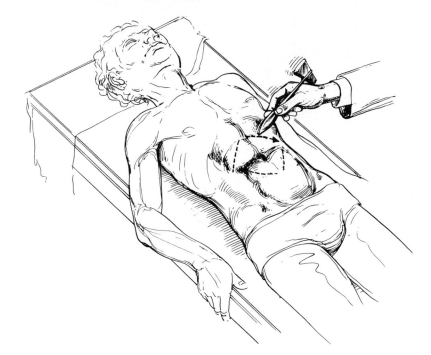

Fig. 33. Testing the superficial abdominal reflex.

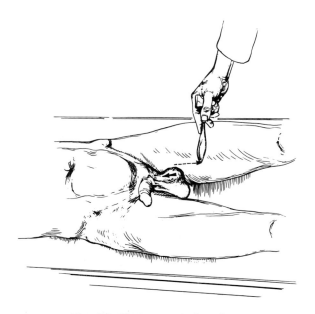

Fig. 34. The cremasteric reflex.

BABINSKI TEST. Run a sharp instrument across the plantar surface of the foot from the calcaneus along the lateral border to the forefoot. In a negative reaction, the toes either do not move at all or bunch up uniformly (Fig. 35). In the positive reaction, the great toe extends while the other toes plantar flex and splay (Fig. 36). A positive Babinski reflex indicates an upper motor neuron lesion usually associated with brain damage after trauma or with an expanding brain tumor. In the newborn, a positive Babinski is normal. However, the reflex should disappear soon after birth.

OPPENHEIM TEST. Run your fingernail along the crest of the tibia. Normally there should be either no reaction at all, or the patient should complain of pain. Under abnormal circumstances, the reaction is the same as for the Babinski test: The great toe extends while the other toes plantar flex and splay.

SPECIAL TESTS

1) tests to stretch the spinal cord, cauda equina, or sciatic nerve
2) tests to increase intrathecal pressure
3) tests to rock the sacroiliac joint
4) segmental innervation tests

Tests to Stretch the Spinal Cord or Sciatic Nerve

STRAIGHT LEG RAISING TEST. This test is designed to reproduce back and leg pain so that its cause can be determined. Instruct the patient to lie supine on an examining table. Lift his leg upward by supporting his foot around the calcaneus. The knee should remain straight. To insure that it does, place your free hand on the anterior aspect of the knee to prevent it from bending. The extent to which the leg can be raised without discomfort or pain varies, but normally the angle between the leg and the table measures approximately 80° (Fig. 37). If straight leg raising is painful, you must determine whether the pathology is due to problems in the sciatic nerve or to hamstring tightness. Hamstring pain involves only the posterior thigh, whereas sciatic pain can ex-

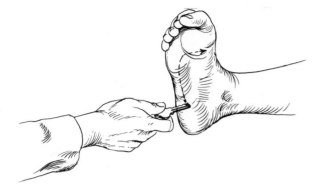

Fig. 35. A negative Babinski.

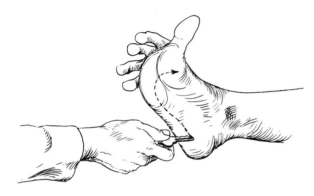

Fig. 36. A positive Babinski.

tend all the way down the leg. The patient may also complain of low back pain, and on occasion, pain in the opposite leg (positive cross leg straight leg raising test). At the point where the patient experiences pain, lower the leg slightly, and then dorsiflex the foot to stretch the sciatic nerve and reproduce sciatic pain (Fig. 38). If the patient does not experience pain when you dorsiflex his foot, the pain induced by straight leg raising is probably due to tight hamstrings. If there is a positive reaction to the straight leg raising test and the dorsiflexion maneuver, ask the patient to locate, as nearly as possible, the source of his pain. It may be either in the lumbar spine or anywhere along the course of the sciatic nerve.

WELL LEG STRAIGHT LEG RAISING TEST. Have the patient lie supine and raise his uninvolved leg. If he complains of back and sciatic pain on the opposite (involved) side, there is further presumptive evidence of a space-occupying lesion such as a herniated disc in the lumbar area (Fig. 39). This test is also referred to as the opposite leg, or positive cross leg straight leg raising test.

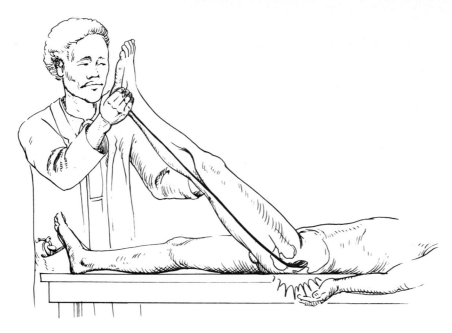

Fig. 37. Straight leg raising.

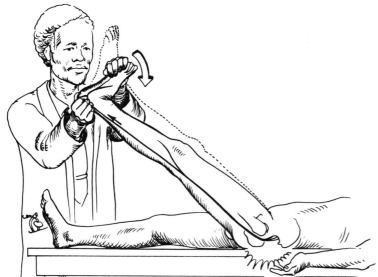

Fig. 38. In this position, dorsiflexion of the foot reproduces sciatic pain.

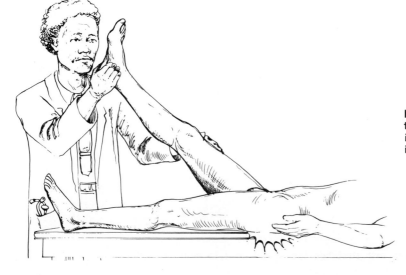

Fig. 39. A positive straight-leg raising test: Back pain on the involved side induced by straight-leg raising the non-involved leg.

HOOVER TEST. This test helps to determine whether the patient is malingering when he states that he cannot raise his leg, and should be performed in conjunction with a straight leg raising test. As the patient tries to raise his leg, cup one hand under the calcaneus of the opposite foot. When a patient is genuinely trying to raise his leg, he puts pressure on the calcaneus of his opposite leg to gain leverage; you can feel this downward pressure on your hand (Fig. 40). If the patient does not bear down as he attempts to raise his leg, he is probably not really trying (Fig. 41).

KERNIG TEST. This is another procedure designed to stretch the spinal cord and reproduce pain. Ask the patient to lie supine on the examining table, and have him place both hands behind his head to forcibly flex his head onto his chest. He may complain of pain in the cervical spine, and, occasionally, in the low back or down the legs, an indication of meningeal irritation, nerve root involvement, or irritation of the dural coverings of the nerve root (Fig. 42). Have him locate the area from which the pain originates so that you can determine its precise origin.

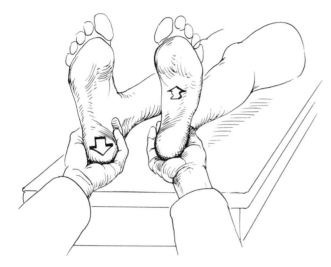

Fig. 40. The Hoover test.

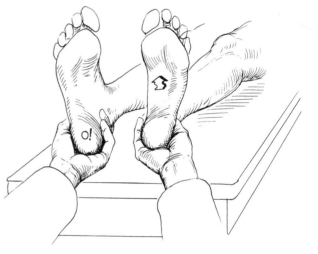

Fig. 41. An absence of downward pressure on the foot opposite the one the patient has been instructed to raise indicates that he is not really trying.

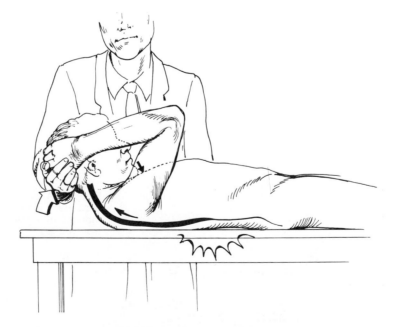

Fig. 42. The Kernig test stretches the spinal cord to reproduce pain.

Tests to Increase Intrathecal Pressure

MILGRAM TEST. With the patient lying supine on the examining table, have him keep his legs straight and raise them to a position about two inches from the table. Then have him hold this position as long as he can. This maneuver stretches the iliopsoas muscle and anterior abdominal muscles, and increases the intrathecal pressure (Fig. 43). If a patient can hold this position for thirty seconds without pain, intrathecal pathology may be ruled out. However, if the test is positive and the patient cannot hold the position, cannot lift his legs at all, or experiences pain as he attempts the maneuver, there may be intrathecal or extrathecal pathology (herniated disc), or pathologic pressure on the theca itself (wrapping of the cord) (Fig. 44).

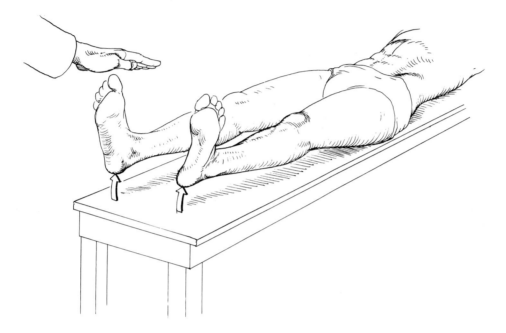

Fig. 43. The Milgram test. If a patient can hold this position for 30 seconds without pain, intrathecal pathology may be ruled out.

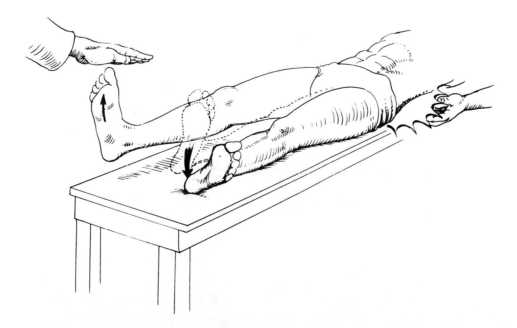

Fig. 44. The inability to hold the position indicates intrathecal or extrathecal pathology.

NAFFZIGER TEST. This compression test is also designed to increase intrathecal pressure by increasing the intraspinal fluid pressure. Gently compress the jugular veins for about 10 seconds until the patient's face begins to flush (Fig. 45). Then ask him to cough; if his coughing causes pain, there is probably pathology pressing upon the theca. Ask the patient to locate the painful area to help determine the source of the problem.

VALSALVA MANEUVER. Ask the patient to bear down as if he were trying to move his bowels (Fig. 46). This, too, increases the intrathecal pressure. If bearing down causes pain in the back or radiating pain down the legs, there is probable pathology either causing intrathecal pressure or involving the theca itself.

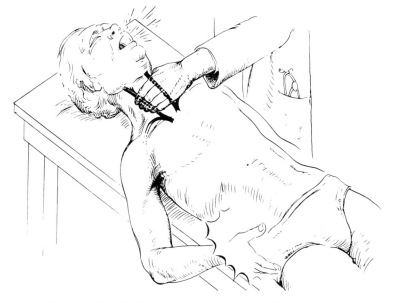

Fig. 45. The Naffziger test increases intrathecal pressure.

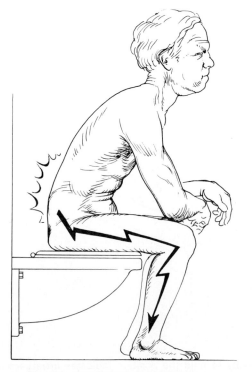

Fig. 46. The Valsalva maneuver.

Tests to Rock the Sacroiliac Joint

PELVIC ROCK TEST. Ask the patient to lie supine on the examining table. Place your hands on his iliac crests with your thumbs on his anterior superior iliac spines and your palms on his iliac tubercles. Then, forcibly compress the pelvis toward the midline of the body (Fig. 47). If the patient complains of pain around the sacroiliac joint, there may be pathology in the joint itself, such as infection or problems secondary to trauma.

GAENSLEN'S SIGN. Have the patient lie supine on the table, and ask him to draw both legs onto his chest. Then shift him to the side of the table so that one buttock extends over the edge of the table while the other remains on it (Fig. 48). Allow his unsupported leg to drop over the edge, while his opposite leg remains flexed (Fig. 49). Complaints of subsequent pain in the area of the sacroiliac joint give another indication of pathology in that area.

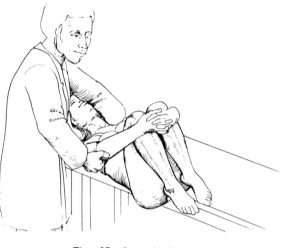

Fig. 48. Gaenslen's sign.

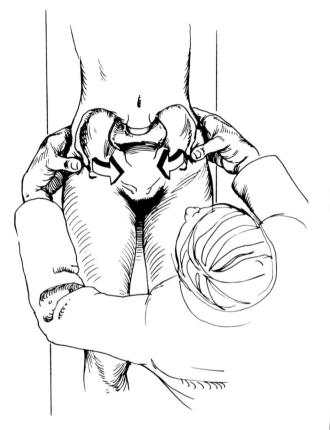

Fig. 47. The pelvic rock test for sacroiliac joint instability.

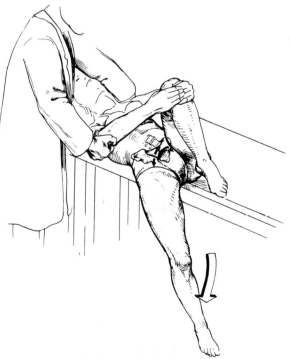

Fig. 49. Pain upon the execution of this maneuver indicates pathology in the area of the sacroiliac joint.

PATRICK OR FABERE TEST. This test can be used to detect pathology in the hip, as well as in the socroiliac joint. Have the patient lie supine on the table and place the foot of his involved side on his opposite knee. The hip joint is now flexed, abducted, and externally rotated. In this position, inguinal pain is a general indication that there is pathology in the hip joint or the surrounding muscles. When the end point of flexion, abduction, and external rotation has been reached, the femur is fixed in relation to the pelvis. To stress the sacroiliac joint, extend the range of motion by placing one hand on the flexed knee joint and the other hand on the anterior superior iliac spine of the opposite side. Press down on each of these points as if you were opening the binding of a book. If the patient complains of increased pain, there may be pathology in the sacroiliac joint (Fig. 50).

Pathology of the sacroiliac joint is relatively uncommon. However, when it is found, it is usually in conjunction with either a severe and massive trauma involving the pelvis or infectious diseases, such as tuberculosis.

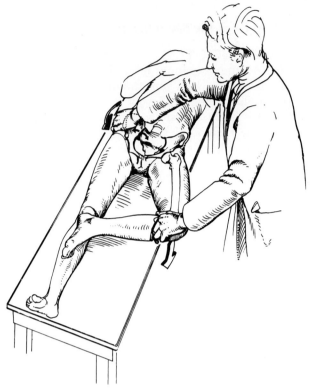

Fig. 50. The Patrick or Fabere test.

Neurologic Segmental Innervation Test

BEEVOR'S SIGN. This procedure tests the integrity of the segmental innervation of the rectus abdominus and the corresponding paraspinal muscles. The rectus abdominus muscles are segmentally innervated by the anterior primary division of T5–T12 (L1). The corresponding paraspinal muscles are also segmentally innervated by the posterior primary divisions of T5–T12 (L1). Ask the patient to do a quarter sit-up, with his arms crossed on his chest (Fig. 51). While he holds this position, observe the umbilicus. Normally, it should not move at all. If, however, the umbilicus is drawn up, down, or to one side, there may be asymmetrical involvement of the anterior abdominal and paraspinal muscles. The umbilicus is drawn to the stronger, or uninvolved, side (Fig. 52). Segmental involvement of one of the rectus abdominus muscles exists side by side with weakness in the corresponding paraspinal muscle. Palpate the muscles of the stomach and the lumbar spine to detect any weakness, signs of atrophy, or asymmetry. The Beevor's sign is frequently positive in patients having poliomyelitis or meningomyelocele.

EXAMINATION OF RELATED AREAS

The hip, rectum, and pelvis may all refer pain to the lumbar spine (Fig. 53). To complete your examination, perform a rectal examination on all patients (see page 169, Hip and Pelvis Chapter). A pelvic examination is also advisable for female patients.

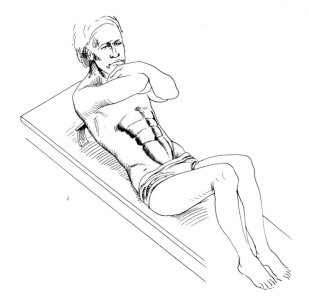

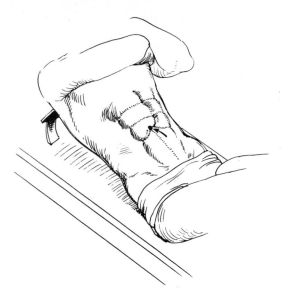

Fig. 51. Beevor's sign: Negative—the umbilicus does not move.

Fig. 52. In this position, umbilical movement indicates a weak segmental portion of the rectus abdominus and paraspinal muscles (positive Beevor's sign).

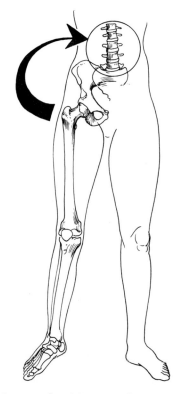

Fig. 53. The hip, rectum, and pelvis can refer symptoms to the lumbar spine.

BIBLIOGRAPHY

AEGERTER, E., KIRKPATRICK, J. A., JR.: Orthopedic Diseases: Physiology, Pathology, Radiology, 3rd ed. Philadelphia, W. B. Saunders, 1968

APLEY, A. G.: A System of Orthopaedics and Fractures, 4th ed. London, Butterworths, 1973

APPLETON, A. B., HAMILTON, W. J., SIMON, J.: Surface and Radiological Anatomy, 2nd ed. London, W. Heffer & Sons Ltd., 1938

BASMAJIAN, J. V.: Muscles Alive, 3rd ed. Baltimore, Williams & Wilkins, 1974

BEETHAM, W. P. JR., POLLEY, H. F., SLOCUMB, C. H., WEAVER, W. F.: Physical Examination of the Joints. Philadelphia, W. B. Saunders, 1965

BUNNELL, S.: Bunnell's Surgery of the Hand, 3rd ed., Boyes, J. H., ed. Philadelphia, J. B. Lippincott, 1970

CRENSHAW, A. H., ed.: Campbell's Operative Orthopaedics, 5th ed. St. Louis, C. V. Mosby, 1971

DANIELS, L., WILLIAMS, M., WORTHINGHAM, C.: Muscle Testing: Techniques of Manual Examination, 2nd ed. Philadelphia, W. B. Saunders, 1946

DELAGI, E., PERROTTO, L., IAZZETTI, J., MORRISON, D.: An Anatomic Guide for the Electromyographer. Springfield, Ill., Charles C Thomas, 1975

FERGUSON, A. B.: Orthopedic Surgery in Infancy and Childhood, 3rd ed. Baltimore, Williams & Wilkins, 1968

GIANNESTRAS, N. J.: Foot Disorders: Medical and Surgical Management, 2nd ed. Philadelphia, Lea & Febiger, 1973

HELFET, A. J.: Disorders of the Knee. Philadelphia, J. B. Lippincott, 1974

HENRY, A. K.: Extensile Exposure, 2nd ed. Baltimore, Williams & Wilkins, 1959

HOPPENFELD, S.: Scoliosis. Philadelphia, J. B. Lippincott, 1967

INMAN, V. T., ed.: DuVries' Surgery of the Foot, 3rd ed. St. Louis, C. V. Mosby, 1973

KAPLAN, E. B.: Duchenne: Physiology of Motion. Philadelphia, W. B. Saunders, 1959

KELIKIAN, H.: Hallux Valgus, Allied Deformities of the Forefoot and Metatarsaligia, Philadelphia, W. B. Saunders, 1965

KITE, J. H.: The Clubfoot. New York, Grune & Stratton, 1964

LEWIN, P.: The Foot and Ankle. Philadelphia, Lea & Febiger, 1958

MERCER, W., DUTHIE, R. B.: Orthopaedic Surgery. London, Arnold, 1964

MORTON, D. J.: The Human Foot. New York, Hafner, 1964

SALTER, R. B.: Textbook of Disorders and Injuries of the Musculoskeletal System. Baltimore, Williams & Wilkins, 1970

SCHULTZ, R. J.: The Language of Fractures. Baltimore, Williams & Wilkins, 1972

SHARRARD, W. J. W.: Paediatric Orthopaedics and Fractures. Oxford, Blackwell Scientific Publications, 1971

SHORE, N.: Occlusal Equilibration and Temporomandibular Joint Dysfunction. Philadelphia, J. B. Lippincott, 1959

SPINNER, M.: Injuries to the Major Branches of Peripheral Nerves of the Forearm. Philadelphia, W. B. Saunders, 1972

STANISAVLJEVIC, S.: Diagnosis and Treatment of Congenital Hip Pathology in the Newborn. Baltimore, Williams & Wilkins, 1963

STEINDLER, A.: Kinesiology of the Human Body. Springfield, Ill., Charles C Thomas, 1955

TACHDJIAN, M. O.: Pediatric Orthopedics, Vols. 1 and 2. Philadelphia, W. B. Saunders, 1972

TUREK, S. L.: Orthopaedics: Principles and Their Application, 2nd ed. Philadelphia, J. B. Lippincott, 1967

Index